HEALTH LIBRARY

CHILDREN'S HEALTH

HEALTH LIBRARY

CHILDREN'S HEALTH

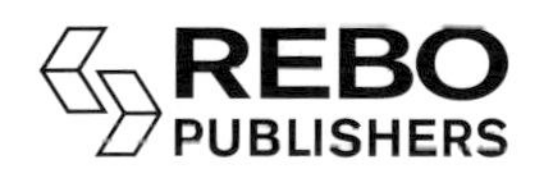

Idea and supervision: Jordi Vigué
Text: Gustavo Villalobos, Myriam Cañas
Editing: Ramón Aymerich
Medical advices: Dr. Gonçal Folch
Photographs: Gorg Blanc photographic archives, Capsa Màgica Studio
Illustrations: Ana Journade, Roger Tallada, David Navarrot, Daniel Martínez
Image processing: Rosa Rigau
Special collaboration: Canica Estudio, Laumar Estética
Graphic design: Celia Valero
Typesetting: Glòria Badia, Manuel Guirado, Marta Ribón, Martín Riveiro
Editorial coordination: Miquel Ridola

Layout: AdAm Studio, Prague, The Czech Republic
Typesetting and pre-press services: A. R. Garamond, Prague, The Czech Republic
Translation: Matthew Clarke for First Edition Translations Ltd, Cambridge, UK
Editing: Laila Friese for First Edition Translations Ltd, Cambridge, UK
Proofreading: Sarah Dunham

ISBN 13: 978-90-366-1907-3
ISBN 10: 90-366-1907-6

CONTENTS

the first month

The first month of life, known as the *neonatal period*, is a critical phase full of changes, not only for the baby but also for the parents. Mutual adaptation marks these first days of life, in which the mother–child bond becomes the vital axis around which the life of the entire family revolves. It is normal to have mixed feelings when expecting a baby: joy and happiness, but also doubt, fear, and difficult moments that demand great tolerance and understanding from all the members of a family.

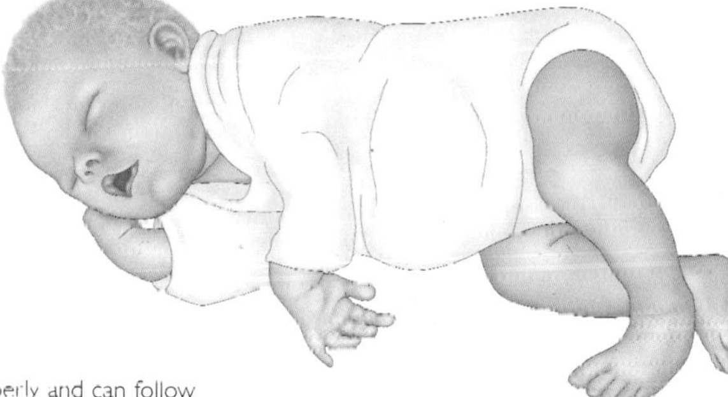

The neck muscles grow stronger, allowing your baby to hold up her head for longer periods.

She starts to murmur and gurgle.

She learns to focus properly and can follow objects with her gaze.

She spends more time awake during the day.

First month

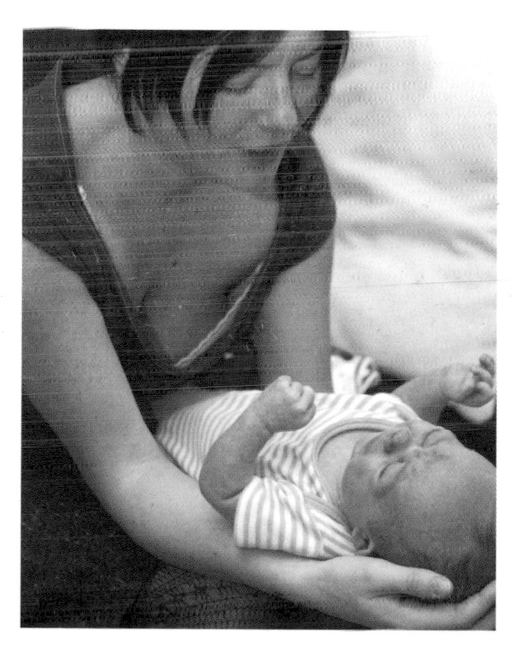

Physical development

- **Posture** A newborn baby retains the fetal posture, i.e. flexed hips, bent knees, and a curved back. When naked on her back, she raises her arms and legs, bends her elbows and knees, but is unable to hold her head upright.
- **Muscle tone** A baby born after 37–42 weeks of pregnancy has robust muscle tone: if a finger is placed on her hand, she will demonstrate a strong gripping reflex . In contrast, a premature baby (born after fewer than 37 weeks of pregnancy) displays much less muscle tone and her legs are straight and limp.
- **Weight** This reflects the baby's nutritional state and development. Tables with mean values relating the weight and gestational age establish the range of normality; if the weight is lower or higher than expected, the doctor will evaluate the

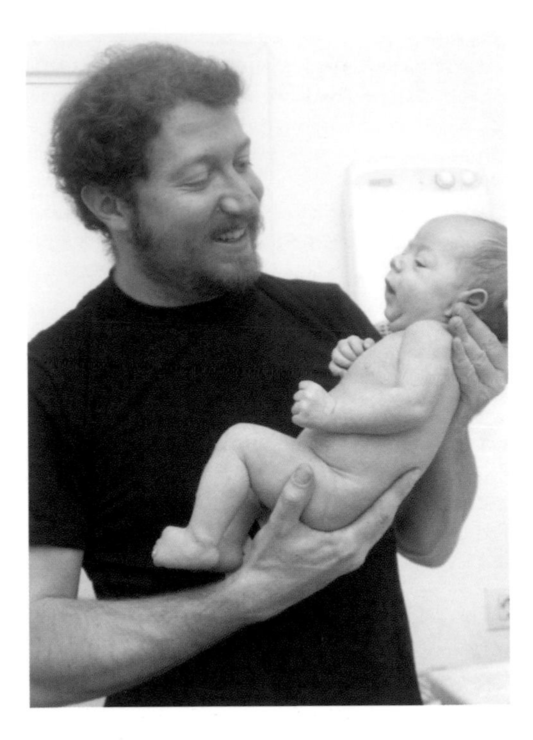

child's condition and, if necessary, prescribe precautionary measures. A baby born after a full term usually weighs between approximately 6 lb and 8½lb (2.7–3.9 kg), while a premature baby will weigh less. Weight loss (up to 10% of the weight at birth) is normal during the first days of life, but if the baby is healthy and develops normally, she will put this weight back on in a few weeks.

• **Height.** A newborn baby can measure 18–20 in (47 cm–52 cm).

• **Head circumference.** As in the case of the other parameters, tables are available to trace the appropriate mean values for a baby's head circumference and its subsequent development.

• **Skin.** This is thin, smooth, and can sometimes be covered with a fine down, which will gradually disappear. It is normal for a baby's skin to flake off in the first week of life.

• **Feeding.** A fetus already displays sucking and swallowing reflexes in the womb. In the first month of life, a baby establishes her own feeding rhythm, which must be respected. She may regurgitate or even vomit after drinking milk.

• **Defecation.** A newborn baby can have up to 6 bowel movements a day. At first, the accumulation of gas makes colic a frequent occurrence, triggering discomfort and crying.

Psychological and intellectual development

• **Sleep.** A newborn baby spends most of the time sleeping, only staying awake for roughly 1 in every 10 hours.

• **Consciousness.** A newborn baby's consciousness is characterized by 6 separate states: subdued sleep, active sleep, sleepiness, subdued alert, agitation, and active crying. The capacity to move from one state to the other indicates maturity and good neurological development. The cardiac rhythm, breathing, muscle tone, and body movements vary with each state.

• **Crying.** This provides a means of communicating and attracting attention. In a few weeks, parents learn to recognize a baby's various ways of crying, and their possible meanings.

The premature baby

Babies who are born before the 37th week of pregnancy are considered premature. The degree of immaturity and the duration of a baby's spell in the incubator will depend on how early the birth occurred. Once your baby leaves the incubator and is discharged from hospital, it is advisable to follow these recommendations at home:

- Avoid any contact with people suffering from any type of infectious disorder (cough, cold, flu, etc.).
- Avoid tobacco smoke and the use of air fresheners and aerosols in the vicinity of your baby.
- Wash your baby's clothes with soft soap.
- Wrap her snugly and make sure that her environment is warm.
- Stick to a routine.
- The doctor may recommend Vitamin D and iron supplements.
- Your baby will gradually acquire a normal rhythm of growth and development. It is important to consult a doctor about any doubts or changing circumstances.

Jaundice in newborn babies

Physiological jaundice is distinguished by a yellow coloring of the skin, mucous membranes, and eyes, brought on by an excess of bilirubin in the blood. This generally appears between the second and fifth day of life and disappears after 1 or 2 weeks. It is a common condition but it needs to be monitored to prevent any more serious pathology or disorder. In normal circumstances, jaundice can be classified as:

- Physiological jaundice. More than 50% of newborn babies get this type of jaundice, which is caused by an immature liver.
- Jaundice in premature babies. This is very common, as these babies take longer to regulate bilirubin, on account of their immaturity.
- Jaundice in suckling babies. This occurs in 1–2% of newborn babies receiving their mother's milk, as some of its components can raise bilirubin levels.

Jaundice does not normally require any treatment and disappears spontaneously within a week, although phototherapy is required if the bilirubin levels are very high or do not fall as expected. This treatment involves exposing a baby to ultraviolet rays for several hours a day, either in an incubator, in serious cases, or in sunshine. Ultraviolet light will hasten the evaporation and metabolization of the skin's pigmentation.

• **Bonding.** The link between a baby and her parents – especially the mother – is very special and close, and this enhances her development. This bond arises instinctively and strengthens over time.

• **Temperament.** Three types have been described: the easy baby, the difficult baby, and the apathetic baby, but every child is different and one baby can display various character traits.

Sensorimotor development

• **Reflexes.** These are involuntary and automatic movements triggered by a stimulus. In the first month, most of a baby's movements are reflexes. A doctor will examine and observe her reflexes to evaluate neurological function and development. The absence of reflexes or the presence of abnormal reflexes can indicate a disorder of the central nervous system.

• **Senses**

– Sight. A baby looks intently at objects or people, opens her eyelids, stops sucking, and observes attentively with both eyes. She distinguishes colors and is capable of following objects in movement.

– Hearing. A baby can hear before being born, but it is only after birth that hearing starts to develop. She distinguishes different tones, although the human voice takes preference.

– Taste. A baby prefers sweet flavors and finds acid, salty, and bitter tastes very unpleasant.

– Smell. A baby recognizes smells and can distinguish that of her mother.

– Touch. A baby seeks closeness, heat, and softness. The sense of touch reassures a baby by helping her to explore and come into contact with the environment.

– Balance. A baby reacts to rocking and changes of position. She tends to convey distaste for abrupt changes of posture by opening her eyes, showing fright, opening and immediately closing her arms, and even crying. This response is the so-called *Moor's reflex*, and it disappears after a few weeks.

Social development

- Almost all of a baby's reactions are instinctive.
- She stares at the faces of her parents.
- She cheers up or calms down when rocked or held in somebody's arms.
- She enjoys being spoken or sung to, as well as following objects and toys with her eyes.
- She may smile in response to certain stimuli.
- There is no adaptation to daily routines.

the second month

After the first month, the complicated initial period of adaptation is overcome and a strong bond is established between the baby and her family. Her mother has now totally recovered from giving birth and increasingly understands her baby's needs and temperament. Moreover, she gradually adjusts to the child's feeding times and periods of sleep and wakefulness. The baby's greater activity and responsiveness, and the parents' greater confidence, mark the start of a period of great joy for the family. Even so, it is normal to have doubts and anxiety about some aspects of a baby's health and development and these should be shared with the doctor.

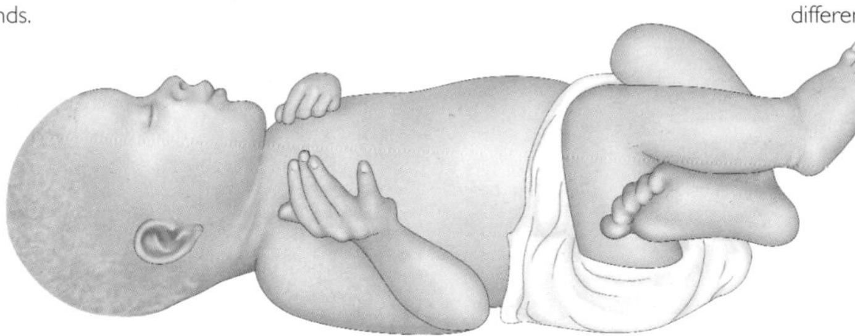

The second month

Physical development

• The baby's movements become increasingly more complex (albeit still uncoordinated). The following are particularly noteworthy:

– Lying face up. She moves her arms and legs, which tend to be bent. Greater mobility is evident.

– Lying face down. She supports herself on her arms and raises her head for a few seconds.

– Pulling with the arms to achieve a sitting position. The head hangs backward but remains raised for a few moments when the upright position is reached.

– Hands. These are often open.

• She keeps her head upright for short periods.

• She holds small objects for brief periods.

For at least the first 6 months of life, your baby must sleep face up, on a stiff surface and without too much covering. Sleeping in the parents' bed is to be avoided.

Psychological and intellectual development

• Your baby is asleep most of the time, but her periods of wakefulness become increasingly longer and can last up to 8–10 hours.

• Her timetable gradually becomes more regular. Nevertheless, in this month it is still advisable to feed her whenever she requires, even during the night.

• She pays attention to other people's faces.

• She can show emotion when she sees certain objects.

• She distinguishes voices and looks for the source of sounds.

• She follows the movements of people and large objects for up to 180°.

Sensorimotor development

• Your baby starts to observe her environment intently.

• She is startled by sudden noises.

• She babbles and emits sounds after pleasurable stimuli.

• She smiles frequently and opens her mouth to imitate the person speaking to her.

Social development

• She expresses pleasure or discontent by means of gestures.

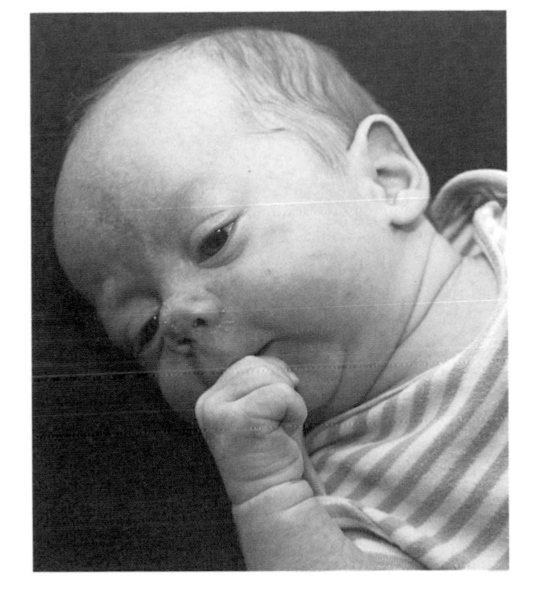

At this age a baby dribbles profusely, due to increased salivary secretion, and also because she is does not as yet mature enough to know how to learn how to swallow her saliva. Her eyes also water frequently. In some cases, the tear duct may be blocked, causing your baby's eyes to stream continuously and become sticky. If the tear duct does not open by itself and the eyes are still streaming after 6 months, consult an eye doctor, who will open the duct with a specially designed instrument.

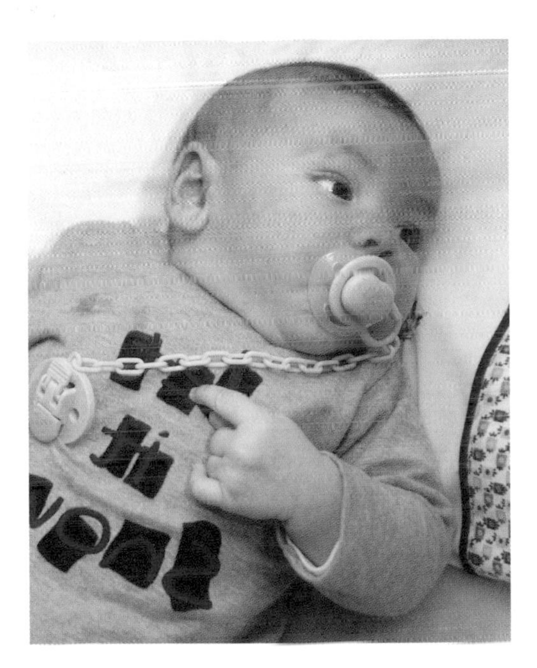

• She is happy in company.

• She moves her arms and legs more, and responds to stimuli from other people, especially parents and close relatives, with more marked gestures.

• A baby usually enjoys bath time, conveying her pleasure with gestures and energetic movement.

Oral thrush

This is characterized by ulcers or lesions in the mouth caused by infection by the fungus *Candida albicans*. These whitish sores can result in discomfort and a dry mouth. It is important to boil pacifiers and feeding bottles regularly, as this prevents the growth of the fungus. If the mother is nursing special care must also be taken in cases where the baby's mother is taking antibiotics or suffers from vaginal thrush, as this could encourage fungi to grow in her baby.

Although oral thrush is not serious, it does require treatment – usually with a liquid or paste applied to the mouth (nystatine is the most common, but there are others). Ideally, this should be given after feeding, as this will allow the medicine to remain longer in the mouth and so be more effective.

Diaper rash

Diaper rash, or inflammation in the areas in contact with the diaper, is very common in the first year of a baby's life. Moisture remaining after a bath, along with contact with urine and fecal matter, causes irritation and makes the skin turn red. This complaint tends to be more frequent in babies with pale skin.

The presence of fungi like Candida albicans also encourages the development of diaper rash. Although this type of fungus usually causes oral thrush, it can also appear in the genital area. In these cases, the irritated, red skin is complemented by small red patches enclosed by a white ring.

Diaper rash can also be caused by feces with a high level of acidity, such as those produced by a baby who cannot tolerate lactose. In these cases, the irritation begins around the anus and gradually extends over the surrounding area.

Good hygiene and thorough drying of the area covered by the diaper is essential to prevent this type of dermatitis, especially in the folds of the skin. There is no need to apply cream every day, as dry skin does not cause irritation. If fungi appear, the doctor will prescribe anti-mycotic medicine. The best creams for such cases are ones that contain zinc oxide; these are usually white and very thick.

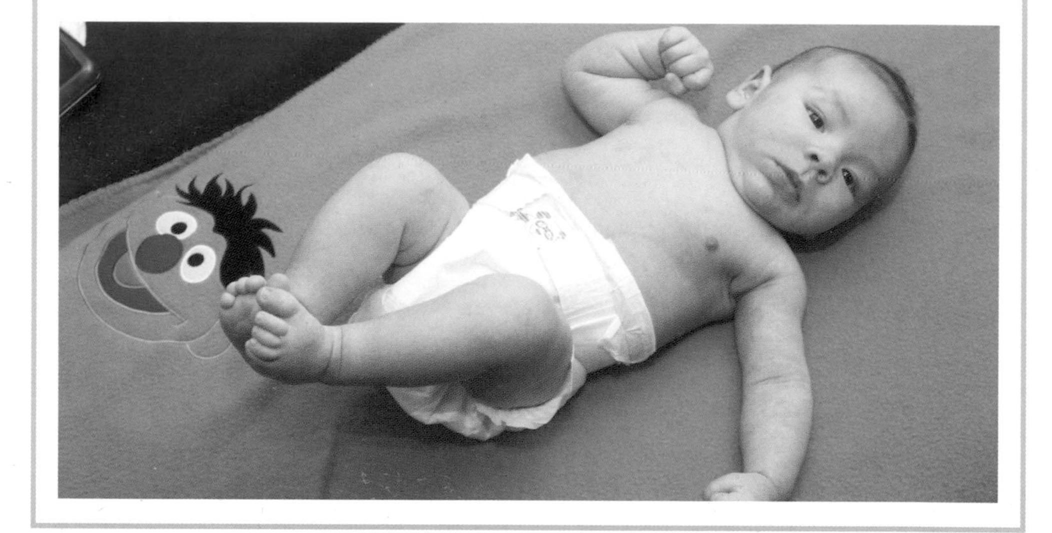

Seborrheic dermatitis (cradle cap)

This is very common in small children. The skin is scaly and yellowish, especially on the head and eyebrows; it can be almost imperceptible, although sometimes thick crusts may form. Seborrheic dermatitis or "cradle cap" spreads rapidly, but it is painless and does not represent a problem (apart from its unsightly appearance). Babies with pale skin tend to suffer from it more often than those with a darker complexion. In mild cases, it can be cleared by softening the skin with almond or olive oil and then gently scraping it off. In more severe cases, a doctor may recommend cream with salicylic acid and other products that help remove the crust.

the third month

Over the course of a month, a baby can make surprisingly rapid progress. This is closely related to a progressive maturing of the neurological system and the stimulation received from the environment. She reacts more often to all kinds of stimuli, as well as laughing more and crying less. She begins to participate in conversations by emitting gurgling sounds, and aspects of her personality start to emerge, in response to both genetic traits and her perception of the home environment.

Your baby socializes with people through smiles and babbling. She responds when called or spoken to.

At the end of the third month, she can usually produce sounds including the following vowels and consonants and combinations of these: R, EJE, AJA, and AJO.

She recognizes herself in a mirror.

She recognizes her mother perfectly and has created a very strong bond with her.

Some babies begin to sleep through the whole night.

The third month

Physical development

• At this age, the mean weight is 12 lb (5.5 kg) and the mean height 24 in (60 cm).

• She acquires greater muscle tone, which allows her to raise her shoulders and head for a few seconds when lying face down.

• She moves her legs and arms vigorously, either separately or together.

• She observes her hands and stretches her arms, as well as hitting objects with a clenched fist.

Psychological and intellectual development

• She recognizes members of her family.

• Her memory begins to be apparent.

• She vocalizes better and continues developing her range of gestures.

• She explores her face, mouth, and eyes with her hands.

Sensorimotor development

• She gradually starts to follow objects shown to her with her head.

• She observes her hands and follows the movements of her fingers.

• She observes and touches objects or parts of her body, and she tries to bring them to her mouth.

• When nursing, she may be distracted by a sound and try to verify its origin.

• She holds objects more tightly in her hands.

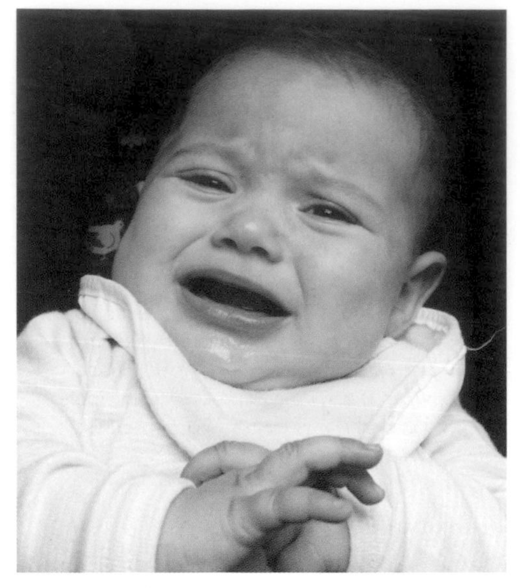

At this age, a baby is continuously bringing her hands to her mouth and sucking on them. The popular explanation is that this is due to teething, which makes her gums hurt. This is not true, however. Teeth do not normally appear before the sixth month – although some children may have a congenital tooth, or a few that grow at the age of 3 or 4 months – and the eruption of teeth does not cause discomfort so long far in advance. Sucking things is simply enjoyable, as well as necessary for a baby. Her mouth complements her sense of touch. She loves nibbling solid objects like toys, plastic keys, rings, and teethers.

Social development

- Increasing regularity is evident in her cycles of sleep–wakefulness–feeding.
- It is easier to make her smile with a variety of stimuli. She cries less often.
- There is wider range of communication and responses to social stimuli.

Around the third month of life, a baby often hits a bad patch. This tends to manifest itself in a greater demand for milk than in previous weeks, as well as irritability and fewer hours of sleep. The child never seems to be satisfied. Remember that critical periods are transitory and are not the fault of either the baby or her parents, and so they do not presuppose any poor upbringing. Such changes are a normal consequence of the development of a baby's neurological and mental structure. These periods demonstrate increasing maturity, and once they are over a baby exhibits new skills and recovers her usual temperament. All of the ages mentioned here with respect to both the breakthroughs and downturns in a baby's development are merely indicative – every child's development is different.

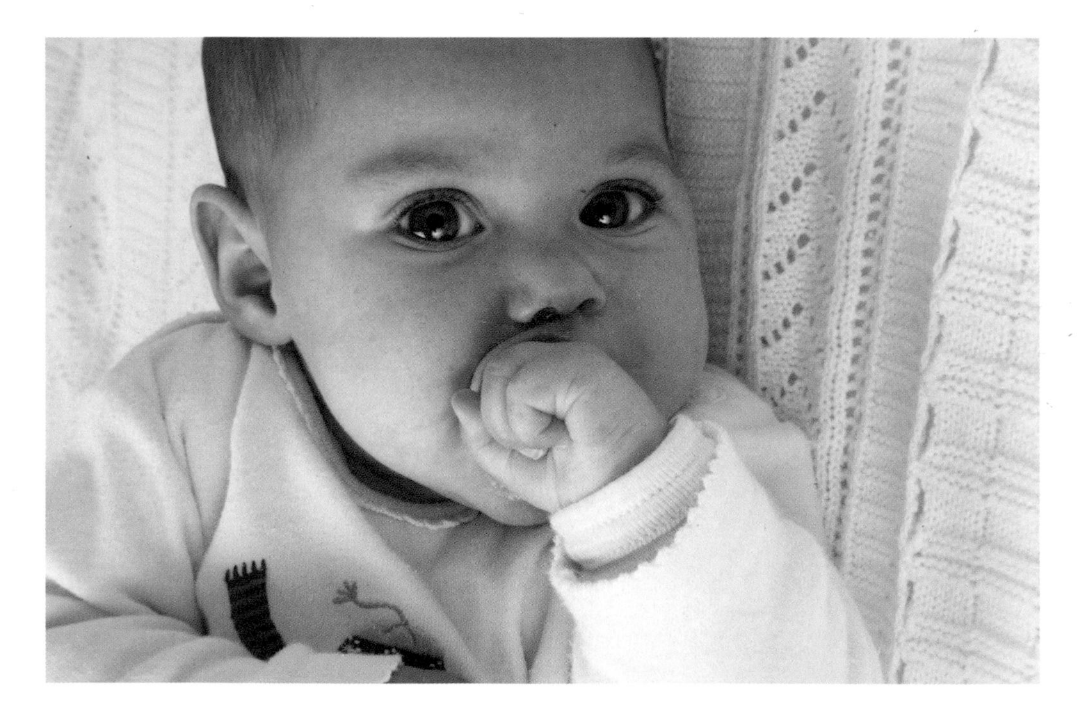

Crib deaths

Sudden infant death syndrome (SIDS, "crib death") is a term used to describe the unexpected death of a seemingly healthy child less than a year old. A sudden death of this type is caused by a cardiac arrest derived from the immaturity of the nervous system and the cardio-respiratory function. Ninety percent of such deaths occur in the first 6 months of life; it is unusual, however, in the first month or after the sixth, and extremely rare in children aged 1 year old or more.

Risk factors

- The male gender: 3 out of every 5 cases are boys.
- The time of day: it normally occurs during sleeping hours, between midnight and 9 am.
- The season of the year: cot deaths are more frequent in winter.
- Sickness: mild respiratory infections and gastrointestinal symptoms during the previous week.
- Family history: the risk is multiplied by 10 if a brother suffered from the syndrome (40% in the case of twins).
- Feeding: cot deaths are more common in babies fed with formula.
- Maternal factors: a young woman who has had several children with short intervals between pregnancies (if the mother is aged under 20 or has more than 4 children, the risk increases fourfold), previous abortions, anemia during pregnancy, alcoholism, tobacco consumption or drug addiction, or no prenatal and postnatal monitoring.
- Environmental factors: low socio-economic level, residence in urban areas, excessive heat.
- History of apnea or apparent life-threatening event (ALTE): the circumstances surrounding infant apnea must be analyzed, including your baby's appearance (color and muscle tone) when it occurs, to be able to anticipate it, and any abnormal posture or movement associated with it.

Prevention

Although the cause of crib deaths is not known, some precautions can be taken to avoid the abovementioned risk factors:

- A baby should not sleep face down during the first 6 months of life.
- Her mother should not smoke during pregnancy or when nursing.
- Keep the baby away from cigarette smoke and aerosols.
- The mother should not take drugs.
- Avoid high temperatures (no more than 68–72 ºF/20–22 ºC), whether from excessive clothing or heating.
- A baby should not sleep in her parents' bed.
- Whenever possible, feed the baby with mother's milk.

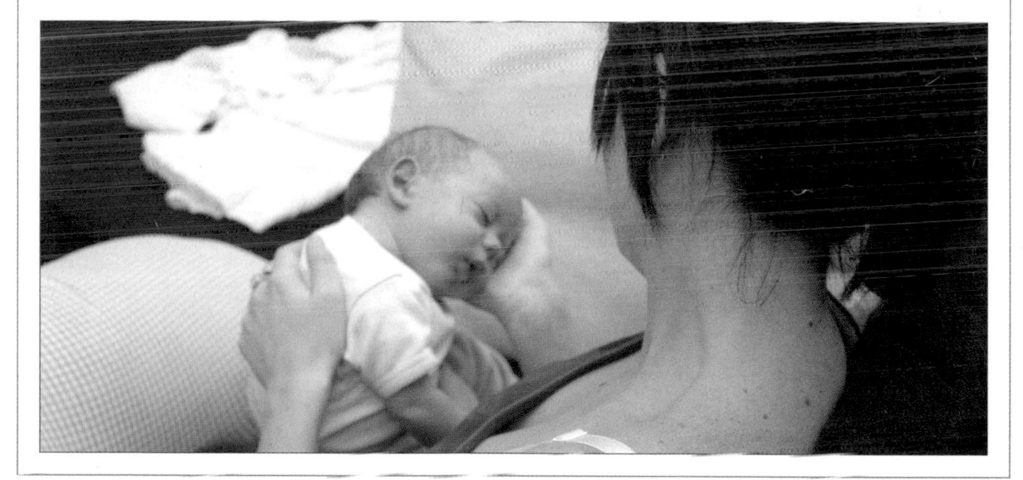

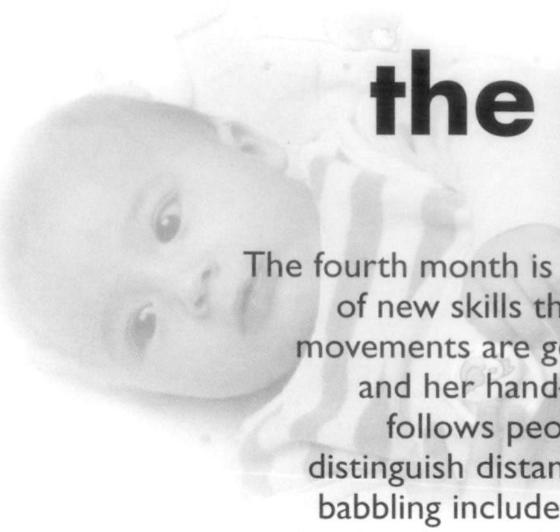

the fourth month

The fourth month is a period of great advances, with the acquisition of new skills thanks to her increased psychomotor ability. Her movements are generally less abrupt and much more controlled, and her hand–eye coordination is also better developed. She follows people and moving objects with an intent gaze, can distinguish distances and colors, and responds to her name. Her babbling includes syllables, she starts to imitate sounds, and her laughter grows louder. Similarly, certain character traits gradually begin to define themselves and this enables her to develop an increasingly close relationship with her family and her environment.

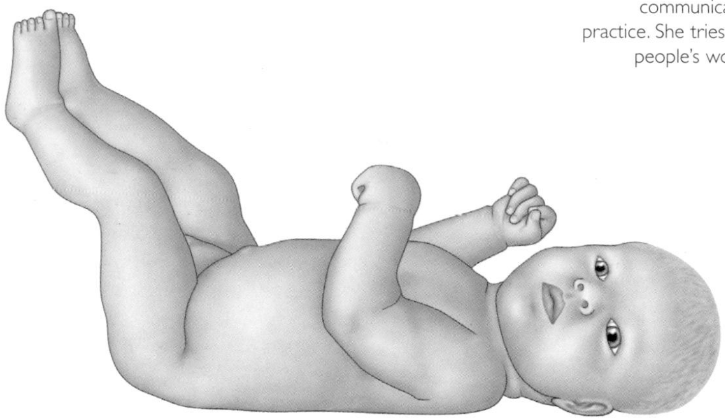

She can raise herself on her arms without any difficulty.

At this age, she can recognize most colors.

She realizes that her primitive language allows her to communicate and starts to practice. She tries to repeat other people's words and actions.

She has a very loud laugh and expresses contentment by smiling and moving her body.

At the age of 4 months, she distrusts unfamiliar people.

The fourth month

Physical development

• She can turn from a face-down to a face-up position on her own.

• If she is face up, she lifts her head and grasps her feet.

• She usually needs to be fed only 4 times a day, although some babies still demand a night-time feed.

Psychological and intellectual development

• The periods of attentiveness are both more frequent and longer.

• She can sleep continuously for 8–10 hours at night and have 3–4 naps during the day.

• She starts to be aware of the reactions she provokes in other people.

• She smiles and communicates in the presence of people she likes.

Sensorimotor development

• When she turns her head, she is capable of coordinating her eye movements.

• She follows the direction of sounds and the movement of objects.

• She adapts her vision to different distances.

• She is capable of recognizing even small objects.

• Music and gentle sounds have a soothing effect and your baby pays attention to what she hears.

Social development

• Your baby expresses displeasure when a game is interrupted, generally through crying.

• Images reflected in a mirror capture her attention and interest.

How to look after a baby's gums and future teeth

In the fourth month, the baby may start to show the first signs of teeth . It is important to take measures to care for these future teeth:

- Never give your baby a feeding bottle to make her go to sleep.
- Carefully wipe her gums once a day with a clean, soft, damp cloth. Do this even before the teeth emerge.
- Some babies' teeth come through when they are barely 4 or 5 months old, but in most cases they appear between the ages of 6 and 8 months.
- When the teeth start to come through, try cleaning them with a toothbrush with soft bristles. (Be sure to use a special toothbrush for babies.) Alternatively, you can continue wiping them every day with a cloth.
- Wash the teeth carefully with water. There is no need to use toothpaste until your baby is about 3 years old; she must be old enough to know how to spit it out after brushing her teeth.

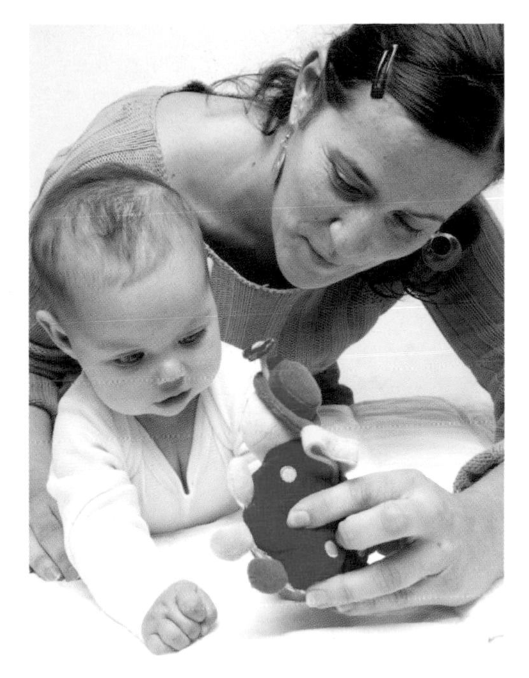

• She likes to be held and cuddled.

• She starts to show a preference for specific toys.

Prevention of accidents

At this age, the most important thing for a baby is to be able to touch and explore everything around her, so it is vital to make sure that nothing dangerous lies within her reach. A few safety rules can be extremely useful for preventing accidents:

• Do not allow her to play with string, paper, or fabric.

• Avoid furry or hairy toys.

• Keep medicines, detergents, cosmetics, lotions, paints, and solvents locked away or out of your baby's reach.

• Never leave a baby alone in the bathtub or on high surfaces like a changing table or bed.

• Always support a baby with one hand while changing her.

• Always check the water temperature before giving her a bath.

• Protect your baby from direct sunlight.

• Do not leave her alone with young siblings or pets.

Food

In the fourth month of life, non-dairy foodstuffs can be introduced, prudently and in accordance with your doctor's advice. These should be prepared in appropriate amounts and at the right consistency, so as not to alter the rhythm of digestive and renal maturing or the progressive neuro-muscular development.

This phase should enhance the development of the senses and encourage your baby to try different flavors and textures. This will allow you to introduce changes in how you feed your baby, from sucking to a spoon, from liquid to purée and, once the teeth have appeared, to diced food. In the fourth month you can start introducing cereals without gluten and fruit purées into your baby's diet.

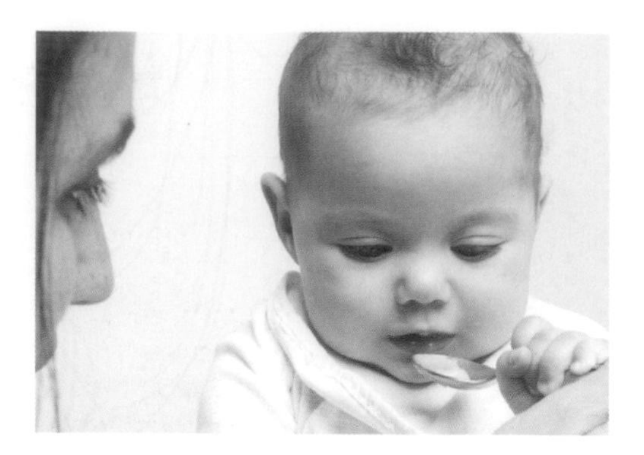

In the fourth month of life, a baby starts to take more solid foodstuffs. It marks the arrival of teatime fruit purées and juices, which provide vitamins and fiber that are vital to a baby's health.

Crossed eyes

This occurs when the ocular axes are not parallel, and so the eyes do not point in the same direction. Crossed eyes are described by a range of technical terms, depending on the type of defect:

- Esotropia: one eye pointing toward the center.
- Exotropia: one eye pointing outward.
- Hypertropia: one eye pointing upward.
- Hypotropia: one eye pointing downward.

- It is common for newborn babies to have crossed eyes.
- In a few weeks, a baby learns to focus properly and synchronize her eye movements.
- If the eyes are still crossed in the fourth month, a children's ophthalmologist should be consulted, as the eyes should be correctly aligned at this age.
- The World Health Organization suggests that the first eye checkup should take place at the age of 4 months.
- If a problem is suspected, or if a baby is born prematurely, this examination should be undertaken at birth.

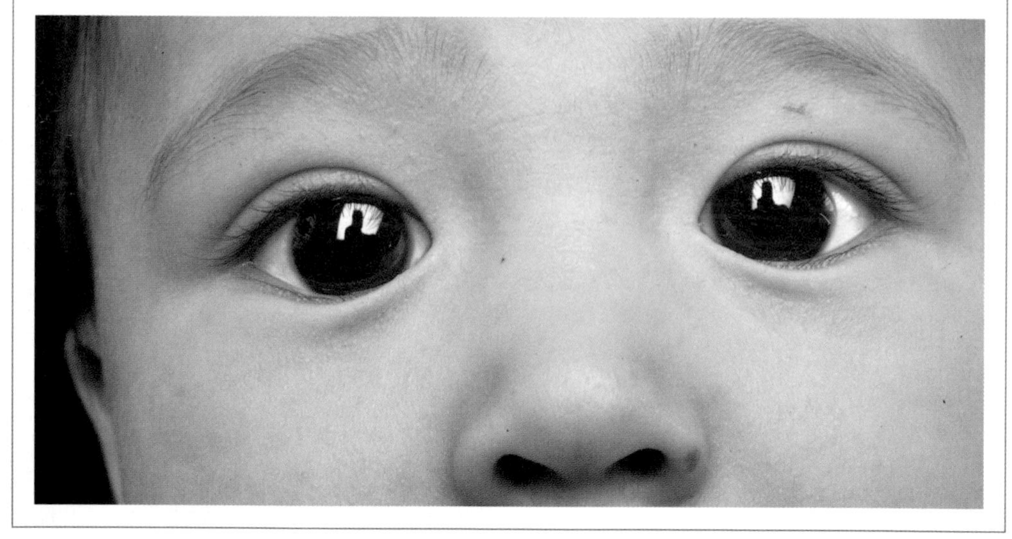

the fifth month

A transitional stage is starting as she will soon learn to move around. Her mobility, dexterity, and capacity for communicating and relating with others all advance in leaps and bounds. She can raise her head and arch her back, and she tries to drag herself about. Her attachment to toys and objects is coupled with a desire to make new discoveries. Every day brings a new discovery.

At the age of 5 months, your baby starts to express her emotions more effusively: she laughs, cries, kisses, hugs, etc.

She starts to babble or make sounds that include the consonants B or M, and she repeats the last sounds she has learned.

She can stand up for a few seconds if supported around the waist or under the armpits.

She takes an interest in everything that moves and has bright colors, and she can follow these objects with her gaze.

The fifth month

Physical development

• The baby is capable of lifting her head and shoulders when stretched out face upward.

• She sucks her toes.

• She is capable of sitting upright with help.

• She touches, holds, and moves objects and brings them to her mouth.

• She passes objects from one hand to the other.

Psychological and intellectual development

• She starts to show fear and distrust in the presence of strangers.

• She pronounces vowels and a few consonants, her gurgling includes syllables such as *pa pa, da da, ma ma,* etc.

• She follows fast-moving objects with her gaze and tries to grasp them.

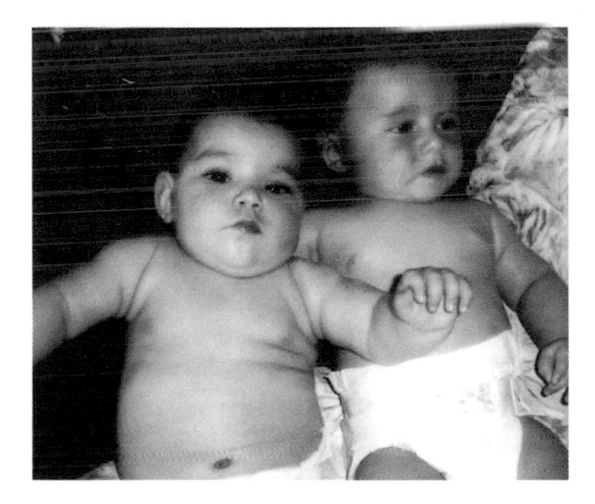

Sensorimotor development

- She grabs objects with greater decisiveness and dexterity.
- She tries to grasp anything that attracts her attention, including parts of her own body, with 1 or 2 hands.
- She entertains herself with the toys within her reach.

Social development

- She smiles and vocalizes, in expectation of a response from the people around her.

Advice for stimulating a baby's learning process

- Lie down on the floor with her and give her something to play with. It is a good idea to put the toy out of her reach so that she has to stretch to grasp it. Alternatively, you can cover part of the toy with a blanket or cushion and see if she can find it. Be sure to make this fun, so that your baby does not lose interest or become exasperated.
- Talk to her and repeat the sounds she makes. When she says *"baa,"* say *"baa"* yourself. She will laugh, smile, and try to repeat the same sound time and time again.
- Read her a book every day, even if it is always the same one.
- Dance with her.
- Sing her children's songs.
- Take her for a walk and describe what you see.
- Show her brightly colored photos, magazines, and images.
- Show her toys with different colors, textures, and shapes.
- When she grows tired of playing or trying to talk, hug and cuddle her. Congratulate her and tell her that you love her.
- A baby loves doing the same thing over and over again. This repetition is an excellent way of learning.

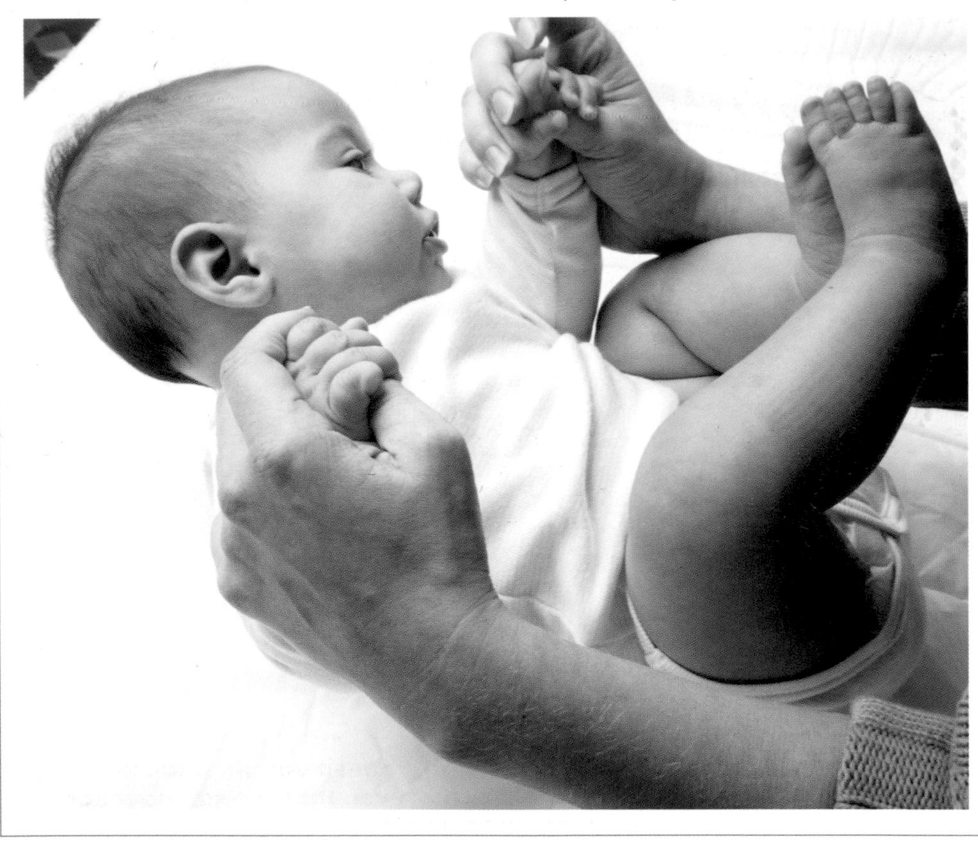

• She stops crying when she is spoken to, recognizes the tone of voice used, and responds accordingly.

• She loses her temper if a toy is taken away from her.

• She shows great curiosity for mirrors.

Sleep

• A 5-month-old baby can sleep for longer spells (5–8 hours), although every child is different and has her own sleep patterns.

• Babies are not always awake when they seem to be. They can shout and make all types of sounds while they are asleep. Even if they wake up at night, they are only awake for a few minutes and can go back to sleep again without any encouragement.

• There is no need to get up if you hear your baby stirring during the night. It is better for her to learn to go back to sleep on her own. If she cries or stays awake for several minutes, however, she must be attended to, as she could be hungry, cold, wet, or even sick.

• If she does require attention, see to her quickly and silently, to avoid stimulating her. Do not talk to her or play with her; it is not even a good idea to switch on the light. Even though she is still very young, she has to learn that night time is for sleeping.

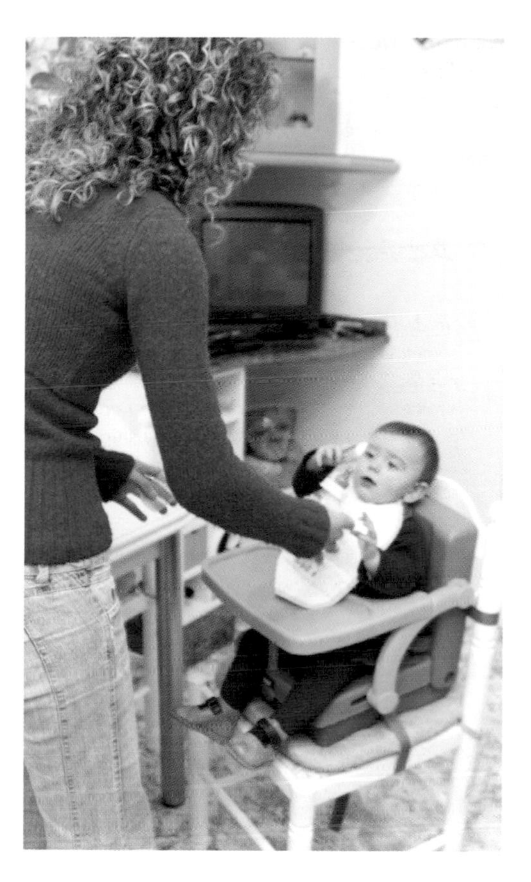

Feeding

A baby can begin to use a high chair whenever she can sit upright and is ready to eat solid foods – normally at the age of 4–5 months.

Choosing a high chair

• A high chair must support a baby securely, with a belt that goes around the waist and a strap between the legs.

• This belt must not be attached to the tray.

• The tray must be secure and your baby must not be able to move it.

• The clasp of the belt must be easy to use.

• The high chair must have the legs sufficiently far apart to prevent it from falling over. You must remember that a baby of this age moves around energetically.

• A folding chair must have a holding mechanism to stop it moving or tipping over.

Using a high chair

• Always fasten your baby's belt. The leg strap prevents your baby from falling out or slipping under the tray.

• Never leave your baby on her own.

• Make sure the tray is securely in place.

• Make sure that your baby's hands are not crossed when you fit the tray.

• There should be no dangerous edges or pieces.

• Put something on the tray to allow your baby to entertain herself.

At the age of four or five months, a baby can sit upright and starts to eat solid food. This does not mean, however, that she can now eat any or everything, prepared in any way.

the sixth month

Although every child is different, at the age of 6 months a baby is usually capable of remaining in a sitting position and starts to drag herself around. Her exploration of her surroundings is still very important, so any object will attract her attention and provide an excuse for play by stimulating her to grasp it and put it in her mouth (or tear it apart!). She may display mood swings at this age. Although she is increasingly aware of her surroundings and her body, her limited ability to get around and grab hold of everything that catches her eye can lead to frustration, tears, and tantrums. She is becoming increasingly sociable, however, and shows a broader range of responses to stimuli.

She starts to open her hand and loses the habit of clenching her fist.

She is capable of supporting herself on one hand and using the other to grab a toy that has attracted her attention. She will bring it to her mouth and pass it from one hand to the other.

It is still very early to know whether a baby is right- or left-handed. At times she may use one hand more than the other, but this may soon change.

She is capable of turning over when lying down.

She likes communicating with other people and immediately relates to anybody who greets her with caresses or a smile.

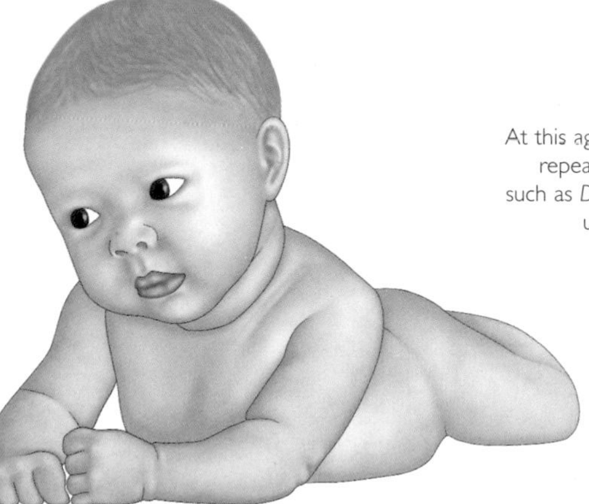

At this age, she starts to continuously repeat chains of identical syllables, such as *DA-DA-DA* or *GUE-GUE-GUE*, using different tones, as if she were singing a tune.

She uses all her senses to explore everything around her. She listens, observes, touches, and smells in order to take in the world around her.

Her hearing is sharper and she can locate the source of a sound without any difficulty, turning her head in that particular direction.

Sixth month

Physical development

• A baby's first means of getting about is by dragging herself, which is the phase prior to crawling on hands and knees.

• She is increasingly able to turn her head in a controlled fashion.

• She sits upright on her own, or with slight support.

• She grabs any object in her path, including the face, ears, glasses, etc. of the person holding her, especially her mother.

• She sleeps for 8–10 hours at night.

Psychological and intellectual development

• The baby closely examines all the objects she plays with.

• She is capable of picking up anything that interests her with precise movements.

• Her changing moods are normally an expression of affection/dislike for somebody in her presence.

• She continues to utter syllables and make gurgling noises to communicate.

• She discovers her own voice and amuses herself by listening to it.

Sensorimotor development

• While holding an object with one hand, she is capable of grasping something else with the other and also turning her attention toward a third object.

• Music calms her down and stops her crying.

• She plays with food and handles it with enthusiasm.

• She spins and turns over objects by moving her wrists. These movements are usually brusque.

Social development

• She enjoys playing and being in contact with other people, but is selective, and she is distrustful of strangers.

• She expresses her feelings (pleasure, discontent) by means of gurgling noises.

• She smiles at her reflection in a mirror and plays with it.

A feeding bottle can cause tooth decay

• If a baby needs a feeding bottle before sleeping, this should be filled with water. Do not use breast milk, baby milk formulas, juices, or sweetened liquids in the night-time feeding bottle. The sugar in milk and juice can accumulate on a baby's teeth while she is asleep, causing tooth decay. Water does not have this effect, however.

• This type of tooth decay is very troublesome; it can cause pain and prompt an emergency. Protect your baby's teeth even before they appear. Delicately clean her gums once a day with a soft, clean cloth.

• When your baby reaches the age of 6 months, try to teach her to drink out of a glass or cup. Apart from forming a habit, this will help to prevent tooth decay caused by a feeding bottle.

• Cuddle your baby before she goes to sleep and give her your full attention; reassurance is better than a feeding bottle. You can also offer her a soft toy to hold and hug; this will relax her before she goes to sleep.

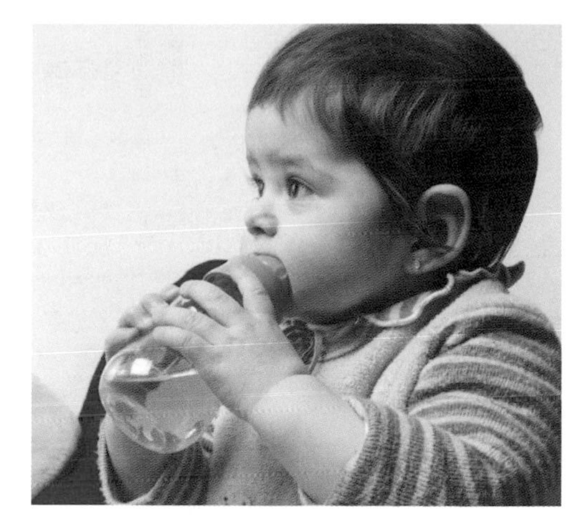

Allowing a baby to eat on her own

• While they are learning to eat on their own, all babies get messy, put their fingers in their mouth, and use their hands to eat and break up more solid foodstuffs. They may also spit out their food. This learning process takes time, but it is a vital one.

• Put a bib on your baby, or allow her to eat wearing only diapers. You can also put a cloth underneath the high chair to make cleaning up easier. Allow her to play with food – this is her way of investigating it and learning to eat. Do not leave her alone at meal times, however, to ensure that she does not choke or hurt herself.

• She may want to play with her toys or spoons, and she may even throw them around. Do not forget that children of this age play all the time, and that this is an excellent means of exploring their environment and communicating.

• You must know what to do if your baby has a choking fit.

• Try to give your baby a little fruit juice, breast milk, or formula milk in a cup. When you give her a cup, help her grasp it. She will find this easier with a cup with 2 handles.

• Babies with a disability or medical problem may need special assistance. It is possible that they have physical difficulties that impede their ability to chew or eat by themselves, or maybe they cannot digest food in the same way as other children. In such cases, ask the doctor the best way to help your child eat non-liquid food.

Your baby moves about without any difficulty and is very frisky; take care that she does not slip out of your grasp when you are changing her, for instance. She is gaining awareness of her body and starting to explore it. Generally speaking, a baby finds her own balance.

The floor is for playing

Babies of 6 months need to spend plenty of time on the floor, so that they can learn to crawl. If your baby does not like being alone on the floor, sit down and play with her.

Some activities to share with your child

In this period, you will find your baby going through big changes. She is maturing at a very fast rate and needs to be constantly entertained and given new skills. Affection is the essential ingredient: the best proof of your baby's happiness is the smiles she gives you, and love is often much more effective than any medicine in overcoming sickness.

- To stimulate all your baby's senses, give her toys and objects with different colors, textures, weights, and sounds (as long as they are safe). Dolls with bells inside, fluffy objects, or a soft rubber ball are some of the toys preferred by babies of this age.
- Allow her to observe her surroundings by sitting her in her crib or stroller, changing the position of objects on a regular basis to stop her growing bored. Show your baby her reflection, to allow her to investigate it; just watch how she laughs when she sees herself in your arms!
- It is still too early for her to crawl, so encourage her to start by putting her favorite toys in front of her, and then pull them away so that she has to reach out for them.
- This is the ideal age for starting to read to a baby, as she will react by looking at the colorful pictures in storybooks; this encourages sociability and communication – vital factors in the future.

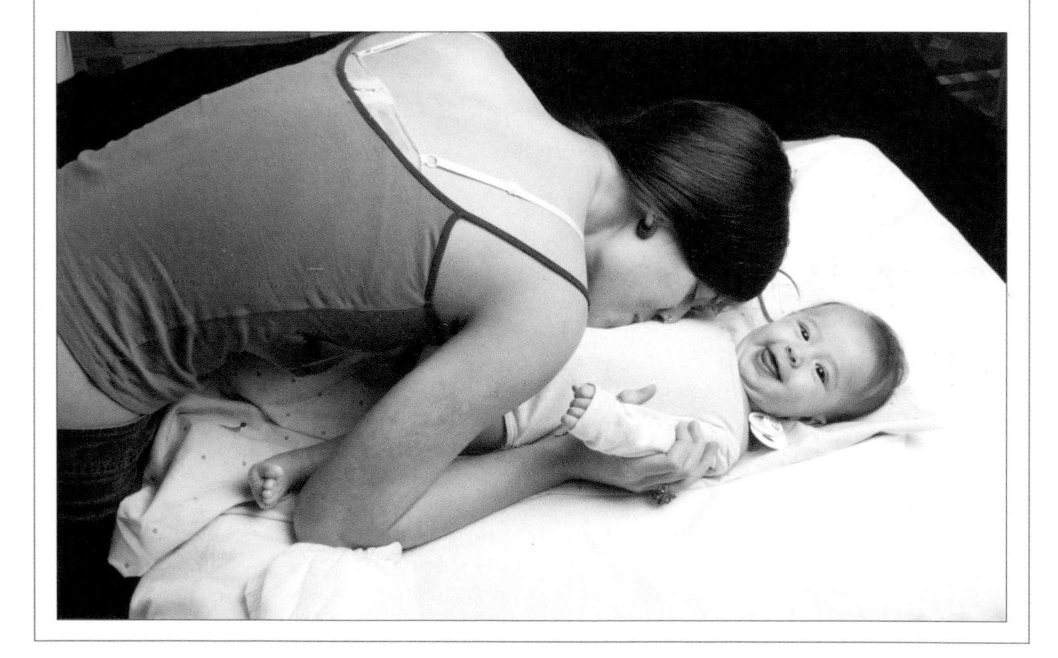

the seventh month

By now, many children are crawling and exploring their surroundings on their own; they cannot stay still for a moment and this can increase the risk of accidents. They need to be continuously accompanied and watched; they need discipline and they also start to distinguish between what they can and cannot do. At the age of 7 months, a baby begins an important period in her verbal development and understands the meaning of some words and gestures. Another important milestone is the appearance of the first teeth – this may make her irritable and nervous.

One of the great advances is a baby's ability to support much of her body weight with her legs. She can also remain seated without any support, enabling her to hold and examine objects with greater freedom. In this period, most babies start to cut their first teeth.

Your baby's curiosity has increased and as a result she requires limits, but she is still disobedient. The best way to teach her at this stage is by simply saying 'no' and then providing a distraction.

She picks up objects with one hand and passes them from one to the other with great dexterity. She is capable of clapping her hands and banging two objects together (great fun!).

At this age, a baby is more perceptive and recognizes small differences in sounds, and she can also understand the different tones in a voice that is addressing her. So, if she is scolded angrily, she may start to cry.

The seventh month

Physical development

• The baby's leg muscles acquire greater tone and strength, to enable her to stand up and try to walk.

• She advances by crawling, maybe with an object in her hand.

• She can sit upright without being supported.

• The lower incisors begin to come through.

Psychological and intellectual development

• She shows interest in details.

• She repeats defined syllables, and gives them meaning.

• She starts to pay attention to colored figures.

• Her memory is more retentive and her attention span is longer. She may try to imitate sounds or simple actions, like applause or saying "bye bye." She likes playing hide-and-seek. If she cannot find a toy that interests her, she moves her head or body to look for it.

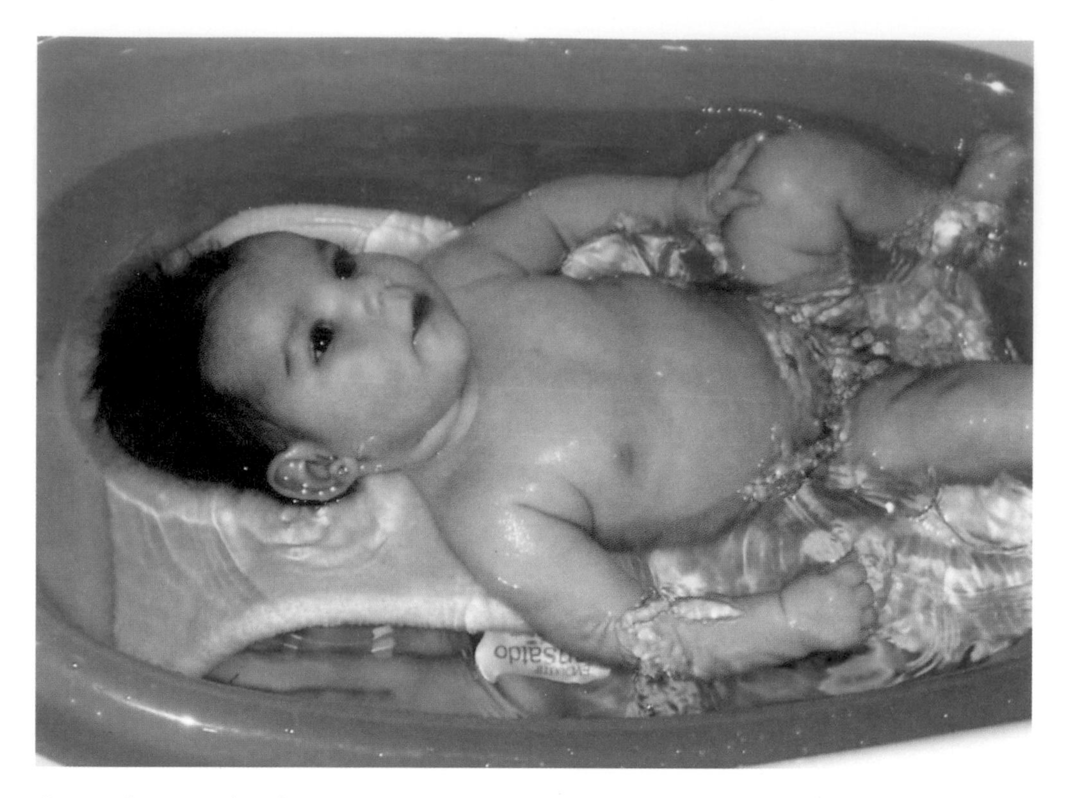

Sensorimotor development

• She can hold a different object in each hand.

• She enjoys playing with objects that make noises, shaking them energetically to produce these sounds.

• She explores her own body.

Social development

• She shows great interest in participating in group activities.

• She plays on her own and with others, having fun in both cases.

• She understands the meaning of "no" from the tone of voice used by an adult.

• She shows affection toward people she knows through caresses, kisses, and hugs.

• She prefers to be picked up by people she likes.

Tips for washing a baby in a bathtub

• At this age, a baby is too big for a child's bath. When she can sit without assistance, she can be washed in a regular tub.

• Prepare everything before bathing her. First, assemble the soap, towels, and toys, then turn on the faucet. Touch the water with your elbow to make sure that it isn't too hot. If it feels very hot on your elbow, it will certainly be too hot for your baby.

• When everything is ready, put your baby in the water. Stay close to her while she is in the tub, not letting her out of your sight for a single moment. It is advisable to hold her, to prevent her from slipping or banging herself against the tub.

• Bath time can be fun for both of you, so enjoy yourselves! Play with your baby and let her revel in the water. As playing in the bath can cause splashing, put mats or towels on the floor to stop it getting wet and slippery.

• Allow your baby to splash as much as she wants. Talk and sing to her while you wash her. Give her a cup or toy that she can fill with water and then empty.

• Put toys in the water so that she can touch them. She will learn to use her hand to reach the ones she likes.

• Give your baby her own sponge to wash herself. With just a little effort, bath time can provide pleasure for the whole family.

Never leave a baby alone in a bathtub, even if it contains very little water. Remember that just a few inches can be enough to drown a baby.

Father and child

Fathers should spend time with their kids too. Lie on the floor with your child, put a toy out of her reach, and encourage her to drag it toward her. Do not over-insist if she is still not ready to do this. Here are some other activities a father can share with his baby:

- Roll a soft ball and let her collect it.
- Play hide-and-seek.
- Smile and applaud when she succeeds in performing a task.
- Hug and reassure her when she is upset because a task proves too difficult for her.

Schedule a time to be with your baby, whenever suits you best: at lunch, bath time, or before going to bed. She will be delighted. You are her father: it is good that you do things in a different way from her mother.

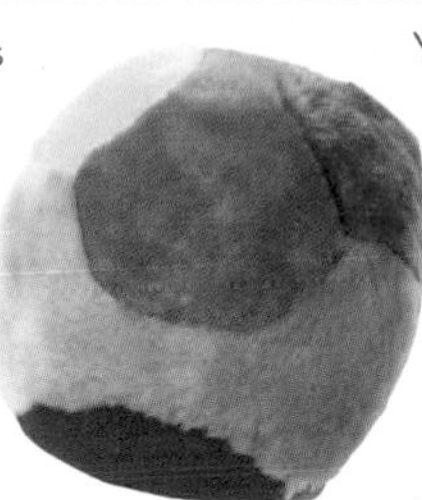

Your seven-month-old baby loves playing. Here are some more ideas for spending time with her:

- Take a toy that makes a noise and produce a sound with it. Now, hide it under a blanket or a cushion, in view of your baby. Encourage her to search for it.
- Bang two toys or objects against each other in front of your baby. Then, let her do the same.
- Put your baby on one end of a towel or scarf and gently pull the other end.
- Cut out large, brightly colored photos from magazines, then stick them on to sheets of paper to make a book for your baby. Sit her on your lap and explain each photo to her.
- Let her play with musical toys, such as bells, a baby's keyboard, or rattles. Always make sure that no toy has any small pieces that could come off.

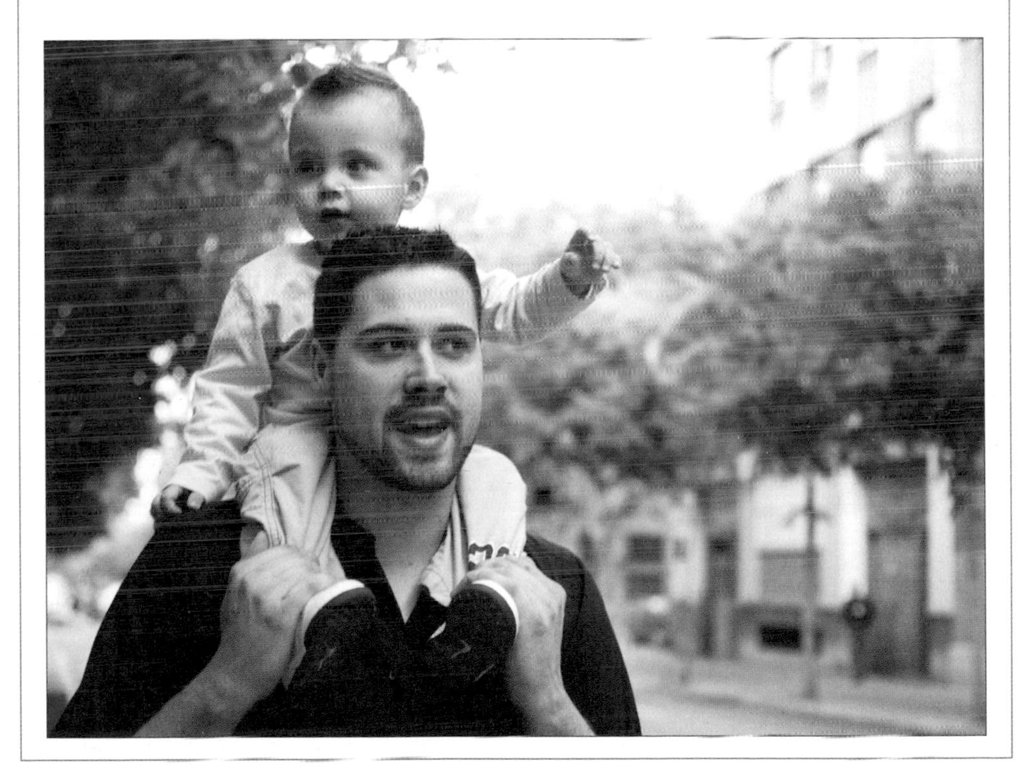

the eighth month

At this age, a child may change some of her habits, especially as regards eating and sleeping: she may not want to be fed but prefer to eat for herself; when her first teeth appear, she may lose her appetite; she may reject food with unfamiliar textures and flavors, etc. It is common for a baby to need a couple of naps every day until the age of 14–15 months. She displays growing dexterity and speed in her movements, as well as a greater ability to get around. Tantrums can be frequent in this phase, so she requirest a firm establishment of limits from her parents. As regards communication, she is still unable to make herself understood, but uses her own vocabulary, which is full of meaning for her.

Your baby can sit on her own, with her legs slightly bent and head upright, for at least one minute, without losing her balance.

She can move about at will by lying on her abdomen and raising the upper part of her body. This movement will soon give way to crawling on her hands and knees.

She acquires greater control of her hands and starts to be more skilful with her fingers. She can point and use her forefinger and thumb as a pincer, allowing her to pick up small objects with greater precision.

She can stand up with the help of furniture (a chair, sofa, or table) or her parents' legs.

Her personality starts to define itself.

All babies go through a period of fearfulness (so-called *separation anxiety*). This occurs as a result of her greater awareness of herself as an individual, and she gets anxious when her mother or another loved one goes away.

She will investigate every object she comes across, as each one produces different results after it has been banged, shaken, flattened, pulled, twisted, bitten, and opened!

Eighth month

Physical development

- She can crawl forward and backward.
- She rocks when kneeling.
- She maintains a sitting position.
- She drags herself across the floor.
- She tries to stand up with the support of an object.

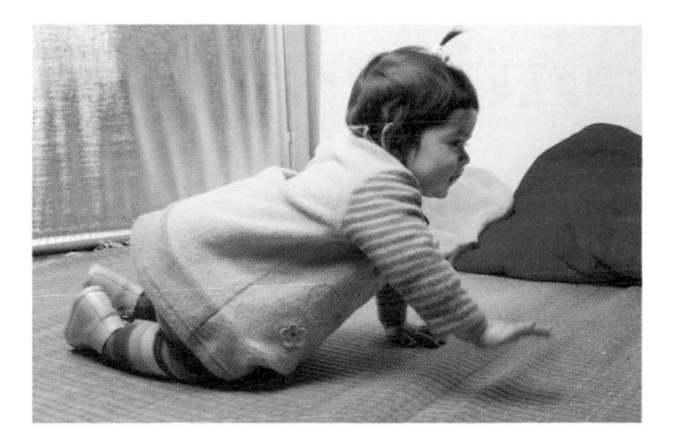

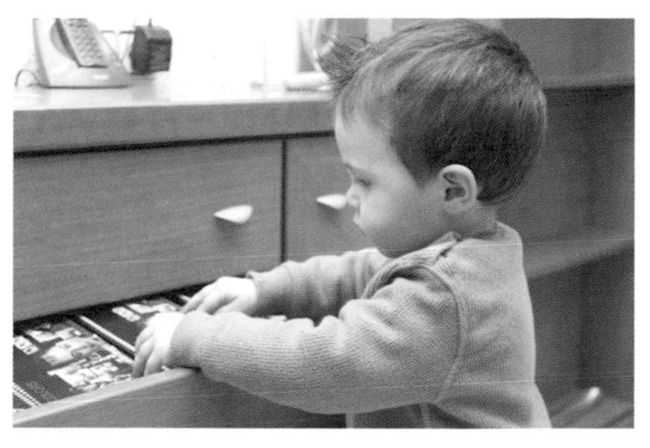

Psychological and intellectual development

• She starts to memorize the faces of the people she sees.

• She is capable of recognizing some words and tries to repeat them.

• She can point at something she wants and follow it with her gaze.

Sensorimotor development

• She holds objects of a certain size with her thumb, forefinger, and middle finger.

• She holds small objects with her thumb and forefinger.

• She points at something that interests her with her finger.

THE APPROPRIATE AGE FOR INTRODUCING VARIOUS FOODSTUFFS INTO A BABY'S DIET

Months	1	2	3	4	5	6	7	8	9	10	11	12
Breast milk	■	■	■	■	■	■	■	■	■	■	■	■
Infant formula	■	■	■	■	■							
Follow-on formula				■	■	■	■	■	■	■	■	■
Cereals without gluten				■	■	■	■	■	■	■	■	■
Cereals with gluten							■	■	■	■	■	■
Fruit juices					■	■	■	■	■	■	■	■
Fruit purees					■	■	■	■	■	■	■	■
Vegetables					■	■	■	■	■	■	■	■
Meat						■	■	■	■	■	■	■
Natural yoghurt without sugar						■	■	■	■	■	■	■

The best way to ensure your baby is safe is by keeping close watch over her. If you leave the room for a moment, make sure your baby is in a safe place, such as the crib or playpen. Keep a list of emergency telephone numbers at hand.

Social development

- She shouts to attract attention.
- She pushes away things she dislikes with her hands.
- She starts to express her feelings. For example, she cries when her mother goes out.
- She does not like being left alone.
- She wants to be with her parents and siblings.

Preventing accidents

A baby has to be safe, but she also has to explore. You have to decide when to say "No," and also when to allow her to discover things for herself. It is important to anticipate everything she may do.

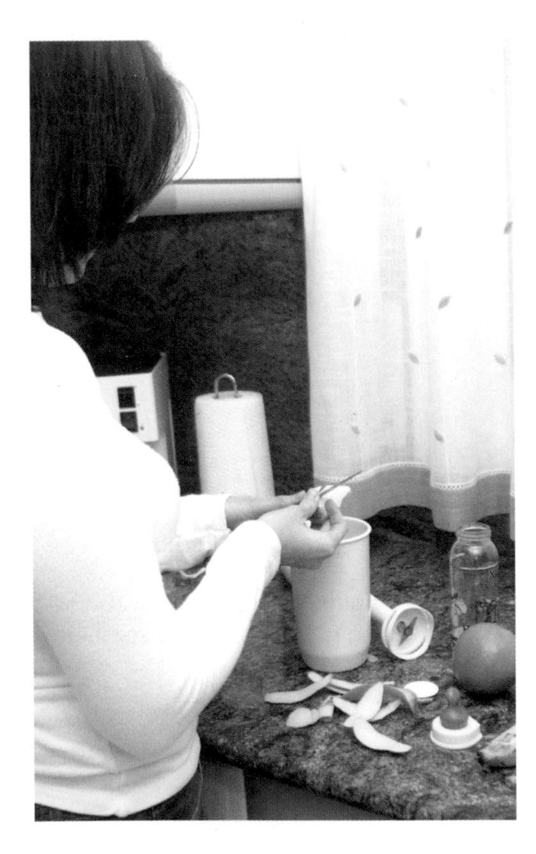

Preventing accidents at home

- Keep all medicines and vitamin supplements under lock and key.
- Be attentive when you receive visitors: they may be carrying medicines or objects that could harm a baby.
- Put all sharp objects out of reach of your baby.
- Cover up all electrical sockets and make sure that all electrical components and cables are beyond your baby's reach.
- Keep your baby away from radiators and electric fans.
- Remove all small objects, as a baby can put them in her mouth and choke. Keep detergents and cleaning products out of her reach.
- Put safety catches on drawers and doors.
- Put tight lids on garbage cans.
- Close the lid of the toilet.
- Try to put protective cushioning on the corners of pieces of furniture in the playing area.
- Do not store toys in trunks or other containers with hinged lids, as these could hurt your baby by dropping down on her.

Preventing falls

- Do not leave your baby alone on a bed, changing table, or chair.
- Make sure that your furniture cannot slide or move. It may be worth adding rubber bases, so that pieces of furniture will not slip when your baby leans on them.
- Install safety gates at both ends of staircases.
- Never leave a baby alone in the bathtub.
- Never leave a baby alone near a swimming pool, or anything else containing water, however little. A baby can drown in even a small amount of water.

Feeding

Your baby is starting to change her diet. At this age, she can be given solid food. Here is a list of things that she can eat and drink (always following the recommendations of your doctor):

- Chicken, beef.
- Bread and cereals.
- Fruit juices and purées.
- Vegetables and potatoes.
- Breast milk, then follow-on formula milk, yoghurt, and cream caramel with no egg.
- Special baby biscuits.

Your baby is still not ready to drink whole milk or eat fish, honey, candies, or whole eggs. Do not add any sugar to purées or juices.

the ninth month

This phase is distinguished by two basic elements: curiosity and mobility. The increasing coordination and dexterity of a nine-month-old baby's movements, her ability to get around by crawling, and her first attempts at standing up and keeping her balance unaided combine to turn her into a veritable whirlwind. She proves more capable of understanding, memorizing, and reasoning, and she also expresses a wider range of feelings: delight and friendliness, as well as fear and loneliness.

She can establish a minimal dialogue: if you repeat a syllable that she can say, she will repeat it in her turn. At this stage, she starts to understand words. She does not know how to articulate them herself, but she tries to do so in her babbling. She understands more from a tone of voice than from the meaning of words, but the more words she hears, the more she will learn and sharpen her intelligence. She understands the meaning of the word "no" even though she disobeys it!

Your baby can crawl up stairs and can walk by holding on to furniture, before succeeding in making her first independent steps.

At the age of 9 months, the separation anxiety of the eighth month becomes even more intense. This makes her stick more closely to her mother and makes her anxious when she sees a stranger.

She likes to throw objects on the floor, not only because of the way they fall but also because of the noise they make and the possibility of repeating this action time and time again. She imitates hand gestures like waving goodbye and clapping.

She also knows when she is being called by her name.

Ninth month

Physical development

- By the end of the ninth month, a baby usually weighs about 20 lb (9.1 kg) and measures around 28 in (71 cm).
- She is capable of crawling on one hand while doing something else with the other.
- She is continuously trying to stand up, and sometimes manages it.

Psychological and intellectual development

- She enjoys playing at finding hidden objects.
- She is capable of remembering a game she played on the previous day; this reflects her growing memory.
- She finds repetitive games boring.
- She understands simple concepts like cold/hot.
- She continues babbling words and syllables that have a special meaning for her.

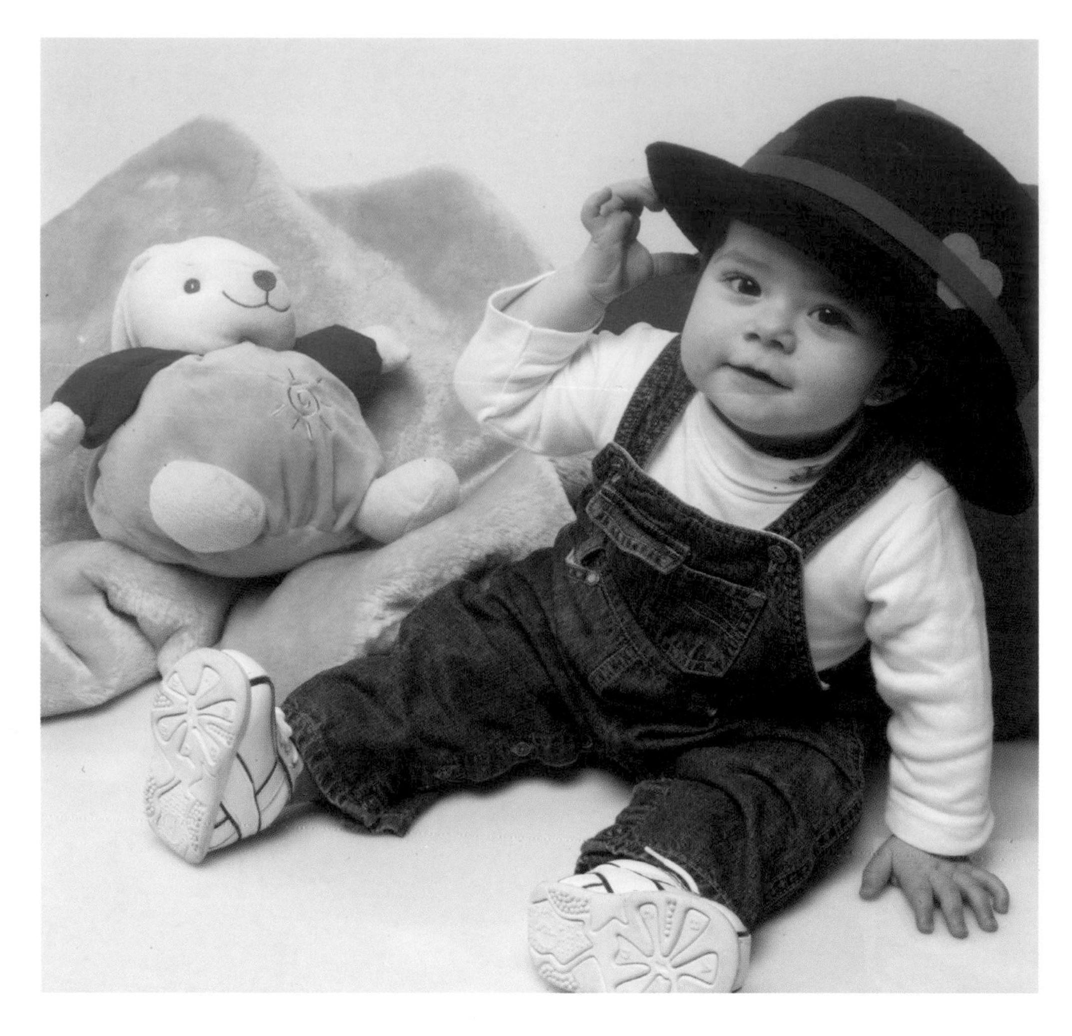

Sensorimotor development

- If your baby has both hands occupied, she will discard one object in order to pick up another.
- She piles one object on top of the other.
- She is capable of building a tower with toy cubes.
- She will hold one object in her hand and hit it with the other hand.
- She feeds herself and is capable of holding a cup in both hands.

Social development

- She seeks the approval of adults.
- She is conscious of the reactions that her behavior provokes in those around her.
- She reacts to other people's comments and actions. She cries if other children cry.
- She enjoys playing hide-and-seek with her siblings and with adults.
- She learns to defend herself and her possessions, as well as growing angry if her toys are taken away from her.
- She learns by imitation. This characteristic is particularly evident if she has older brothers or sisters.

Sleep patterns

Generally speaking, at this age, most babies sleep for about 13 hours a day, spread over 3 phases: 10 hours at night, a short nap in the morning, and another longer one in the afternoon. She may also still be awake after her normal bedtime, when she is excited or occupied, or simply when she does not want to be separated from adults.

Sleeplessness can be avoided by establishing a routine that helps a baby make the transition from playing to sleeping.

- Dim the lights and turn down background noise, such as the television and music, to avoid her thinking that she is going to lose out on something interesting.
- Certain activities can help form routines that indicate the arrival of bedtime: a relaxing bath, reading a story, asking her to give a goodnight kiss to the members of her family, and giving her a soft toy, a blanket, or another comforting object.
- Encourage your baby to help in the preparation of her crib or bed.
- Do not be surprised if she does not go to sleep straight away. She may babble away on her own before falling asleep. Allow her to form her own habits to lull herself to sleep, such as rocking or sucking a finger.

Games to stimulate the development of skills

- **Physical skills.** To help your baby grow strong muscles and improve her balance, pile pillows on the floor and encourage her to crawl over them. Sit down on the floor to help her keep her balance as she climbs.
- **Social skills.** Sing with your child and dance with her to the rhythm of music. Make gestures with your fingers or arms in keeping with the lyrics of a song.
- **Emotional skills.** Your baby starts to become self-aware and recognize herself. Encourage her to look at herself in a mirror and talk to her about what she sees.
- **Linguistic skills.** At the age of 9 months, a baby babbles, imitates sounds, and will soon articulate words. Talk to her frequently and urge her to repeat sounds.
- **Intellectual skills.** Hide objects and encourage her to look for them, to stimulate her capacity to discover something she cannot see and form a clearer idea of reality.

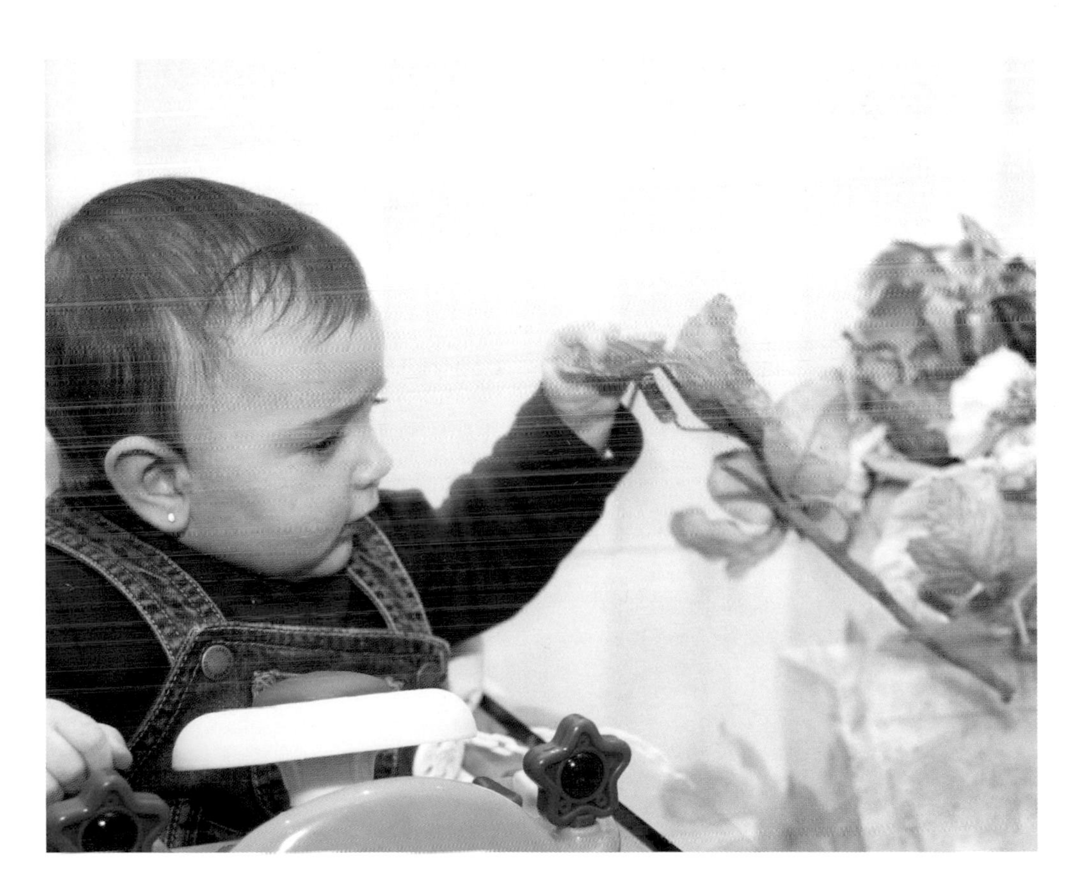

Starting to go to the toilet

The changes in your baby's diet at this age affect her defecation habits. The increased presence of solid food slows down the digestive process and gives rise to firmer stools and, therefore, less frequent bowel movements. Some babies defecate once or twice a day, or even once every two days. This can be normal for some children, but if evacuation is arduous and painful, you should consult your doctor.

It is still early for a baby to learn to go to the toilet herself. You usually have to carry on using diapers until your baby has turned 2, or even later. If you try to teach her before this, both of you will end up frustrated. You should begin to prepare her, however, by talking to her when you change her diaper, saying, for example, "Look! The diaper is very wet this morning. Let's change it so that you'll be clean and dry." In this way, your baby will gradually understand the words "wet" and "dry," and she will associate the latter with being clean and comfortable.

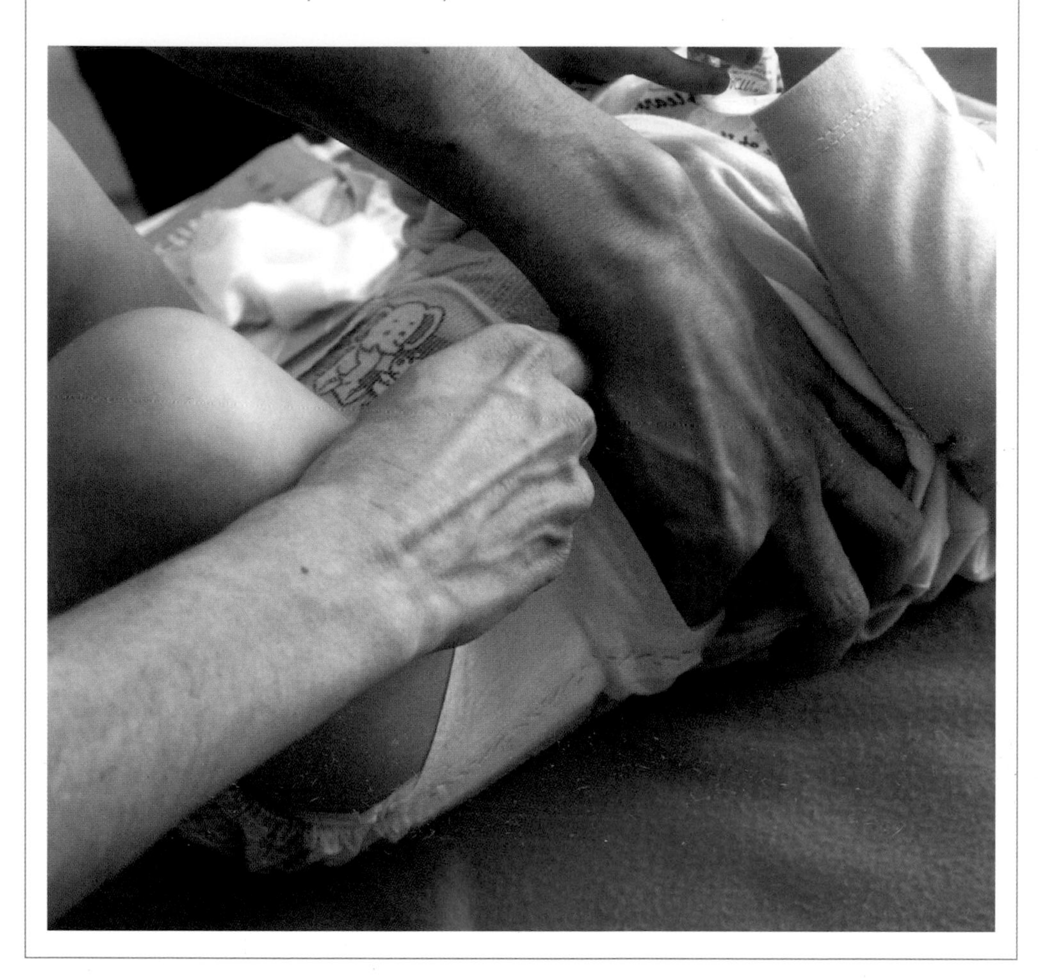

Now that your baby can not only move around but also get about by herself, she loves exploring the space around her. You should ensure that there is nothing on the floor apart from toys and furniture, which provide her with support when she stands up, although her balance will still be uncertain.

the tenth month

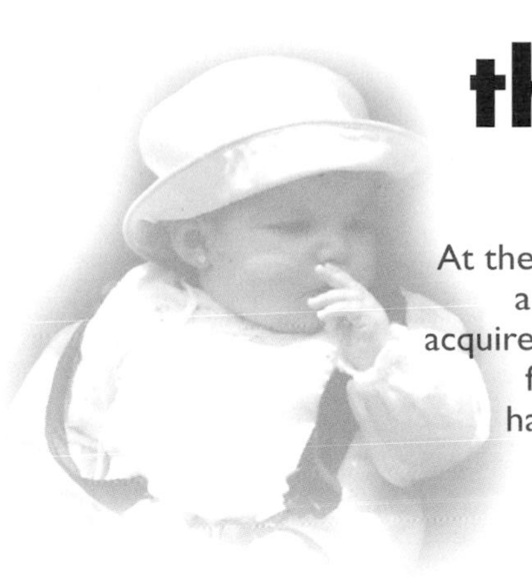

At the age of 10 months, a baby's house starts to look like a battlefield. She gets in everywhere, her crawling has acquired a new agility, and, moreover, she starts to take her first steps. Her curiosity has no limits, causing her to handle everything around her and explore by opening drawers and doors. She needs constant attention.

She can now crawl freely on her hands and knees. Her first crawling is irregular and uncertain, but then it becomes easier as her legs become sturdier and her back aligns itself in parallel to the floor.

At this age, she can sit with her legs outstretched and her back straight, keeping perfect balance even when she is pushed or her legs are gently raised.

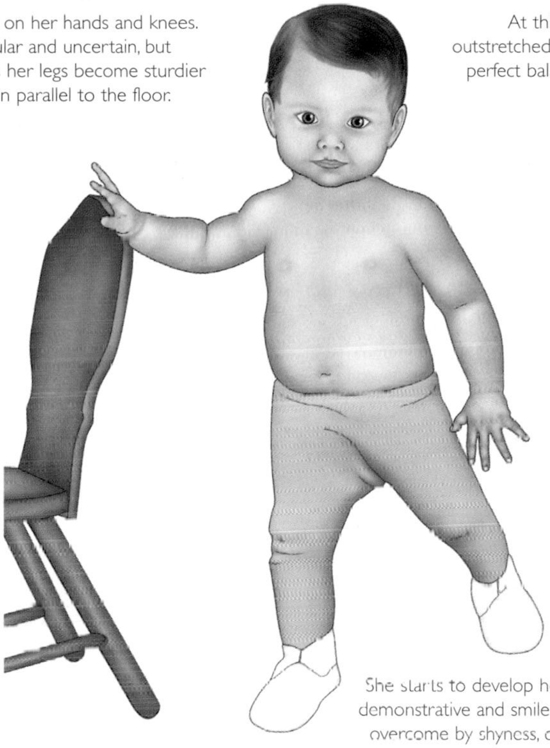

As her fingers are increasingly skilful, she can not only pick up small objects with her hands but also hold them by forming a pincer with her thumb and forefinger, with her wrist totally unsupported.

If you put your baby down she may try to walk, although her steps are still tentative and irregular.

She may be frightened by the unknown, or even by things that did not previously bother her, such as a car horn honking in the street or a door slamming abruptly in a gust of wind.

In this month she can use her hands, unaided, to eat cookies, cheese, or any other foodstuff that she can squash with her gums.

She starts to develop her personality. She can be very demonstrative and smile at strangers, or, in contrast, be overcome by shyness, covering her head and showing unease when approached by a stranger. She also protests about things she knows she dislikes. Her memory is maturing with every day at this stage.

Tenth month

Physical development

• Your baby finds it increasingly easy to stand upright.

• If she is helped or supported, she is capable of taking a few steps.

• She helps you dress her.

• She is capable of crawling up a staircase.

• She can get on or off a chair or bed by herself.

Psychological and intellectual development

• She tries to eat on her own and enjoys offering food to others with her spoon.

Clean teeth are healthy teeth

- At the age of 10 months, you can start accustoming your child to cleaning her teeth. She will learn how to do this by watching and imitating the people around her. Set an example by brushing your teeth after every meal and letting your baby watch you. Next, clean her teeth with a clean, soft, moist cloth to remove any microbes. Do this after every meal. Do not use toothpaste until she is older and knows how to rinse her mouth and spit out toothpaste.
- Make cleaning teeth fun, as this will encourage her to try to do it for herself. Make a puppet with an old (but clean) white sock. Draw eyes and a mouth near the toes, then put your hand inside and pretend to clean the puppet's teeth. Allow your baby to repeat your actions. You could also use a soft toy.

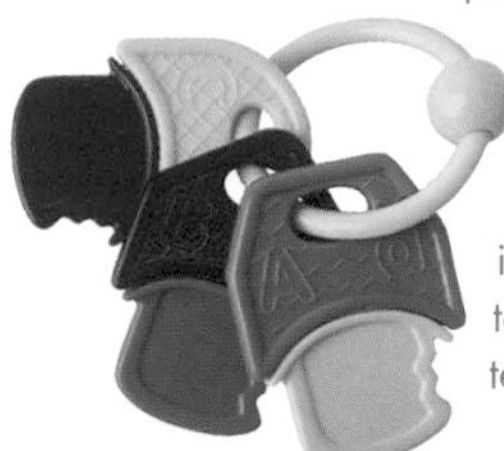

- Sing while you clean her teeth. Make up the words or use the lyrics of a well-known song.
- Use dental hygiene to expand your baby's knowledge. Point to her teeth and say, "Teeth." Ask your baby, "Where are your teeth?" Use related words like toothbrush, clean, tongue, up, down, forward, and backward. She has to be familiar with these words when she starts to clean her teeth.
- White patches on a baby's teeth can be a sign of decay. If you notice any such marks, consult your doctor.

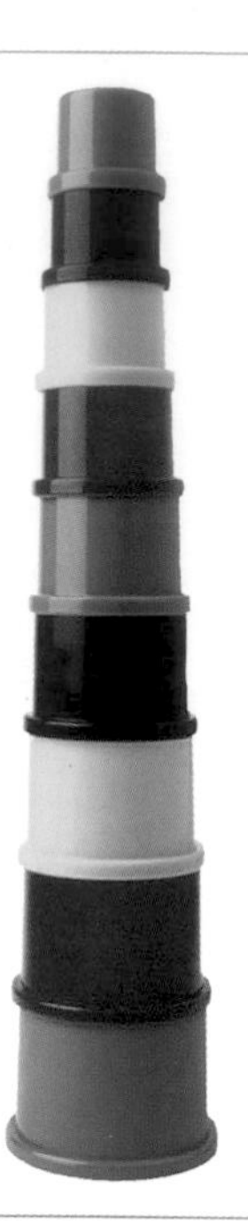

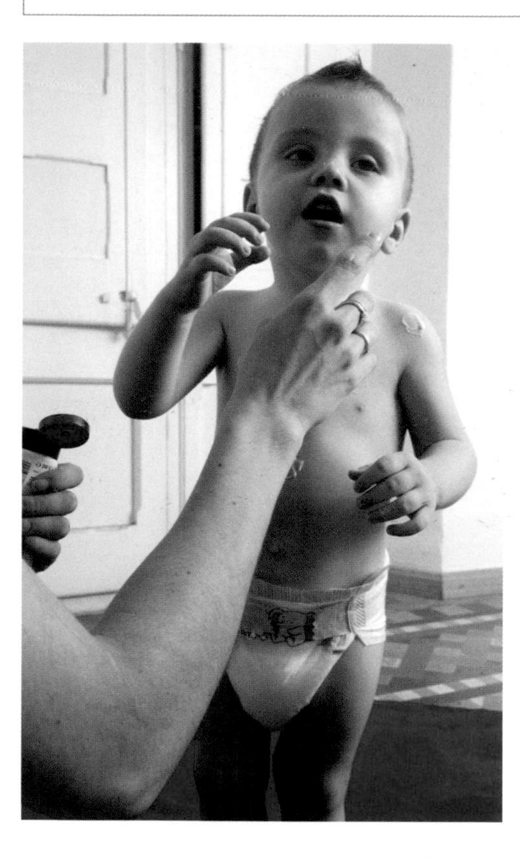

• She can recognize and point to the various parts of her body.

• She obeys orders and follows simple instructions.

Sensorimotor development

• She starts to understand and differentiate between opposites: big/small, near/far.

• She shows a preference for one particular side of her body, which she turns into her main instru-

At the age of ten 10 months, some babies scream, hide, or cry in the presence of strangers. A baby needs time to adapt to new places or unfamiliar faces. Take her in your arms and allow her to look round, while you talk to her softly. Tell your friends and relatives not to force their relationship with her but rather allow her to take the initiative; she will soon feel at ease. Sometimes her curiosity will get the better of her wariness and she will decide to climb down from your lap to explore new, uncharted territory.

Favorite things

If your baby has a favorite blanket, cushion, or toy that serves as a comforter – it is not a sign of weakness. On the contrary, it will help her learn to be apart from her parents by consoling her and providing a sense of security; it could even help her to sleep.

Some tips:

- Encourage your baby to choose a favorite toy; give it to her when she is upset or seeking comfort.
- Establish a bedtime routine. Do not forget to give her the favorite toy or blanket. For example, say: "It's bedtime, let's go and get your teddy bear."
- Do not hide her favorite toy or stop her playing with it. Never use it for rewarding or punishing.
- Show your baby where to keep this toy when she does not need it.

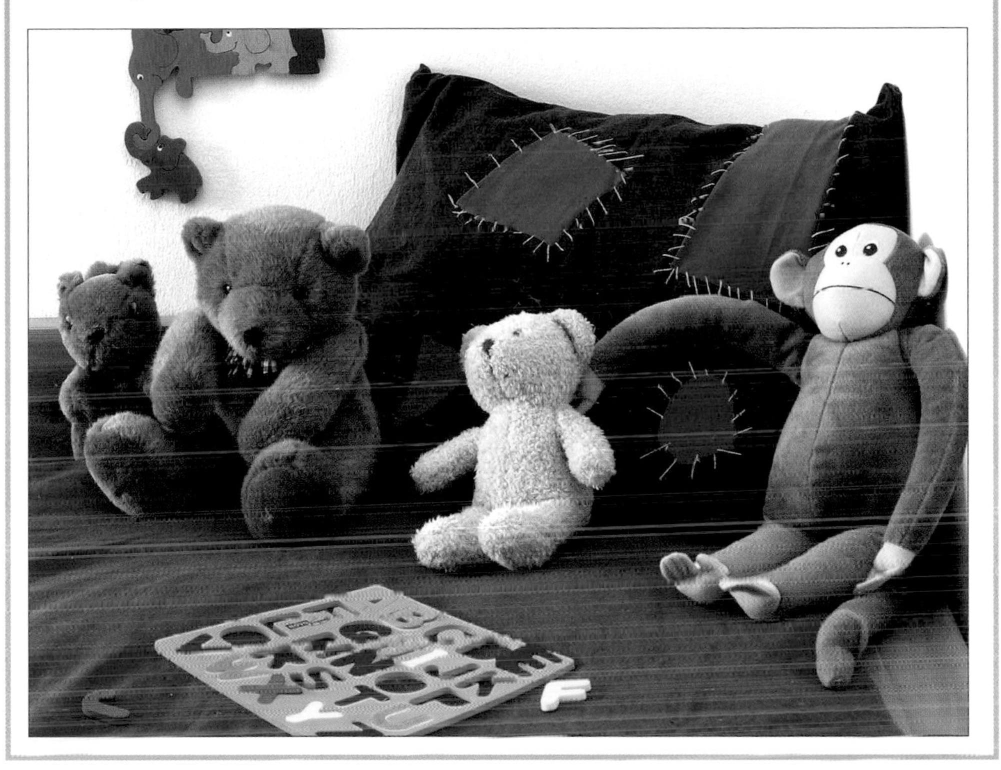

ment. So, you will notice that she habitually uses her right or left hand and foot more than the other.

• She examines more closely all the objects that come her way, and she is capable of distinguishing between them.

• She can use toys involving simple assemblage without any problem.

• She dances or sings when she hears music.

• She recognizes the voices of the members of the family without needing to see them.

Social development

• She craves company and seeks attention through eye-catching actions.

• She understands the difference between approval and reprimand.

• She likes new and unfamiliar places, although she can sometimes react fearfully and seek comfort from the person accompanying her.

• She tries to test the limits imposed on her.

the eleventh month

At 11 months a baby can usually remain standing upright on her own and can probably take her first steps without the help of any objects or people. Even so, she still uses crawling to move around. She gets on and off chairs and beds with some agility, although there are still frequent falls. At this age, a baby is a great imitator of postures, gestures, and sounds. Her powers of comprehension continue to develop at startling speed; this is echoed by a similar enrichment in self-expression, not only as regards her wishes and needs but also her singling out of objects and people _ all this with rudimentary language skills (although progress in this respect can vary greatly from one child to another). An 11-month-old baby is extremely provocative, with defiance of established restrictions and a capacity for refusal (through the recently learned "no") as two of her distinguishing traits.

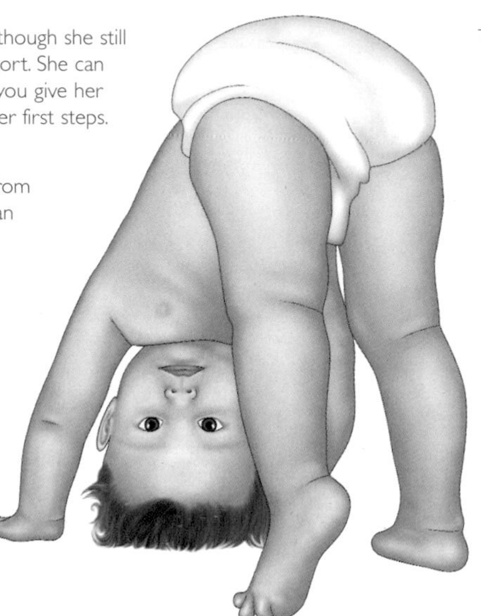

She is increasingly independent, although she still requires substantial care and support. She can stand up without any help and, if you give her your hand, she will start to take her first steps.

She is capable of drinking water from a glass or cup with handles and can eat on her own with her hands.

At this age, she shows interest in books and stories; she likes turning over the pages to see what comes next.

The vocal utterances she emits to identify objects are increasingly longer; this is the real start of language.

The front lobe of the brain develops quickly at this stage, leading to cognitive advances that stimulate reasoning and speech.

She can also imitate sounds and actions, as well as understanding simple orders.

Her memory is still underdeveloped, so it is important to establish limits in this period and teach her what is good and what is bad.

Eleventh month

Physical development

- At the end of this month, a baby will usually weigh about 21 lb (9.8 kg) and measure around 29 in (74 cm).
- She can stand upright without any help.
- She can bend over and raise herself up again.
- She can take one or two steps without supporting herself with furniture and she can go up stairs, either by dragging herself or by crawling.
- Most 11-month-old babies like coming into contact with different textures, although they do not always feel confident walking on sand or grasping sticky substances in their hands.

Psychological and intellectual development

• She still expresses herself in a confused manner, although her use of language is progressing.

• She fits together dismountable toys, piles up objects and makes towers with 2 or 3 elements. She can calculate dimensions.

Baby walkers

Some parents are anxious for their baby to start walking and think that a baby walker will speed up the process. In fact, the opposite is the case. Baby walkers slow down progress, as they strengthen the lower leg muscles but not those of the thighs and hips. Moreover, as they allow a baby to move around very simply, they do not help her learn balance and coordination.

Not only that, baby walkers are also dangerous. They can tip over very easily and increase the risk of falling down a staircase or straying out of bounds.

Baby walkers are a classic example of something a baby does not need at all. A better alternative is a carriage that she can push around: this will help her develop the muscles and coordination that she needs to walk.

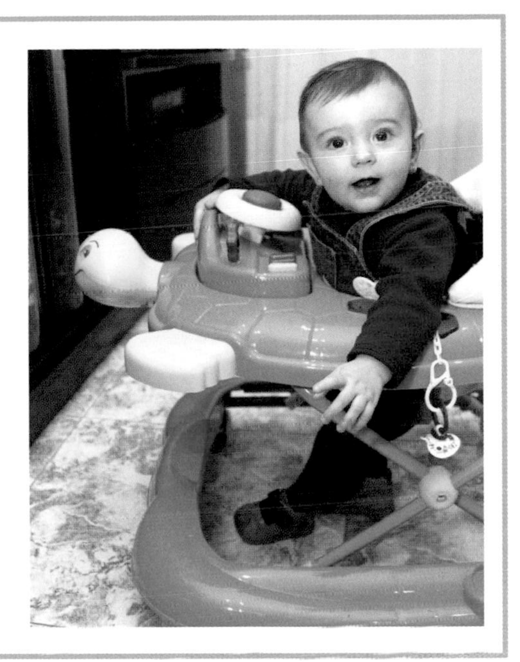

Developing skills through play

Help your baby to develop the skill of learning. Try some of the following activities, involving objects you probably have around the house:

- **Physical skills.** Up and down. Your baby is discovering that she is changing in size; she is now too big to fit into spaces where she once had room. Furthermore, she can now reach things that were formerly beyond her grasp. Help her explore dimensions. Make a tunnel with cardboard boxes stuck together with sticky tape and encourage her to crawl through it. Put a toy on the couch, just out of her reach, and ask her to stretch and grab it.
- **Linguistic skills.** The sounds of animals. Cut pictures of animals out of old magazines and show them to your baby. Tell her the name of the animal and point out its characteristic features. Say things like, "This is a blue bird. It flies. Can you see its feathers?" Imitate the sound made by each animal. Encourage your baby to repeat the sound.
- **Emotional skills.** Trying on hats. Gather together several hats, plastic pots, and light saucepans. Teach her how to put them on your head. Put her in front of a mirror. Laugh and talk to her during this fashion show.
- **Social skills.** Cooking together. Give her a saucepan and wooden spoon. Whenever you empty a receptacle, pass it on to your baby. She will imitate you by emptying and mixing. Do not be surprised if she also makes a racket!
- **Intellectual skills.** Balls in a pie mold. Give her a tray for baking small pies and several balls the size of a tennis ball. Teach her how to put the balls into the individual molds, and encourage her to move them from one mold to the other. You can also play this game with an egg box and plastic eggs.

Sensorimotor development

- She brings a spoon to her mouth by herself.
- She is capable of taking off her shoes and socks.
- She uses different boxes and containers to store objects.
- She can put rings round a stick.
- She leafs through the pages of a book.

Social development

- She is a willing helpmate (some of the time!)
- She seeks approval and tries to avoid reproaches.
- She has a greater capacity for concentration when she plays.
- She knows the names of objects and is capable of following simple instructions. This is a good time to teach her the use of "please" and "thank you" every time she wants to ask for something.
- She can imitate the meowing of a cat and point to the sky when she hears the noise of an airplane.
- She can imitate with greater ease the language and facial expressions of those around her, even though she does not fully understand their meaning.

The ideal toys for this age

- Toys that fit together, in a variety of shapes, sizes, and colors.
- Unbreakable mirrors.
- Toys with wheels, such as cars and trucks made of flexible plastic.
- Balls of all sizes.
- Cardboard books with realistic photos.
- Telephones, music boxes, and other toys with sounds.
- Rubber dolls.
- Toys that come apart but have no small pieces.
- Toys that open and close.
- Toys made of resistant material that can be bitten.
- Toys that imitate objects that your baby can see at home: saucepan, wooden spoon, receptacles for water, etc.

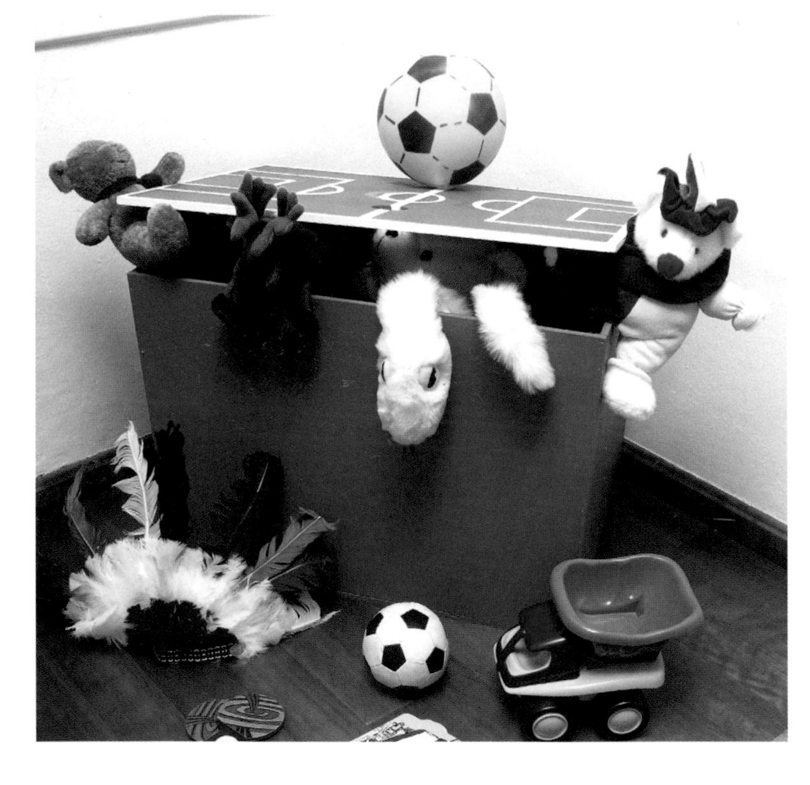

A child not only learns to sharpen her awareness and amuse herself with toys but also starts to create her private world, in which she is the boss and feels at ease.

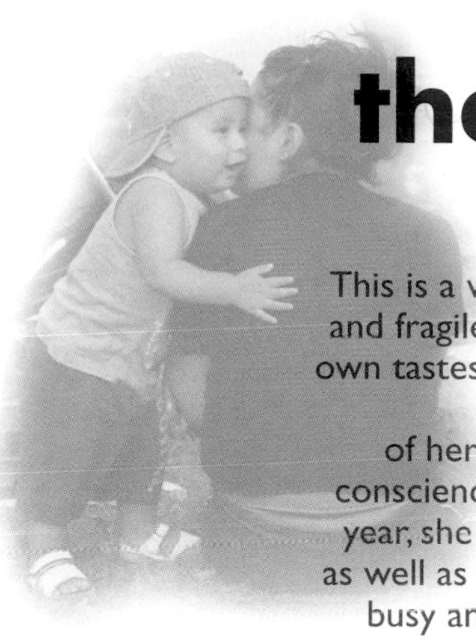

the twelfth month

This is a very important stage: whereas once she was dependent and fragile, she is very nearly a person in her own right, with her own tastes, even though she still depends on her parents. She can distinguish good from bad, and in the depth of her being she is starting to develop a rudimentary form of conscience, although she still behaves capriciously. After her first year, she acts with greater awareness, as she is starting to think, as well as talk to communicate what she is thinking. She is always busy and full of energy. She is sometimes capable of playing on her own but becomes upset if things do not turn out the way she wants, or if she feels tired.

For the next 6 months, your baby will devote all her energy to learning how to walk freely.

Most children start walking on tiptoes, with their feet pointing outward.

She loves to push, pull, or hit anything that crosses her path, because she is discovering her own strength and finding that her actions provoke reactions that she had not seen before.

It is difficult to get a 12-month-old baby to sleep, as her restlessness will take away any desire to go to bed, even when she really feels tired.

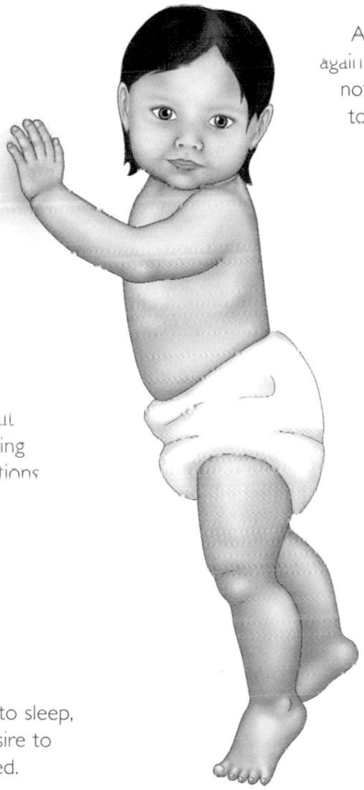

At this age, most babies can experience once again the anxiety typical of the eighth month. It is not easy to leave her alone, because she starts to cry inconsolably and feels vulnerable in the absence of her parents.

She now speaks what sounds like a proper language, although only her parents can understand it. Generally speaking, at this stage a baby can clearly say the words *Mom* and *Dad* as well as some others.

She replies correctly to simple questions, as she associates people and objects with their names.

Twelfth month

Physical development

• The average weight and height are 22 lb (10 kg) and 30 in (75 cm), respectively.

• She stands and takes steps with ever greater confidence, but still crawls when she wants to move about quickly.

• She generally eats without any help.

• She remains awake for most of the day, with only one nap (in the afternoon).

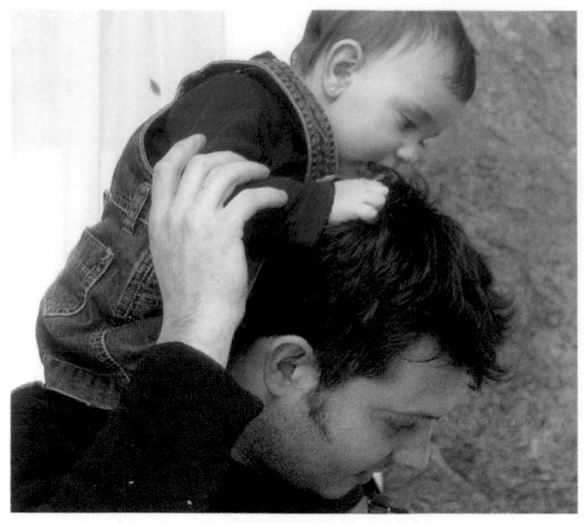

When a baby reaches the age of 1 year, she closes one period and crosses a very important threshold; her fragility and dependency gives way day by day to greater autonomy and independence.

Psychological and intellectual development

- She can group together objects by classifying them in different categories.
- She recognizes animals in images and tries to imitate their voices.
- She speaks in short phrases, although these are still unclear or incomprehensible.
- She understands the concept of action and reaction.
- She has a good memory for recalling people or events from previous days.

Sensorimotor development

- She piles up toys and objects more quickly and dexterously.
- She is capable of picking up objects while looking in another direction.

Starting to use the toilet

- After 12 months of dealing with diapers, many parents want their baby to move on to a new phase. Whatever the parents may want, however, this transition will only occur when your baby is ready. The problems associated with giving up diapers almost always occur as a result of acting too soon. Generally speaking, girls are ready for this change before boys. Some boys are ready after about 18 months, but others may need to wait until the age of three years, or even more.
- How do you know when to give up diapers? Your child is ready to use the toilet when she has acquired the following skills:

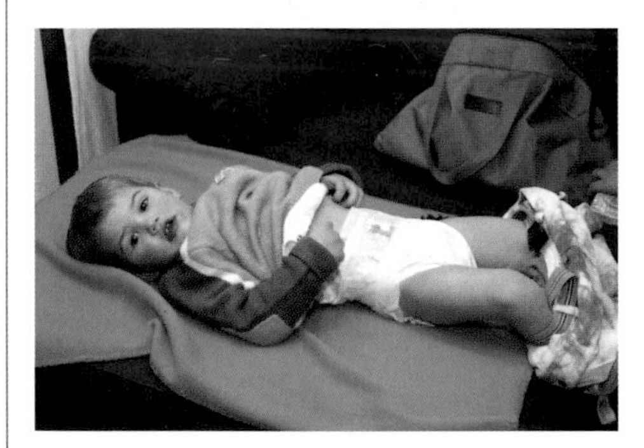

Physical skills:

- She can walk.
- Her bladder is bigger and she urinates fewer times a day.
- She wakes up after a nap with a dry diaper.
- She can control her sphincter.
- She knows to put on and take off her underwear.

Mental skills:

- She understands when her body is telling her she needs to go to the toilet.
- She understands the meaning of the words pee, poop, and toilet or whatever words are used in the home to indicate these.
- She understands what is required of her: what to do, and when and where to do it.

Social and emotional skills:

- She can express her needs, such as a change of diapers.
- She wants to learn how to use the toilet.

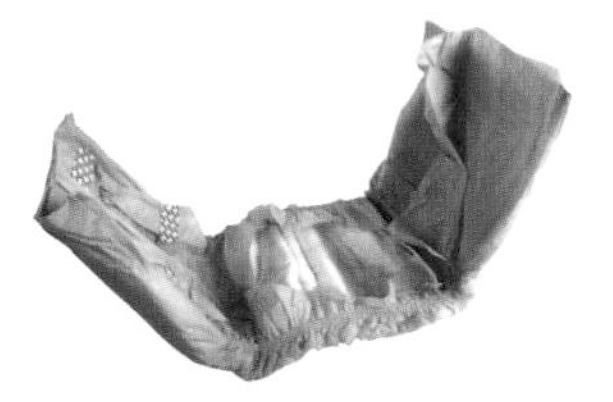

• She enjoys noisy games and toys.

• As she acquires greater control over her steps, she can also push or pull toys or other objects while walking.

• She still sleeps with her favorite toy.

Social development

• A 12-month-old baby expresses many emotions and is capable of recognizing them in other people.

• She clearly expresses affection for her most cherished people and objects.

• She resists going to sleep and becomes angry when she is obliged to go to bed.

• She becomes upset when separated from her parents and she demonstrates this by crying.

• She says 'no' and disobeys with greater frequency.

• She shows great interest in the activities of adults and, when performing a task, she may ask for more help than she really needs, as she knows this will lighten her workload.

Helping your child to learn

When your child is ready to use the toilet, you can enhance this learning process by following some of these suggestions:

- Talk with the person who looks after her. Parents and minders have to agree about when a child is ready and when she is capable of using the toilet.
- Supervise your child while she learns to use the toilet. Put a seat with a potty in the bathroom, or leave a sturdy seat by the toilet. Make sure the toilet paper is readily accessible.
- Dress her with clothes that are easy to remove.
- Use disposable underwear; your child will think that disposable underwear is the same as diapers.
- Help the child lose her fear of the toilet.
- When she urinates or defecates in the toilet, say "Well done!" but do not overdo it. Children have to learn to use the toilet for themselves, not to please other people.
- Never scold or humiliate a child when she has an accident. You are dealing with natural body functions and it easy for children to forget or be distracted.
- If your child has frequent accidents, use diapers again for a while. Try using the toilet again when she seems ready.
- Do not rush things. She will take her time to learn the skill of going to the toilet on her own.

When she has all these skills, your child will give up diapers without any problems. A child who is not ready may resist learning and become frustrated (along with her parents). Do not pressure her!

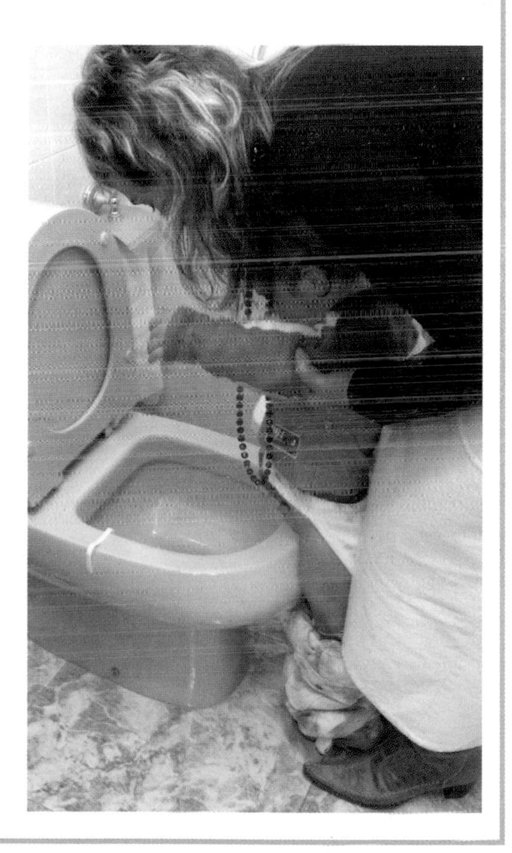

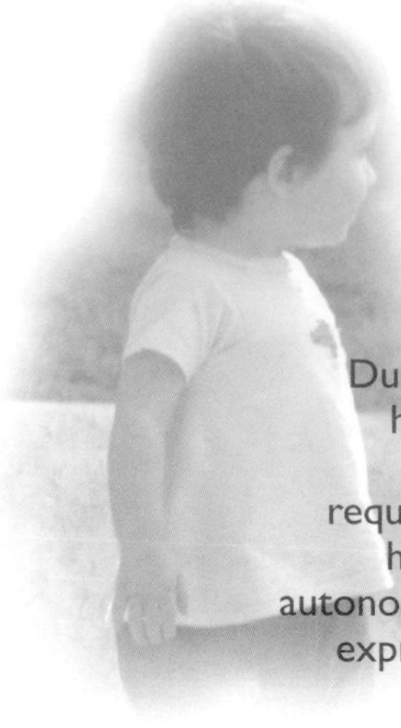

the second year of life (1–2 years)

During the second year of life, a child masters two basic aspects of human behavior: walking and speaking. This can be an exhausting period for parents, as their child becomes intensively active and requires constant supervision. It is also an extremely exciting phase, however, as the child develops her relationships and extends her autonomy. Curious and tireless, she assesses her influence on adults by expressing rejection and using her favorite words: no and mine. It is the ideal time to start establishing rules of conduct.

She likes walking on her own and makes great use of the pincer formed by her forefinger and thumb.

If you give her an object, she lets go of it voluntarily.

At the age of 15 months, she climbs the stairs and can walk backward.

When playing with cubes, she can make a tower with 2 or 3 of them, in imitation of the person playing with her.

At the age of 18 months, she runs with agility.

She is capable of throwing objects when standing, without falling over.

She builds towers with a height of 2 or 3 cubes.

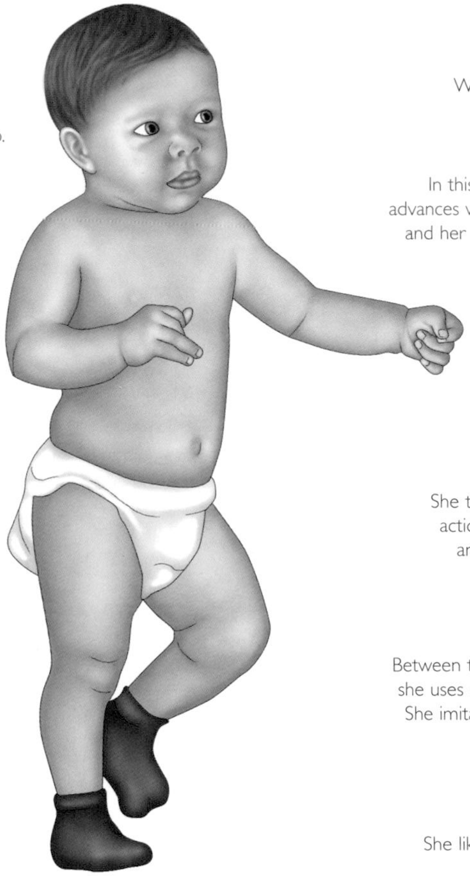

When reading a book, she turns 2 or 3 pages at a time.

In this period, the child makes great advances with respect to her vocabulary and her interaction with other people.

She goes from using 2 words (apart from Mum and Dad) to using 7–20 words (at about 17 months).

She tends to imitate other people's actions, she responds when called, and she cooperates when being dressed.

Between the ages of 15 and 18 months, she uses a spoon and a glass by herself. She imitates adults (sweeping, dusting).

She likes playing with other children.

13–18 months

The second year of life

Physical development

• Her weight is between 24 and 27 lb (11 kg–12.5 kg), her height between 33 and 34 in (83–87 cm).

• She walks on her own, forward and backward, and knows how to climb stairs.

• At the age of 18 months, she runs with agility.

• Some children start going to a playschool, where they play, learn, and share with other children.

Psychological and intellectual development

• She acquires greater control over language, both in the number of words and the clarity of expression.

• She puts together higher and more complex constructions.

• When given a pencil, she can copy a line.

Sensorimotor development

• She displays greater dexterity and can use the forefinger and thumb as a pincer.

• She is capable of throwing objects when standing, without falling over.

• She takes off her shoes and undresses by herself.

• When a book is read to her, she is capable of turning the pages.

Social development

• She makes great advances in her use of language and her interaction with other people, especially children.

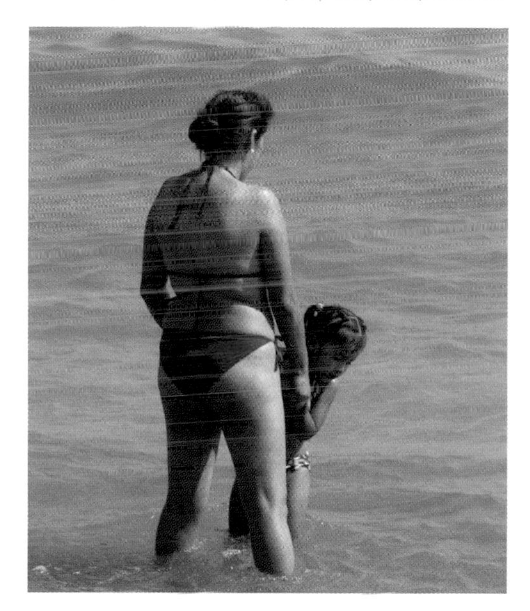

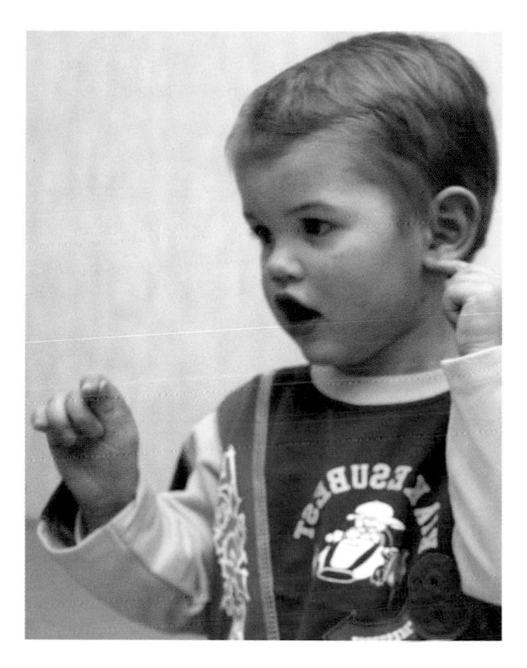

• She imitates adults.

• She enriches her vocabulary to a total of 7–20 words.

• At the age of 17 months, she recognizes 5 parts of the body; a month later, she recognizes 8 parts.

• She tends to imitate actions performed by other people, she answers when called, and she cooperates when being dressed.

• Between the ages of 15 and 18 months, she can use a spoon and glass by herself.

• She lets people know when she is hungry or needs to go to the bathroom.

Feeding and nutrition

• From now on, the doctor will recommend that almost everything the child eats is cut into pieces, according to her ability to chew.

• Parents should encourage good eating habits, starting by only offering food at mealtimes.

• A child has less appetite at this age, due to her slower rate of growth, and she may make a fuss by refusing to eat at mealtimes. She should not be forced to eat a dish, but neither should she be offered an alternative or given an extended eating period.

• Your doctor will tell you when she can start taking cow's milk. Once she does, she should drink at least 2 glasses a day, in addition to other dairy products like yoghurt and cheese.

Preventing accidents

- Take precautions: never leave a child alone in the bathtub, or near staircases or windows.
- Make sure that your child cannot reach any medicines, alcoholic drinks, cleaning products, plastic bags, irons, or heaters, and cover up or block electrical sockets.
- Use cleaning products with safety caps.
- Check that toys fulfill safety standards and are suited to your child's age. It is important to check that they are not toxic and have no detachable pieces that are small enough for a child to swallow, choke on or put up her nose.
- When she travels by car, she must use a safety chair that conforms with prevailing regulations.
- When she is out on the street, let her walk alone on the sidewalk but do not let her out of your sight for a second.

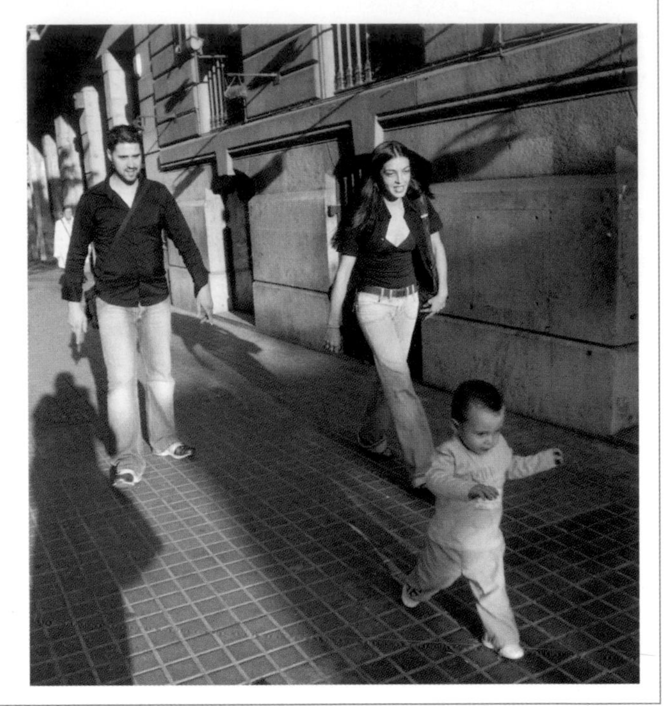

Stimulating a child

- You should speak to her correctly and clearly, without mangling any words.
- She needs help to become acquainted with the world around her: her objects, her house, her neighborhood, animals and plants, contrasts between day and night, large and small, etc.

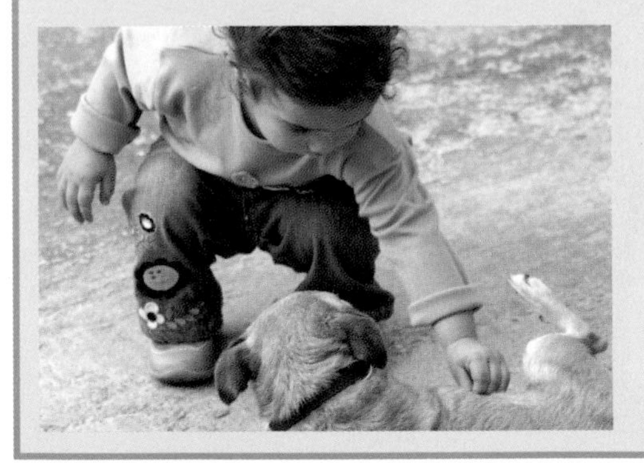

- Her fantasy and imagination are developing in leaps and bounds: they can be stimulated by games, stories, and songs.
- To help her control her sphincter in the future, she has to become familiarized with the potty or toilet from the age of 18 months.
- During the second year of her life, the child discovers the existence of constraints, which she has to understand and experience within the family circle, above all; you should answer her with the confidence and authority you consider appropriate, firmly setting a few very clear limits. Always praise positive behavior. A child will stop having tantrums if she realizes they fail to make adults change their attitudes.

pre-school age (3–5)

During this pre-school phase, a child undergoes significant physical and cognitive changes (albeit more gradual than those experienced before this). Her comprehension, expressiveness, and memory are enhanced, giving her greater autonomy. Although she still needs supervision, she knows how to wash her face, go to the bathroom, eat, put on her shoes, and dress herself. And, although there are frequent tears and temper tantrums, she starts to leave behind her egocentricity, knows what she can and cannot do, and understands when she is being scolded or praised.

3 years

She sings songs.

She can hop on one foot.

She plays with a ball, catching and throwing it.

She can go down stairs on her own.

She draws people with three different body parts.

She builds towers of 10 blocks.

She understands the difference between fantasy and reality.

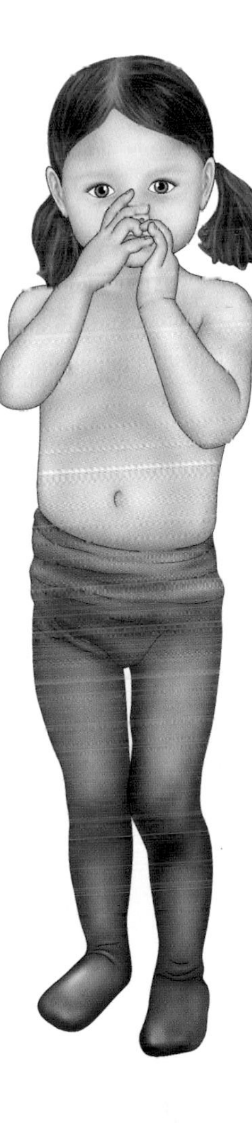

5 years

She skips with a rope.

She sometimes confuses the order of syllables in a word.

She can keep her balance on one foot with her eyes closed.

She uses scissors.

She starts to learn to tie her shoelaces.

She copies shapes when she draws.

She dresses herself.

She knows her address and telephone number.

She can recognize letters and recite the alphabet.

Her permanent teeth may start to come through.

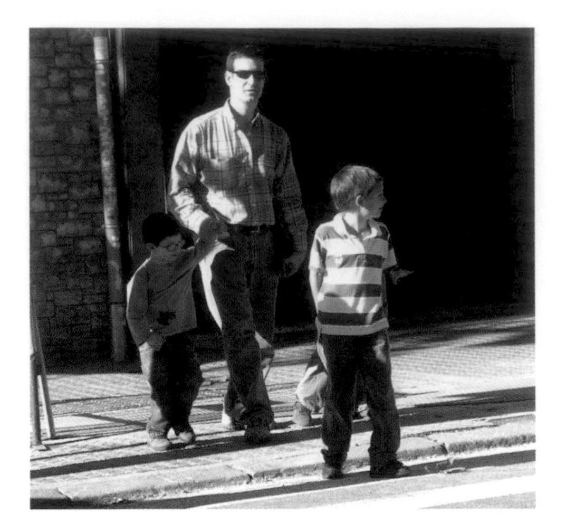

Pre-school age (3–5 years)

Physical and sensorimotor development

• The growth rate is slower than in the previous phases. In the third year, her weight will increase by about 5 lb (2.3 kg) and her height by 3 in (9 cm); after her fourth year, these parameters will have increased by merely another 4 lb (2 kg) and 2 in (6.5 cm), respectively.

• Her build becomes more slender and athletic.

• At this age, boys tend to be taller and heavier than girls. Boys have a greater muscular mass, girls more fatty tissue.

• These physical changes, along with the development of the brain and nervous system, stimulate motor functions (long and short muscles).

• The maturity of the circulatory and respiratory system gives the child greater physical vigor which, in conjunction with the maturing of the immune system, leads to a more healthy and athletic physical condition. It is common to find that some conditions such as allergies and repeated infections, which were once frequent, disappear at this stage.

• At around the age of 3, it becomes clear whether a child is right- or left-handed, although this will not be confirmed until she is 5. It is vital to respect her preferences and never impose the use of a particular hand; a child has to follow the natural process of cerebral development.

Psychological and intellectual development

• The child will gradually develop her capacity for handling symbols (talking and starting to write).

• She understands the relationship between cause and effect.

• She is more emphatic.

• Her capacity for classification and numerical comprehension is greater.

• She is still very imaginative and has difficulty in distinguishing the real from the unreal.

• She has yet to develop the capacity to think of several ideas at once, and this can lead her to illogical conclusions and a failure to understand that something can be done in more than one way.

Social development

• A child's personality and sense of self-esteem become stronger.

• She has a greater capacity for experiencing and conveying emotions.

• She develops a concept of gender, i.e. she can identify the social and cultural aspects that correspond to a man or woman.

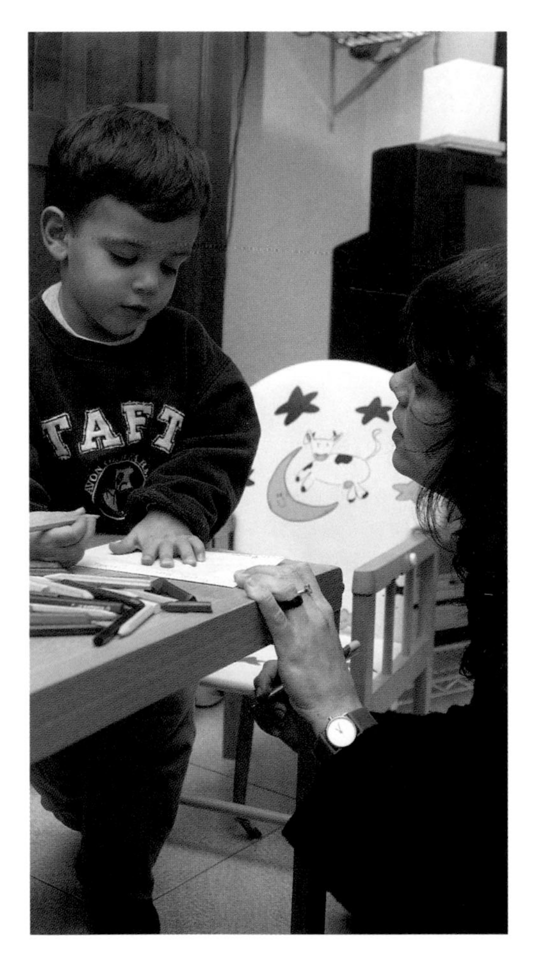

Language

- The development of language stimulates the capacity to reason and optimizes the use of speech.
- At this age, children are capable of talking about things that are not present, remembering aspects of the past, planning the future, talking of imaginary objects, and using plurals and the past tense.
- Between the ages of 3 and 5, children normally learn several new words in a day, but they do not always use them like adults; the word tomorrow, for example, can be used for any time in the future. At this age, sentences tend to have an average of 4 or 5 words.
- It is common for children of this age to talk aloud to themselves, without any intention of communicating with another person. You need to be attentive, however; if this behavior does not disappear over time (as is usually the case), it may indicate a problem, or that something is worrying the child.
- During their first years of life, children receive a host of verbal instructions, orders, and constraints, so, once they start to master speech, it is normal for them to try to impose their wishes through words. As a result, children aged 4 usually test the power of words by being very bossy, especially with younger children. It is important to realize that this is only a transitory phase that contributes to the formation of their character.

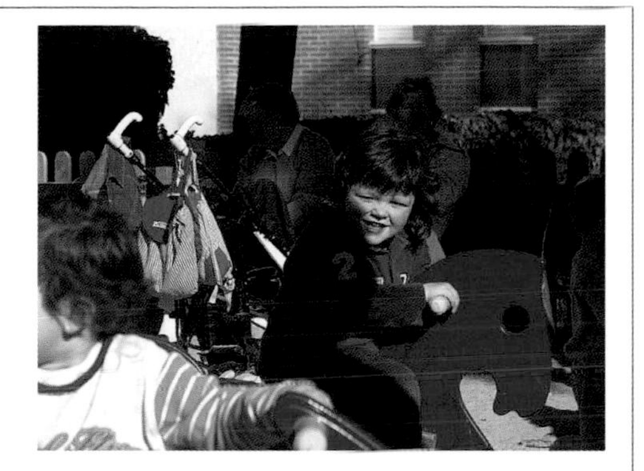

- At around the age of 3, your child will feel the need to know the names of things and understand how they work, ushering in the phase of the constant Why? Parents have to try not to become exasperated but give short, simple answers that the child can assimilate, without dismissing her capacity and need for learning.
- The onset of this phase is a clear sign that a child is developing, and although her questions may sometimes seem impossible to answer, they must receive a sensible reply.

- She starts to interact with her siblings. Parents should encourage harmonious relationships, based on affection, mutual respect, and acceptance and avoid any unfavorable comparison of different children.
- At around the age of 3, a child starts to form friendships. She learns to share through companionship and casual acquaintances with other children. She starts to see different forms of behavior and relate to others by seeing their point of view.

Discipline starts to be important. A child has to be capable of dominating her impulses and her own body. As learning and discipline are basically achieved through imitation, the example of her parents is crucial. They should be a model and reference for behavior and so their words and their actions and what they ask of their child have to be compatible.

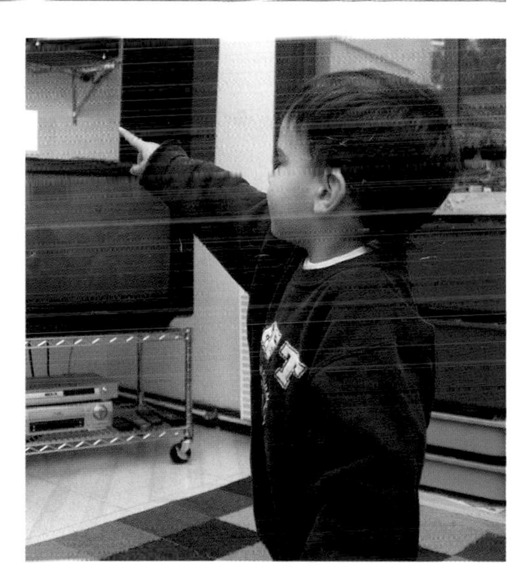

primary school age (6–12)

This is a phase marked by the child's schooling; now she is more mature intellectually and is ready to discover new concepts and fields of knowledge. At school she encounters new companions and learns how to live with them. She feels the need to test herself, to perform tasks, and achieve success, inducing a sense of competence and a capacity for effort and work. As regard physical development, this continues (albeit more slowly) throughout this phase, until the arrival of puberty (at the age of 10–11 in girls and 11–12 in boys), which heralds a new period of rapid changes.

The differences between the two sexes become more marked in the course of these years: girls reach puberty first and overtake boys in terms of weight and stature; later on, this situation is reversed, as boys go on to display greater growth curves.

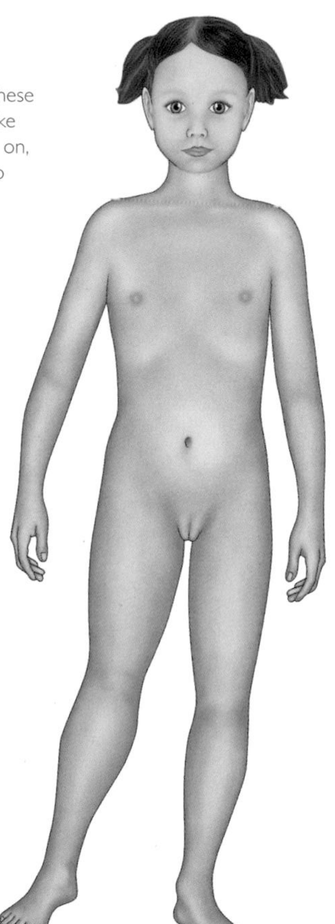

6–7 years

She enjoys many activities and keeps herself busy.

She likes painting and drawing.

She may lose her first tooth.

Her vision is as sharp as that of an adult.

She practices her skills in order to perfect them.

She skips with a rope.

She rides a bike.

8–9 years

She displays greater elegance in her movements and manual tasks.

She jumps, skips, and plays hide-and-seek.

She dresses and washes herself entirely on her own.

She can use tools (e.g., a hammer, a screwdriver).

10–12 years

She grows the rest of her adult teeth.

She likes painting and handicrafts.

She can read well.

Primary school age (6–12)

Physical development

• In this period, children grow by an average of about 2 in (6 cm) and 4–6 lb (2–3 kg) a year.

• The nervous and musculoskeletal systems continue to mature and develop more motor functions.

• There is a greater capacity to control mobile body parts separately, and coordination between the latter to perform more complex movements.

• Confirmation of the predominance of one side with respect to hand-eye-foot, first apparent at about the age of 3.

• At around the age of 8, the sexual differentiation starts to become more marked, apart from the external genitals. The first signs of puberty appear earlier in girls than in boys.

Psychological and intellectual development

• **From 6–7 years of age.** She understands the concept of numbers and can distinguish day from night, and her right hand from her left. She can copy complex shapes like that of a diamond. She can tell the time. She can understand orders with three separate instructions. She can describe

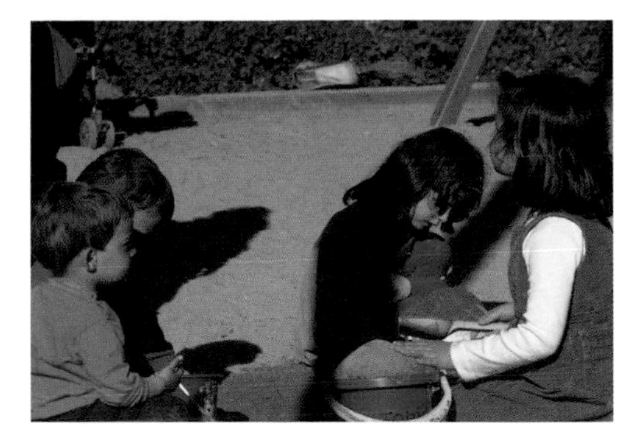

objects and explain their use. She can read books and/or material appropriate for her age.

• **From 8–9 years.** She can count backward. She reads more, and enjoys it more. She understands fractions and the concept of space. She can recite the days of the week and the months in order, and she understands dates. She draws and paints. She enjoys collecting objects.

• **From 10–12 years.** She writes stories. She likes writing letters. She reads well. She likes talking on the telephone.

Sensorimotor development

• **From 6–7 years of age.** She enjoys numerous activities and occupies herself. She likes dra-

Enuresis (bedwetting)

Enuresis is the medical term for bedwetting in children of an age at which they should be capable of controlling their bladder. Girls usually learn to control their bladder before boys. A diagnosis of enuresis can be established in girls over 5 and boys over 6 who still have problems controlling their urination.

There are several factors that may be involved, and many theories have been put forward to explain urinary incontinence in children. These are some of the possible causes of this condition:

- Inadequate toilet training.
- Delay in the capacity to hold in urine (this can apply to children under the age of about 5).
- A small bladder.
- Bad sleeping habits or the existence of a sleep disorder.
- Psychological disorders, fear, or stress.
- Hormonal disorders.

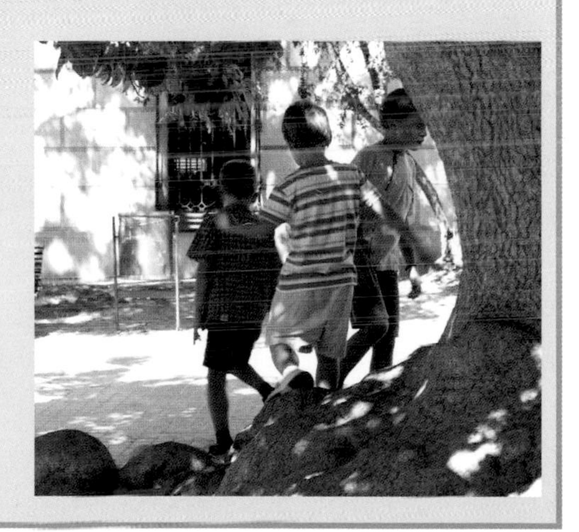

Tips for stimulating a child's social aptitude at primary school age.

- Praise your child whenever she is cooperative or achieves a personal goal.
- Help your child choose activities that help to develop her capabilities.
- Encourage her to talk and be sincere about her feelings.
- Encourage her to read.
- Encourage her to take up hobbies and other activities.
- Encourage physical activity.
- Foster self-discipline and expect your child to obey rules.
- Teach her to respect and listen to adults in positions of authority.
- Encourage her to talk about peer pressure and help her to establish ways of handling it.

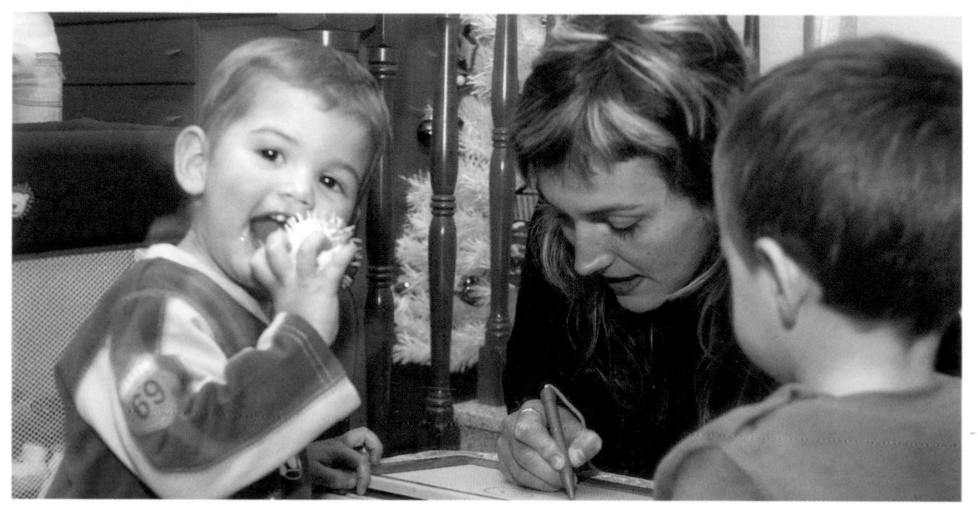

wing and painting. Her vision is as sharp as that of an adult. She practices her skills in order to perfect them. She skips rope and likes riding a bike.

• **From 8–9 years.** She displays greater elegance in her movements and manual tasks. She jumps, runs, and plays tag. She dresses and washes herself entirely on her own. She can use tools (e. g., a hammer or screwdriver).

• **From 10–12 years.** She likes painting and handicrafts. She plays sport and likes playing in a team.

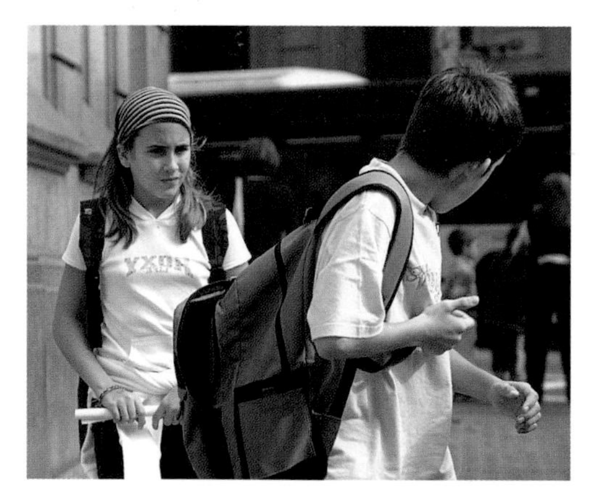

From 6–7 years, she collaborates and shares. She cheats, if she has the chance. She is jealous of her siblings and other people. She likes copying adults. She likes playing on her own, but her friends are becoming important. She plays with children of the same sex. She can have tantrums. She is shy about her body. She likes playing board games.

adolescence (ages 13–18)

Adolescence, heralded by the first signs of puberty, is a period marked by changes. The child's body starts its journey toward its adult form, both physically and functionally. Leaving childhood behind and reaching maturity is a difficult process involving drastic changes that also extend to an adolescent's brain and psyche. New behavior patterns, fads, relationships in family and social circles, feelings and moods are used experimentally by adolescents to strengthen their identity and develop their character.

Sexual characteristics

The anatomical differences between a man and a woman are determined by primary and secondary sexual characteristics.

- Primary These correspond to the internal and external genital organs: the penis and testicles in boys, the ovaries, uterus, and vagina in girls.
- Secondary. These emerge at the start of puberty and eventually constitute the definitive differences between the bodies of males and females.

Phases of adolescence

Early adolescence (10–13 years)

- The child's thoughts are still focused on immediate ends, with little capacity for analysis, and this manifests itself in the strong bonds that still exist with her parents.
- Although there may be a rebellious attitude, this does not result in introverted aloofness.
- In this period, a child tends to have friends of the same sex and places great emphasis on the group, and very little on boy/girlfriends.
- There are frequent tantrums and displays of rudeness, often aimed at parents.

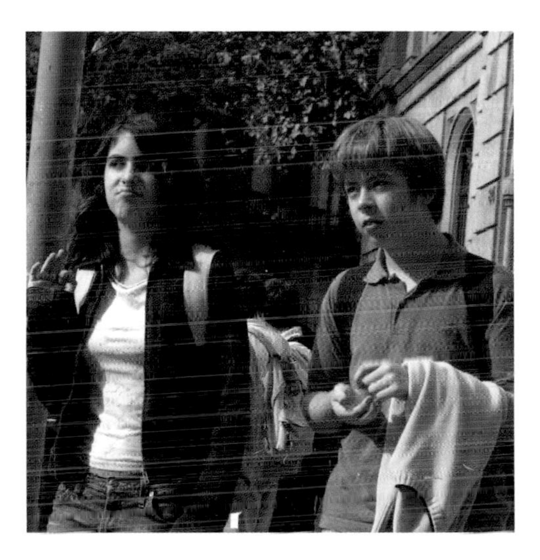

The physical changes that appear in puberty are so fast and intense that adapting to them poses a real challenge for an adolescent. Adolescents' bodies stretch and widen, the face and voice change ... and, to top it all, sexual characteristics make their presence felt.

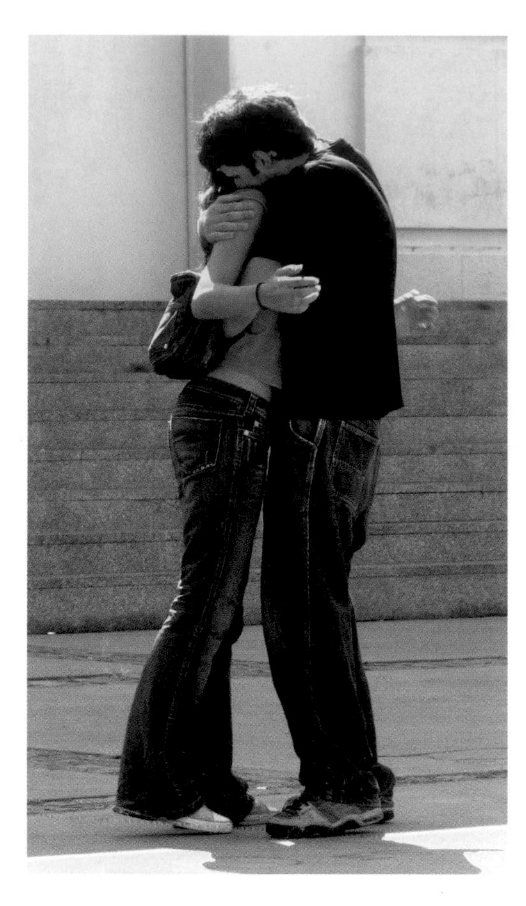

Sexual characteristics in girls

- Development and spread of pubic hair.
- Development and maturing of the breasts.
- Appearance of the first menstrual flow.

Sexual characteristics in boys

- Development and spread of body hair.
- Growth of the penis and testicles.
- Changes in the voice.
- Changes in the muscular mass and body structure.

Pubertal development in girls

- 10–11 years: appearance of the first sign of breasts; acceleration of growth.
- 11–12 years: appearance of pubic hair.
- 12–13 years: clear development of internal and external genitals: menstrual cycles without ovulation; further breast development; increase in pubic hair and appearance of underarm hair.
- 14–15 years: regular periods and fertile ovulatory cycles; complete development of the breasts.
- 17 years: welding of the cartilages; cessation of growth.

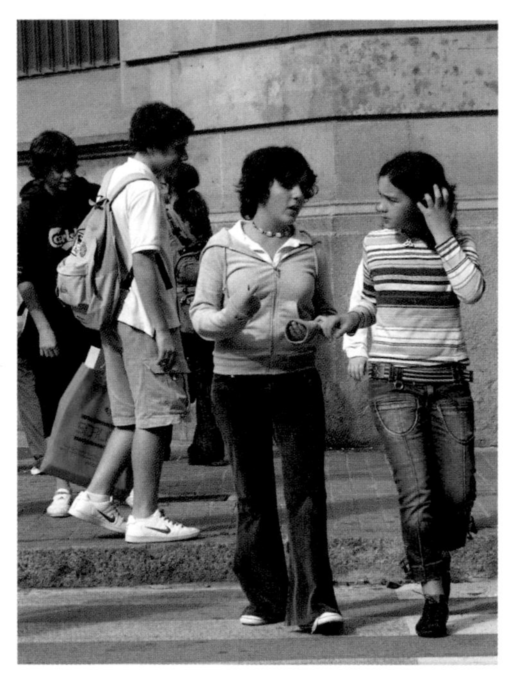

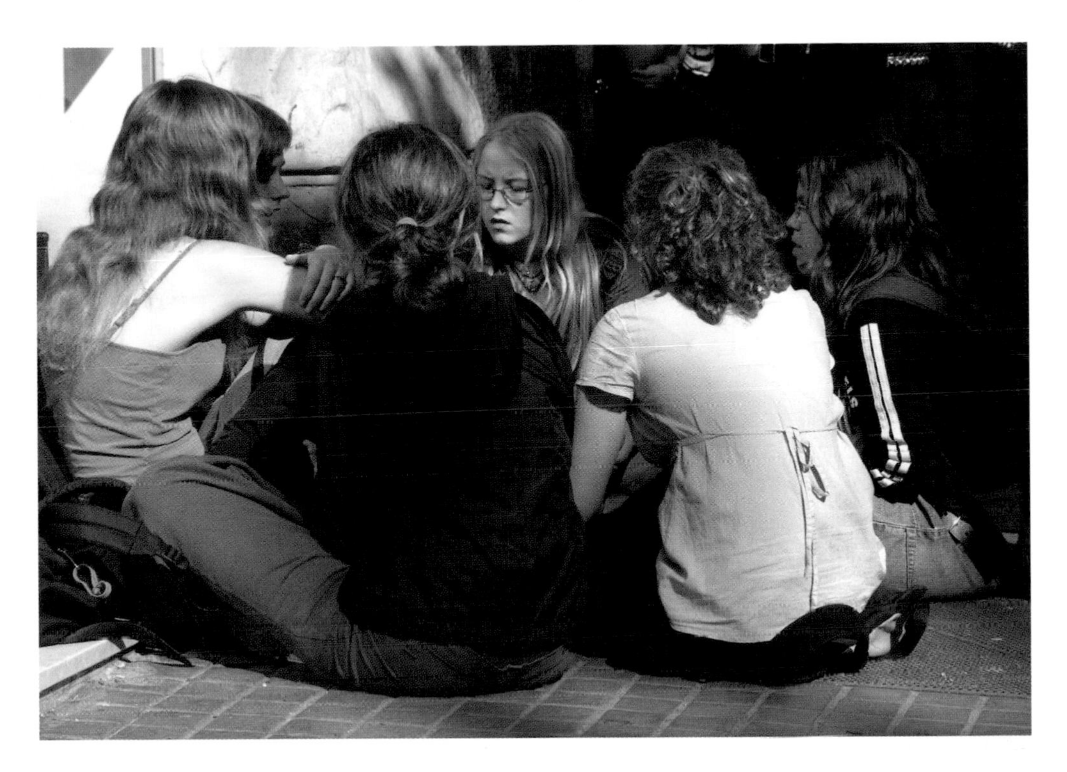

Pubertal development in boys

- 11–12 years: growth of the penis and testicles.
- 12–13 years: appearance of pubic hair; acceleration of growth.
- 13–14 years: clear development of the penis and testicles.
- 14–15 years : appearance of moustache and underarm hair; maximum increase in growth.
- 15–16 years: change of voice; complete development of the penis and testicles; mature spermatozoids.
- 17–19 years: growth of the beard; welding of the cartilages; cessation of growth.

Middle adolescence (14–16 years)

• Separation from the family is more evident.

• They are more selective about their friends and some activities may be shared with a friend from the opposite sex.

• Abstract thought starts to develop, so an adolescent constantly needs to know different points of view and new alternatives.

• Excessive preoccupation with the changes she is experiencing gives rise to a special attention to personal relationships.

Late adolescence (17–19 years)

• Relationships with boy/girlfriends become more stable.

• The capacity for abstraction makes it possible to plan studies, work, or life with a partner.

• The relationship with the family calms down again and the attitude to parents is less critical and aggressive. Negativity does appear sometimes, however: adolescents rebel against family values and explore new ideas and approaches.

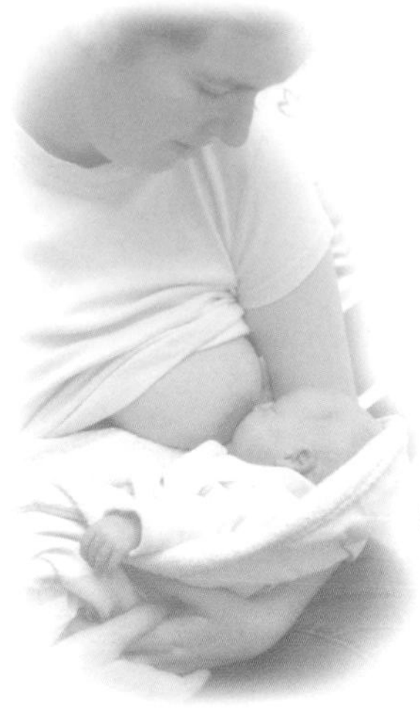

feeding a baby

In the first year of life, a baby's diet is basically comprised of milk, whether from his mother or from formulas. It is very important to know about the essential aspects of feeding a baby, following your doctor's advice, as it in this stage that a human being has the highest growth index, at the greatest speed, in proportional terms. It is also important to establish the foundations of a healthy diet right from the start.

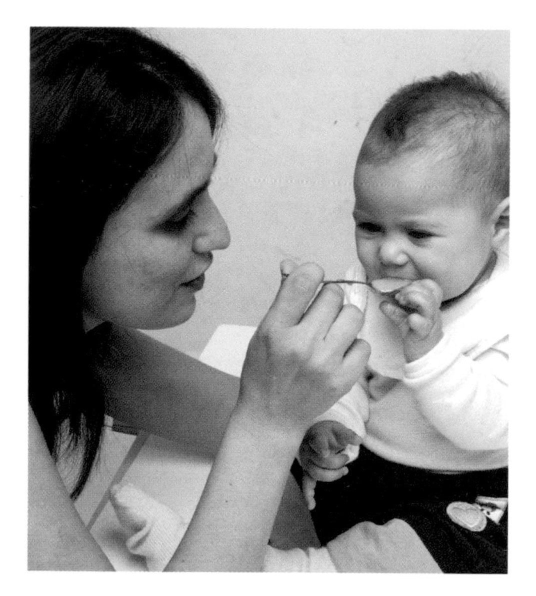

Starting to nurse

• It is very important for a baby to be nursed at once, half an hour after being born. Although he will not suckle at first, the contact with his mother's skin is very beneficial. This first contact means that when the baby is ready to feed, his mother can offer him her breast straight away.

• During the first days, the milk is yellowish (colostrum) and contains a lot of proteins and antibodies. Mature milk will come in later. There is no such thing as low-quality mother's milk; it is always capable of satisfying a baby's needs.

• The main stimulus for milk production is the baby's sucking, so the more often he suckles and leaves the breast empty, the more milk will be produced. So, the amount of milk produced will correspond to the quantity consumed by the baby and the number of times the breast is emptied every day.

Nutritional recommendations according to the baby's age (these recommendations should never override those of a doctor)

• First 4–6 months
- Nursing (exclusively, if possible).
- If this is not possible, an early infant formula.

• 4–6 months
- Follow-on formula.
- Gluten-free children's cereals.
- At 4 months: fruits (apple, banana, pear, orange).
- At 5 1/2 months: vegetable puree with chicken.

• 7–8 months of life
- Children's cereals with gluten (in the 7th month).
- At 7 months: introduce beef.

Dietary model 1

- Breakfast (8–9am): follow-on formula plus gluten-free flour (in a feeding bottle or puree).
- Lunch (noon–1pm): vegetable puree with chicken.
- Snack: (4–5pm): fruit puree.
- Dinner (8–9pm): follow-on formula plus gluten-free flour (in a feeding bottle or puree).
- Night-time complement (optional): follow-on formula.

Dietary model 2

- Breakfast (8–9am): follow-on formula plus flour with gluten (in a feeding bottle or puree).
- Lunch (noon–1pm): vegetable puree with beef.
- Snack: (4–5pm): fruit puree.
- Dinner (8–9pm): follow-on formula plus flour with gluten (in a feeding bottle or puree).
- Night-time complement (optional): follow-on formula.

- **8–9 months**

• If there is no previous history of allergy, introduce white fish (e.g. hake, monkfish, sole, etc.).

- **10–12 months**

• 10 months: hardboiled egg (first the yolk and then the whole egg), once or twice a week.

• 12 months: plain, thoroughly cooked omelet, with one egg.

Tips for a suitable diet in the first year of life

1. Mother's milk, if possible, until the 4th–6th month.
2. Early infant formula until the 4th–6th month if nursing is impossible.
3. Follow-on formula from the 4th–6th month until the age of 3.
4. Introduce the gluten after the 6th month.

It is very important to sterilize drinking bottles and teats in the first 6 months of a baby's life.

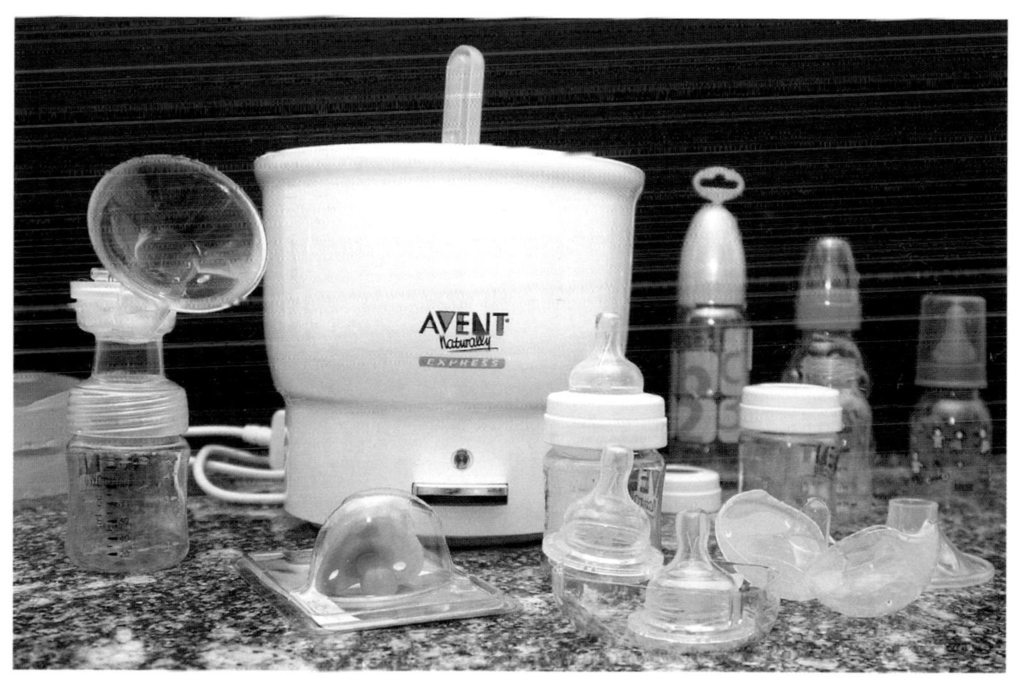

Dietary model 3

- Breakfast (8–9am): follow-on formula plus flour with gluten (in a feeding bottle or puree).
- Lunch (noon-1pm): vegetable puree with chicken or beef.
- Snack: (4–5pm): fruit puree or follow-on formula, alternating with the dinner-time milk.
- Dinner (8–9pm): vegetable puree with fish (3–4 times a week) or follow-on formula.
- Night-time complement (optional): follow-on formula.

Dietary model 4

- Breakfast (8–9am): follow-on formula plus flour with gluten (in a feeding bottle or puree).
- Lunch (noon-1pm): vegetable puree with chicken or beef.
- Snack: (4–5pm): fruit puree or follow-on formula, alternating with the dinner-time milk.
- Dinner (8–9pm): vegetable puree with fish/egg (once a week) or follow-on formula.
- Night-time complement (optional): follow-on formula.

5. Provide approximately 17–30 fl oz (500–900 cubic cm) of milk per day.
6. Ensure a source of Vitamin D.
7. Sequence of introduction of foodstuffs: fruit (4th–5th month), chicken (5th–6th month), beef (6th–7th month), fish (8th–9th month), egg (9th–10th month).
8. New foodstuffs and changes to the diet must be introduced gradually.
9. Food for babies must not be reheated or prepared more than 8–12 hours before serving.
10. Take great care over hygiene and sterilize drinking bottles and teats in the first 6 months.

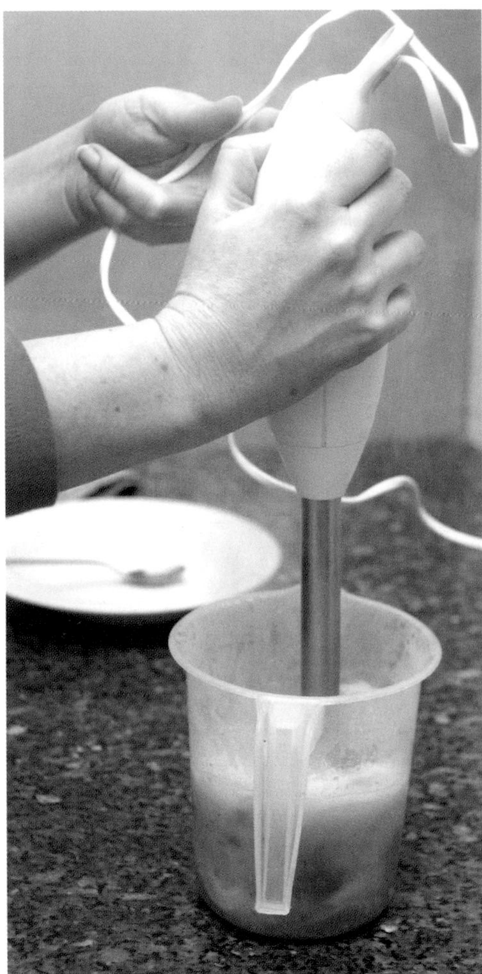

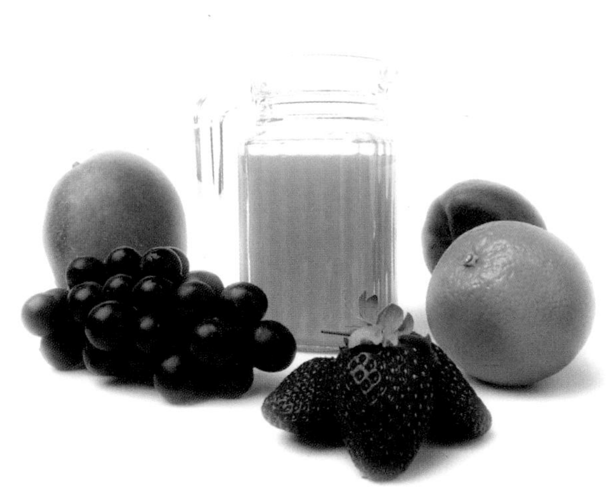

nursing and weaning

Nursing is the safest, most natural, and most convenient way to feed a baby in his first year of life, as maternal milk contains the appropriate balance of proteins, vitamins, minerals, fats, and carbohydrates, as well as supplying antibodies from his mother's immune system. Modern experts advocate maintaining this type of diet for at least the first 4–6 months of life whenever possible, and providing the baby's growth and development are normal for his age and characteristics at birth. The final decision of whether or not to breast-feed a baby is the mother's, however, as maternal milk is only contraindicated in a few situations, i.e. in the case of certain diseases or where the mother is taking certain types of medication.

Reasons for recommending nursing

- Mother's milk is the best food that a mother can offer her newborn baby – not only for its nutritional value, but also for its emotional value, as the bond established between a mother and her baby is a unique and intense experience.
- Mother's milk contains everything a child needs during the first years of his life.
- Mother's milk is always preferable, because of the protection it provides against many diseases: catarrh, bronchitis, pneumonia, diarrhea, ear infections, meningitis, urinary infections, colitis, or crib death.
- It also protects against future illness: asthma, allergy, obesity, diabetes, Crohn's disease, ulcerative colitis, and heart attacks in adulthood. Nursing is also good for a baby's intellectual development.

To be certain that you are producing enough milk, observe whether your baby is putting on weight, wetting more and more nappies every day, and appears happy. A newborn baby will feed 8–10 times over a period of 24 hours. This rate will drop as the baby grows older.

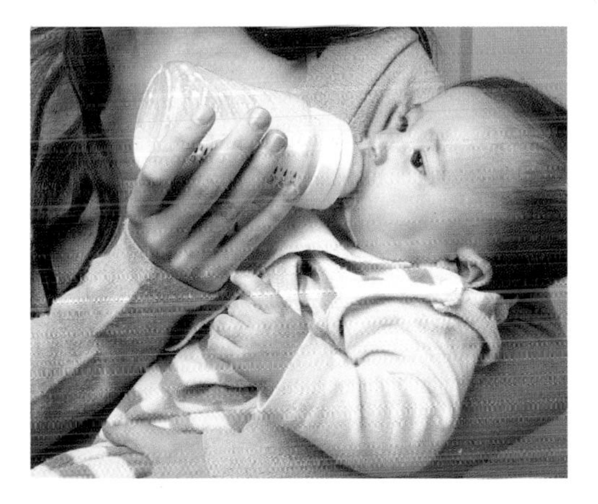

- A nursing mother loses the weight put on during pregnancy more quickly; she is less likely to suffer anemia after giving birth and also has less risk of suffering from postnatal depression and high blood pressure. Similarly, breast and ovarian cancer, as well as osteoporosis, are less frequent in women who breast-fed their children.
- Furthermore, mother's milk is a cheap, ecological food that allows a family to make considerable savings in its shopping budget.

NURSING TECHNIQUE

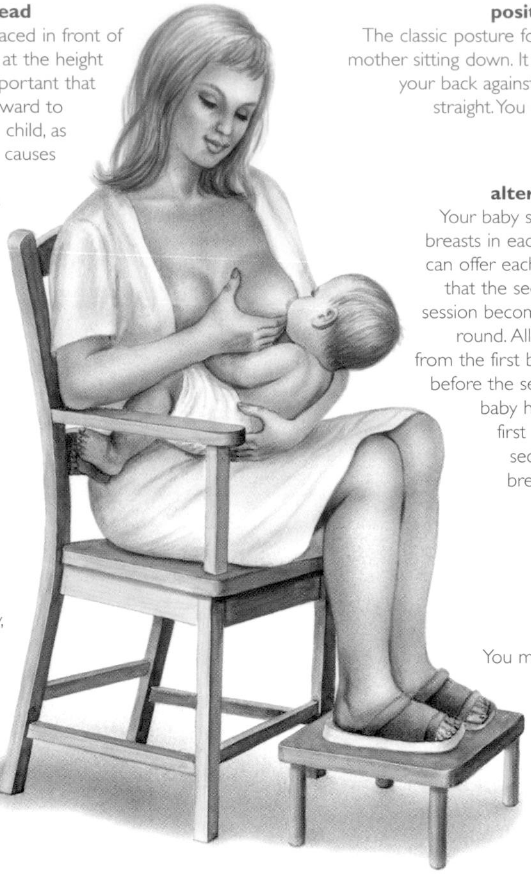

positioning your baby's head
The baby's head should be placed in front of the breast, so that his nose is at the height of his mother's nipple. It is important that the mother does not lean forward to bring her breast closer to the child, as this is a stressful position that causes backache and does not allow the nipple to meet the baby's mouth efficiently.

holding the baby
The mother holds the baby with one of her arms, so that her hand supports his buttocks, his head rests on the crook of the elbow, and his back rests on his mother's forearm.

position of your baby
The baby's head and body should face his mother's body, so that the baby's abdomen comes into direct contact with her body. If the baby were facing upward, he would have to look up and turn his head to search for the nipple, which would make sucking difficult.

position of the mother
The classic posture for nursing involves the mother sitting down. It is a good idea to rest your back against a support, to keep it straight. You can also use cushions.

alternating the breasts
Your baby should feed from both breasts in each nursing session; you can offer each breast alternately, so that the second breast from one session becomes the first next time round. Allow your baby to feed from the first breast until it is empty, before the second is offered. If the baby has had his fill with the first breast and rejects the second, offer the second breast first the next time

feet slightly raised
You might find it convenient to have your feet slightly raised on a stool or pillow.

Tips on how to nurse

1. Hold the baby close to your breast, with his stomach against you.
2. Rub the baby's cheek with your nipple, to make him turn toward you.
3. As far as possible, put the dark area around your nipple into the baby's mouth.
4. Allow the baby to suck for 10–15 minutes.
5. Use your finger to press the lower part of your breast close to the baby's mouth, to make him stop sucking.
6. Feed him with the other breast for another 10–15 minutes.
7. Allow your breasts to dry in the air.

Feeding with a bottle.

When it is not possible to give a baby mother's milk or when nursing cannot be re-established for some reason, the alternative is feed a baby with a bottle containing early infant or follow-on formula, according to the baby's needs and the doctor's advice.

In this case, you will need the following feeding equipment:

• Several feeding bottles; they come in various shapes and sizes.

• Teats. A range of models is available on the market. You have to decide which is most acceptable and suited to your baby: anatomical, universal, anti-colic, with a wide base for disposable bottles, etc.

• Brushes for feeding bottles. Remember that hygiene is essential to prevent the growth of germs and bacteria.

• A plastic spoon and knife for measuring and leveling, respectively, the amount of milk to add to the feeding bottle.

• Sterilizer. Cold-water models use sterilizing pills or liquids. They should have a tray or floater to help submerge all the elements. You should wait until the pills dissolve before inserting all the elements and make sure that there are no air bubbles, as these will impede the sterilization. Hot-water models look similar but they do not require sterilizing pills or liquids, although their materials must be able to resist high temperatures, as they must be left on a burner in boiling water for at least thirty minutes if they are to work properly.

• Other elements: scissors, plastic funnel, a jug for preparing milk, etc.

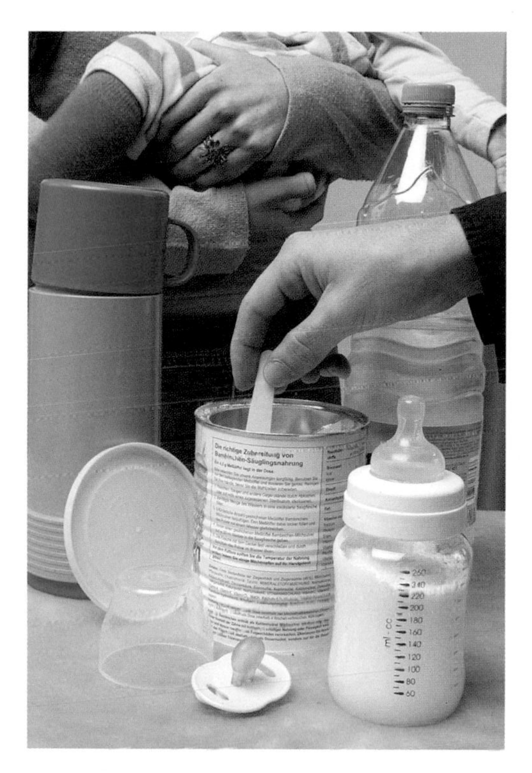

Weaning

This transition can be a source of conflict and has to happen gradually, step by step, to give your baby time to adapt to the new situation. The process is usually sparked off by a baby's need to broaden his diet. Weaning does not, therefore, imply a complete stop to nursing or drinking milk from a bottle, but rather a gradual replacement of some of the feeding sessions.

The following measures can be used as guidelines for the weaning process, always remembering that none of them should supplant or contravene any of your doctor's recommendations:

• 1st -2nd week of weaning: try a few small tests with purées at midday, to complement the feeding session.

• 3rd -4th week: introduce the new food as half of the breakfast session and increase the amount at midday.

• 5th–6th week: introduce solid foods as half of the snacktime session. A few days later, offer your baby two dishes at lunch (e.g. vegetable purée followed by fruit puree), giving him 3 spoonfuls of each one. Add a cup containing his drink; he will not use it yet, but he will play with it.

• 7th- 8th week: offer him solid food as the first part of lunch and then fill him up with mother's milk. He can now be served two dishes at snack time, but you should continue nursing him first at breakfast and snack time. Encourage him to drink from the cup, helping him to hold it.

• 9th–10th week: once your baby has eaten solid foods, offer him formula milk to drink from his cup, instead of nursing him or using a bottle. Stop nursing him at lunch time in favor of solid food only.

• 11th–13th weeks onward: from now on, offer him drinks in a cup and purées 3 times a day, apart from his formula milk.

It is recommended that the mother nurse for the first 4–6 months of life.

diet during infancy

In the second year of life, a child leaves behind the eating habits of babyhood and his diet becomes increasingly similar to that of an adult. Bearing in mind that these early years establish behavior that will probably endure throughout the rest of his life, it is essential to instill good eating habits in infancy. Furthermore, the rapid growth rate in childhood and adolescence impose nutritional criteria that will allow a youngster to develop normally. Dietary deficiencies can result in irreversible disorders.

General recommendations

• It is common for an infant to prefer particular foodstuffs that he is always prepared to eat and equally to invariably reject others. To counteract this tendency, you should persistently encourage him to try unappealing items of food essential to a balanced diet by seeking new combinations and different ways of preparing or presenting them.

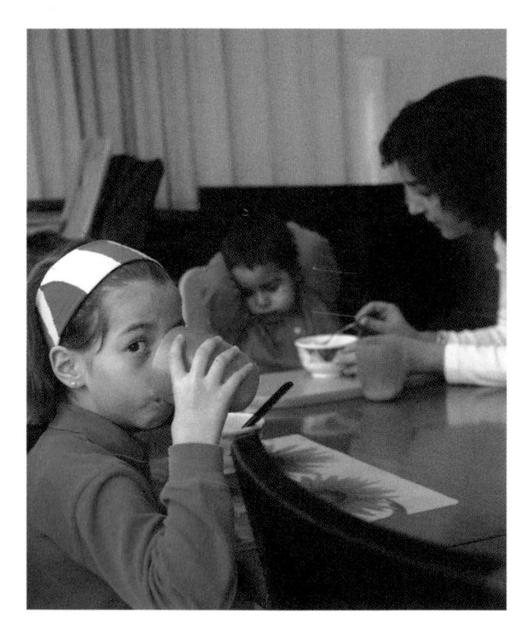

• Forget about rewards and punishment when it comes to food. A healthy diet is important in its own right and should not be modified in accordance with a child's reactions.

• It is vital to convey the positive values of a balanced diet by telling your child that eating properly will make him healthier, stronger, taller, and cleverer. You can experiment with the presentation, preparation, and garnishing of foods to ensure that a particular ingredient is accepted (or at least tolerated). Food should be a source of pleasure, and never one of stress.

• You have to be very cautious about special diets followed by other parents, whether for reasons of health or ethics. Restrictions on any type of food – as in vegetarianism, dissociated diets, or diets low in cholesterol, fat, salt, etc. – endanger the correct development of children, as they need a greater supply of nutrients than adults.

• It is important to spread out meals over the course of the day. The younger a child, the lower the capacity of his digestive system to adapt to

It is a proven fact that the preferences of parents influence those of their children, as it is unusual for children to crave food that is not found in the home environment.

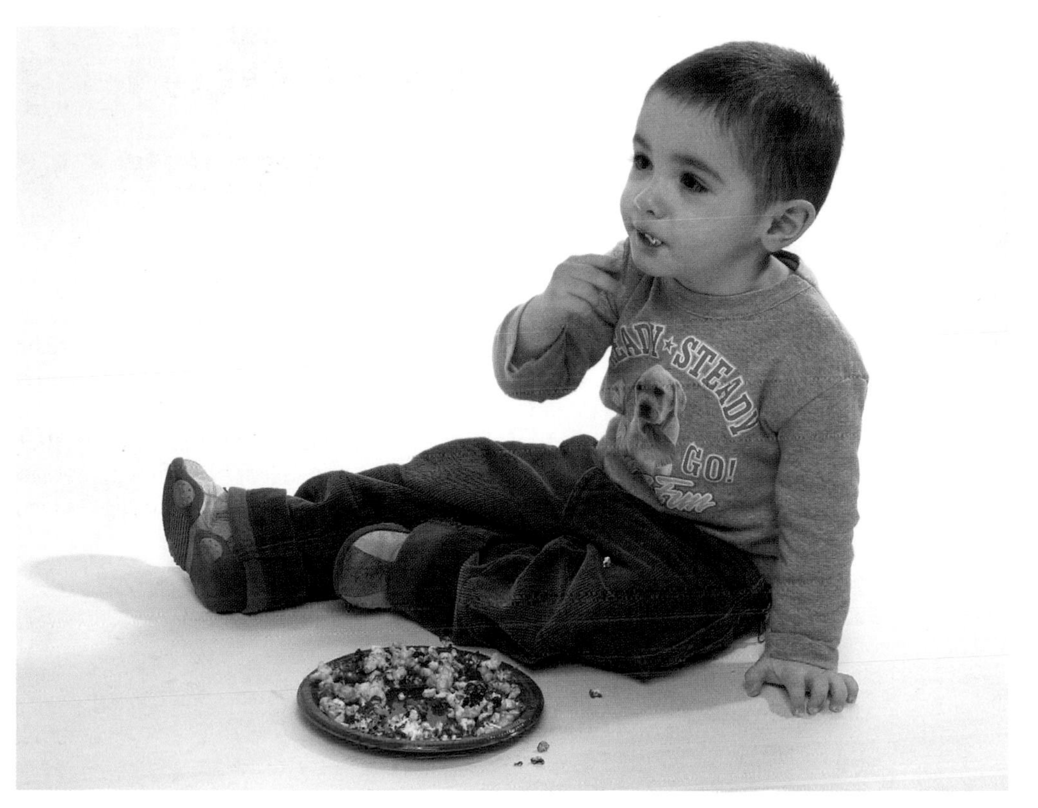

It is inevitable that children will eat candies, pastries, and junk food. The problem with these products lies in the quantity, rather than the quality. They can be eaten in small amounts in exceptional circumstances, but they should never be offered on a daily or regular basis.

long spells without food. It is better to divide up meals and serve them in 4 or 5 daily sessions, rather than concentrating them into 2 or 3. Breakfast should be the main meal of the day.

PROTEINS. The protein requirement is 2 g/kg of body weight in the first year of life, and half that amount during the rest of infancy and adolescence.

VITAMINS AND MINERALS

- During childhood, the intake of appropriate amounts of calcium, iron, and Vitamins A and D is vital.
- As regards other vitamins and minerals, the recommended levels are the same as those found in all balanced diets.
- A child needs 3 times more calcium than an adult. Dairy products are the main source.

DAILY CALORIE REQUIREMENTS		
	Age (years)	**Calories (kcal/day)**
Children	1-3	1,300
	4-6	1,700
	7-10	2,400
Boys	11-14	2,700
Girls	11-14	2,200

• Vitamin D is needed for the absorption and use of calcium in the bones, and any deficiency can lead to rickets. Vitamin D is obtained from food, but it can also be produced by the skin after exposure to sunlight.

• A greater need for iron is also typical of this stage of growth and development. Meat is the main nutritional source for this.

Generally speaking, it is advisable to prevent any possible dietary imbalances by increasing the consumption of cereals, fruit, vegetables and dairy products, as well as cutting down fats and serving salt, sugar, and sweet snacks in moderation.

Vitamin and mineral supplements are not recommended, except when required because of illness or on a doctor's prescription. Their indiscriminate use can create an imbalance, which can be equally harmful to a child's health.

Guide to child nutrition

Recommended daily consumption of each food group

Cereals/pulses: 6–8 portions/day

One portion is the equivalent of:

- Bread: 1–1 1/3 oz/30–40 g.
- Breakfast cereals: 1–1 1/3 oz/30–40 g.
- Rice: 3 1/2–5 oz/100–150 g.
- Pasta: 3 1/2–5 oz/100–150 g (when cooked)
- Pulses: 3 1/2–5 oz/100–150 g (when cooked)

Vegetables: 3–5 portions/day

One portion is the equivalent of:
3 1/2–7 oz/100–200 g (when raw).

Fruit: 2–4 portions/day

One portion is the equivalent of:

- One piece of medium-size fruit.
- A glass of juice (one third of a pint/150 ml).

Meat/fish/eggs: 2–3 portions/day

One portion is the equivalent of:

- Meat: 3 1/2–4 1/2 oz/100–125 g.
- Fish: 3 1/2–4 1/2 oz/100–125 g.
- One egg.

Dairy products: 2–3 portions/day

One portion is the equivalent of:

- Milk: 7 02/200 ml.
- Yoghurt, fermented milk, or curds: 4_ oz/125 g.
- Fresh cheese: 1–1 1/2 oz/30–40 g.
- Other cheese: 1/2–1 oz/15–30 g.

Sweet and fatty foods should be eaten in great moderation

diet during adolescence

Puberty and adolescence are marked by an increase in height and weight, as well as by significant modifications to the amount and distribution of body fat. These changes demand alterations in some eating habits, to guarantee a sufficient supply of energy and nutrients. Nutritional deficiencies during this phase of maximum growth can have negative consequences, such as smaller stature, diminished bone mass, and delayed onset of puberty. Proteins, iron, calcium, Vitamin C, and zinc are the key nutrients in adolescence. The psychological and social changes of adolescence can lead teenagers to reject family customs and the eating habits acquired in childhood. Adolescents start to prepare their own meals and eat outside their home more frequently; consequently, there is a greater risk of following an unbalanced and inappropriate diet.

Nutritional recommendations

It is very difficult to make standardized recommendations for adolescents, as each one is different. The following recommendations are based on guidelines designed to promote healthy living.

• Carbohydrates. These should provide 50% of the daily calorie requirements.

• Proteins. Around 15-20% of the total daily energy supply, especially those from vegetal sources.

• Fats. These should represent 30–35% of the total calories, with a suitable distribution of saturated, monounsaturated, and polyunsaturated fatty acids. Don't forget that an appropriate fat intake involves satisfying the body's requirements with respect to essential fatty acids (needed for the formation of various metabolites) and fat-soluble vitamins.

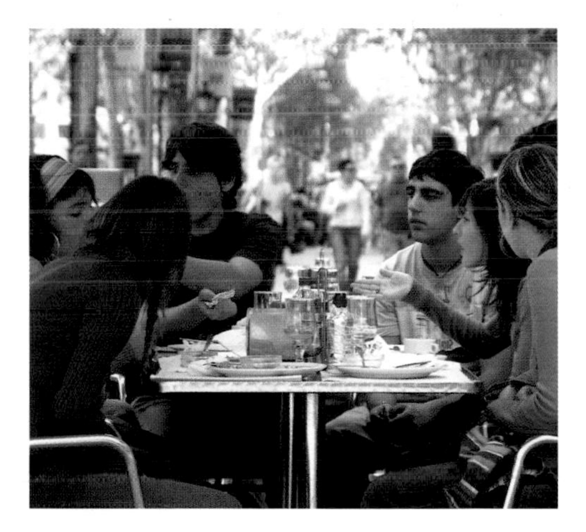

The body mass practically doubles during puberty. This causes an increase in the child's requirements of energy, proteins, and minerals, so any deficiency in this period can have negative consequences. Both sexes reach their adult height between the ages of 18 and 20, although the bone mass continues to increase until the age of 25.

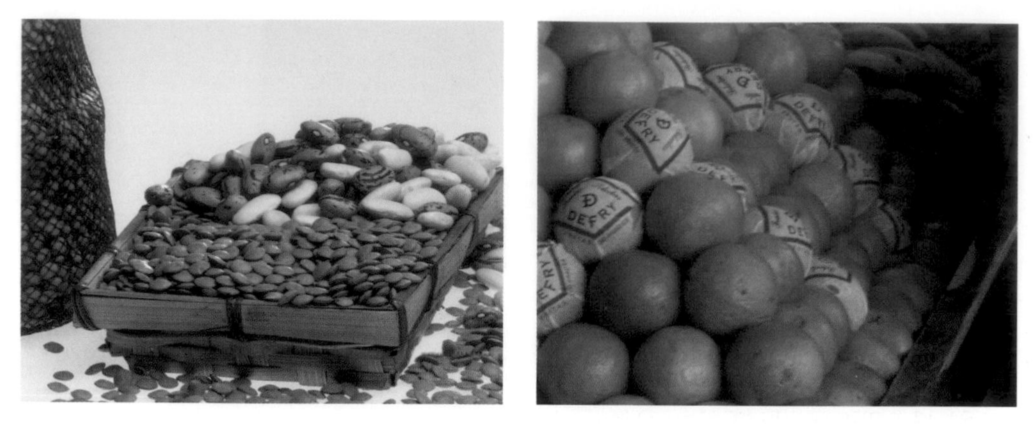

Main natural sources of calcium: *milk and its derivatives, sardines, dried fruit, seafood, soya, chickpeas, vegetables, and pulses.* Main natural sources of zinc: fish, spinach, cabbage, Swiss chard, oysters, liver, and pulses. Main natural sources of iron: *meat, oranges, raisins, dates, seafood, tripe, egg, celery, cauliflower, broad beans, asparagus, and almonds.*

• Minerals. The body has a particular need for calcium (1,200 mg/day), iron (2 mg/day for males and 5 mg/day for females after onset of the menstrual cycle), and zinc (12 mg/day for females and 15 mg/day for males).

• Vitamins. It is important to cover an adolescent's needs for Vitamins A, D, folic acid, B12, B6, riboflavin, niacin, and thiamin. Fruit and vegetables are the main sources of all these elements.

Nutritional tips for adolescents

• Foods with a plastic function. These are rich in proteins and constitute two of the seven groups that make up the food wheel: milk and its derivatives and meat/fish/eggs.

• Milk and its derivatives: 21–28 fl oz/ 650–850 ml, apart from a portion of cheese (5–7 oz/150–200 g) at least once a day.

• Meat or fish: 5–7 oz/150–200 g per portion (once a day).

• Eggs: once a day (four times a week). When they substitute a portion of meat or fish, use two.

• High-energy foods. These include cereals, flours derived from them, and their by-products, such as bread, pasta, cookies, rice, sugar, and pastries. All these are rich in carbohydrates. Many of

DIETARY GUIDELINES, IN ACCORDANCE WITH AGE, SEX, HEIGHT, AND BODY WEIGHT				
Age (years)	**Height (ins/cm)**	**Weight (lb/kg)**	**Proteins (g per day)**	**Energy (kcal/day)**
Females				
11-14	62/157	101/46	46	2,200
15-18	64/163	121/55	44	2,200
19-24	64.5/164	128/58	46	2,200
Males				
11-14	62/157	99/45	45	2,500
15-18	69/176	145/66	59	3,000
19-24	70/177	158/72	58	2,900

the processed foods in this group (bread, pasta, cookies, etc.) are made with refined or white flour obtained from cereals, particularly wheat. Sugar and the sweetened products in this group are neither basic nor necessary foodstuffs: they are empty calories.

- It is essential to eat at least two, not overly copious meals and ensure the intake of sugars and carbohydrates (potatoes, rice, pasta, bread, etc.), especially at breakfast time.
- Regulatory foods. These are distinguished by being a source of vitamins, minerals, and water. They also have high levels of fiber.
- It is very important to eat fruit and both raw and cooked vegetables. One salad a day is recommended, along with 3–4 items of fruit.
- Drinks. There should be a sufficient intake of water (around 2 liters per day), and only a moderate consumption of sweetened drinks. It is important to make adolescents aware of the harmful effects of any alcoholic drink.

Recommended daily intake of the various food groups for adolescents:

- 3–4 portions of milk and dairy products.
- 2 portions of meat, fish, or eggs.
- 6–8 portions of cereals and pulses.
- 2–4 portions fruit.
- 3–5 portions of vegetables.
- Moderate consumption of oil, fat, sugar, and sweet things.

The group of high-energy foods includes fat of animal origin (butter, pork and beef fat, etc.) and oils (olive, corn, sunflower, etc.). These are needed in a balanced diet, as they not only provide calories but also fat-soluble vitamins and essential fatty acids.

Foods rich in saturated fatty acids should be avoided because of their association with high levels of blood cholesterol. These foods include oils used to make pastry products, disguised under the heading of vegetable fat. By contrast, olive oil has a high proportion of unsaturated fatty acids, known to provide protection against cardiovascular disease.

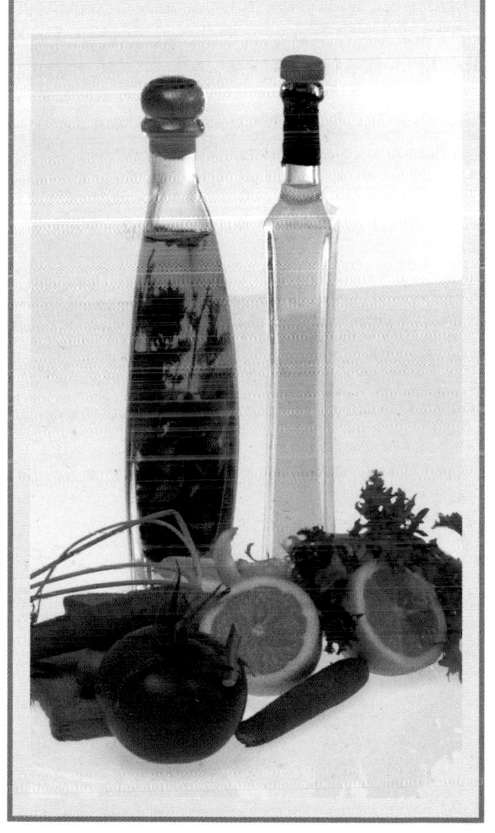

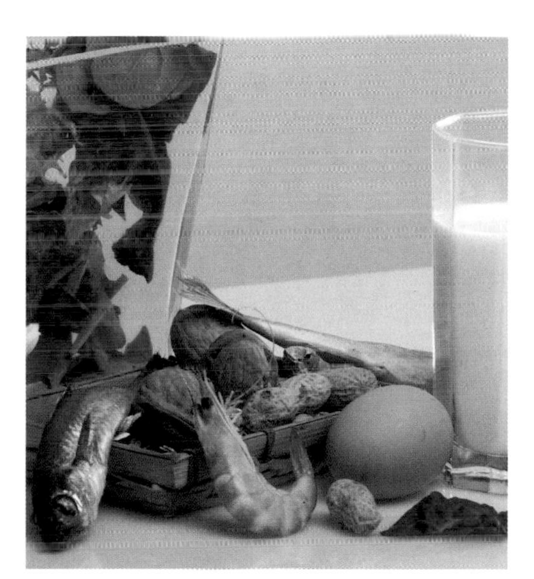

anemia in babies and children

Anemia can be defined as a reduction in the number of red blood cells or their hemoglobin content, resulting in inadequate transportation of oxygen to the tissues. In 90 percent of cases, anemia in a baby or child is caused by insufficient iron in the diet (ferropenic anemia). Iron is vital to the formation of hemoglobin, so any deficiency produces, first, a reduction of its deposits in the body and, secondly, a drop in the rates of its synthesis. It is normal to find fluctuations in hemoglobin levels, depending on age, gender, and the altitude of the home environment, so these factors should be taken into account before confirming a diagnosis of anemia.

Normal variations in the levels of hemoglobin in the blood

- A baby is born with a high level of hemoglobin – generally over 15 g/dl; this slowly drops down to 9 g/dl by the third month.
- It then starts to increase gradually, so that by the end of the first year the normal value is 12 g/dl or more.
- In adolescence, the normal value for boys is over 13 g/dl, while in girls it is approximately 12 g/dl.

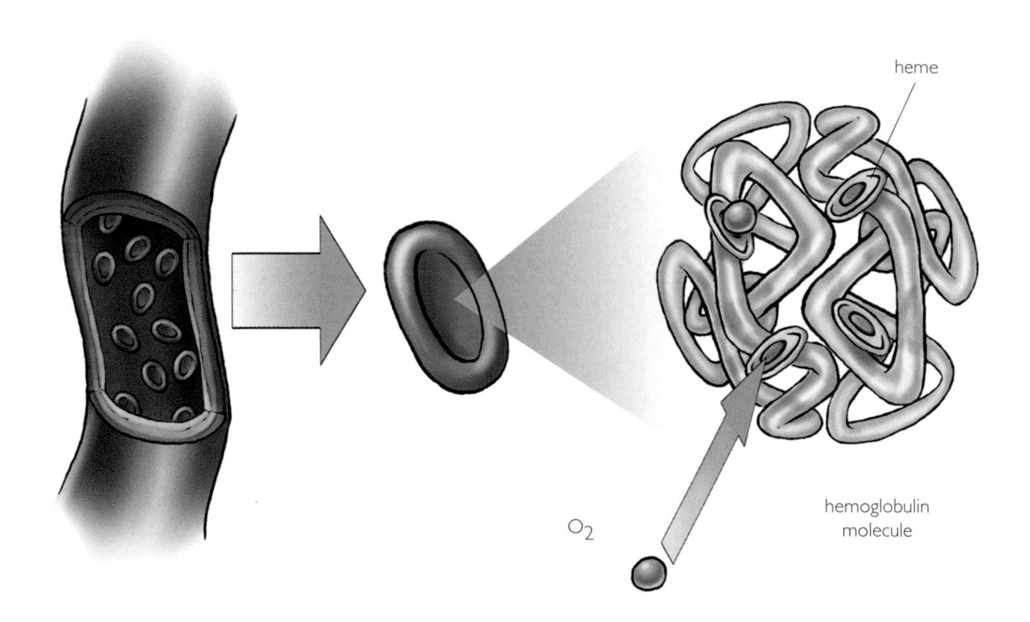

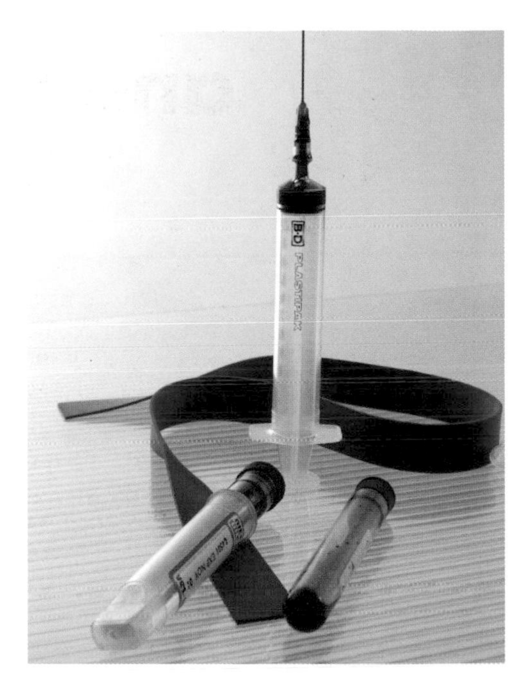
A diagnosis of anemia is confirmed if the levels of red blood cells and hemoglobin in a blood sample are lower than normal.

It is normal for hemoglobin levels to vary with age, gender (after adolescence), and altitude above sea level; it is lower in people living on a coast, and it goes up with an increase in the altitude of a person's home. All these factors must be considered in the analysis of a blood sample before confirming a diagnosis of anemia.

General recommendations

Experts are unanimous about the measures required to prevent ferropenic anemia in babies: they should receive extra iron in their diet at the age of 4 months if they are taking formula milk, at 6 months if they are feeding on mother's milk, or after one month if they were born prematurely.

- Babies fed with formula milk receive iron from the milk itself, as it comes enriched with minerals

Hemoglobin is one of the most important elements in red blood cells, and iron is the main mineral involved in its formation. Hemoglobin is responsible for the transportation of oxygen to the tissues and the elimination of carbon anhydride resulting from metabolic processes.

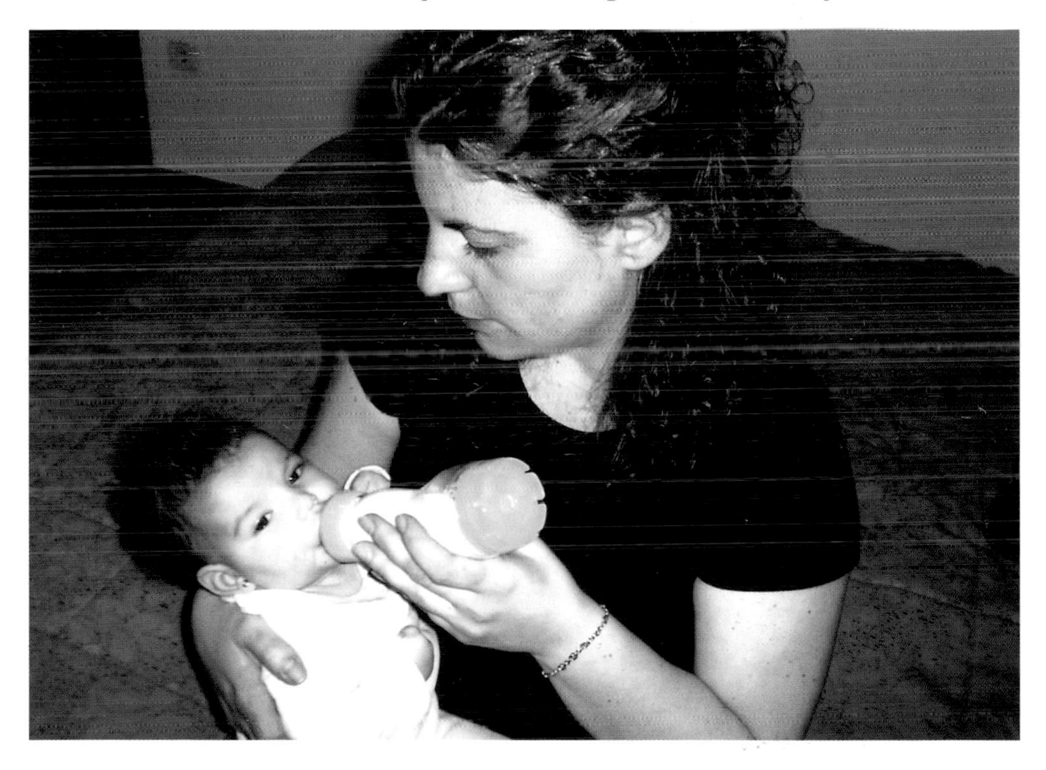

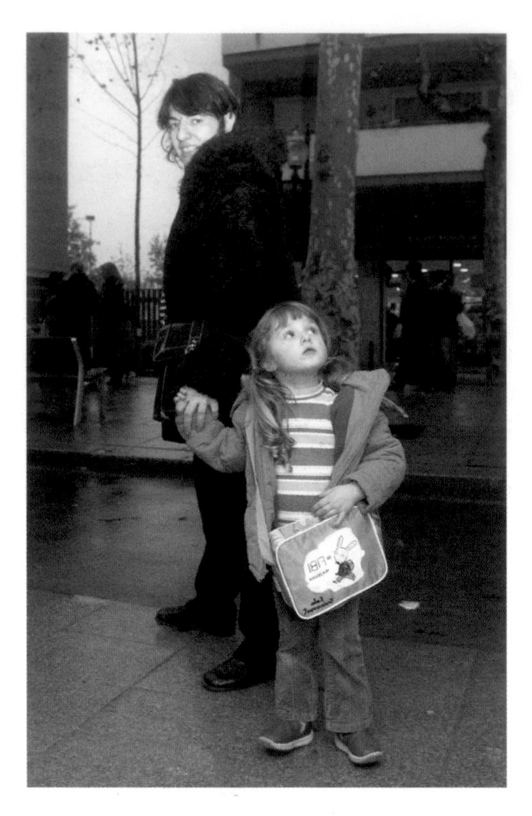

Children need an appropriate amount of iron in their diet, especially during periods of rapid growth, such as the first 2 years of life and adolescence.

• It is important to avoid ferropenic anemia in a baby, as numerous studies have demonstrated that it can affect a child's development.

• Ferropenic anemia is easier to prevent in an adolescent, as her diet is more varied and virtually without restrictions – unless she is suffering from another condition that contraindicates certain foods. It can be treated satisfactorily with iron supplements, if a doctor considers them appropriate.

and vitamins. In some cases, a doctor may consider iron supplements necessary.

• If a baby is breast-feeding, she receives iron from her mother (albeit to a lesser extent than formula milk, although it is absorbed better). Even so, she should receive extra iron from the age of 6 months, whether from iron-enriched cereal or from iron drops, according to your doctor's advice.

• Iron-enriched cereal is a good option, but you should make sure that the quantity is appropriate. A baby's iron requirement is usually equivalent to 6–8 spoonfuls of cereal per day.

• A baby should not drink cow's milk in the first year of her life as it has been proven to cause small intestinal hemorrhages, aggravating any anemia.

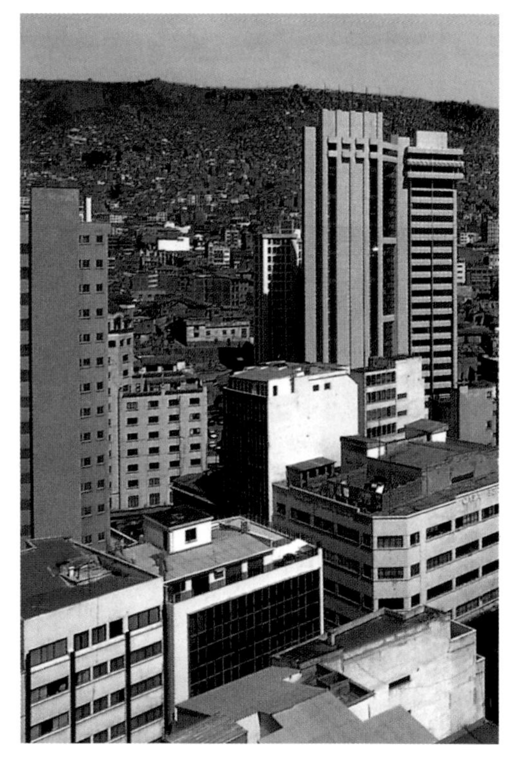

The higher the altitude, the less oxygen there is in the atmosphere. This reduction in oxygen molecules means that people who live at high altitudes have higher counts of red blood cells and hemoglobin, allowing them to make efficient use of the limited supply of atmospheric oxygen. This is the case, for example, in the Bolivian city of La Paz, which is situated 12,140 ft (3,700 m) above sea level.

constipation in children

Constipation is common in childhood; it is thought to affect between 1.5 and 7.5 percent of children of school age. Constipation means that the stools turn hard and dry, making bowel movements difficult and painful. A child may express a desire to defecate but fail to do so, even after making an effort. This situation may be detected by a child's tears or complaints after going to the toilet. It is more difficult to identify a baby with constipation, as it is normal for the frequency of her bowel movements to vary considerably. A baby is considered to be constipated when she defecates less than 3 times a week.

Most frequent causes of constipation in children

- The most common cause of constipation in a child is a diet low in fiber, i.e. lacking in fruit, vegetables, pulses, cereals, and dried fruit. To a large extent, it can be cured by changing the child's diet and eating habits.
- Excess of astringent foodstuffs that cause constipation, such as potatoes, bananas, rice, cooked carrot, etc., or the consumption of products to which she is unaccustomed, such as chocolate, candies, or other sweet things.
- Insufficient intake of liquid. Water and fruit juice help defecation by moistening the intestine.
- Inadequate hygiene in school toilets can affect a child by making her reluctant to go to the bathroom at school.
- Negative factors in training a child to control her sphincter – such as insistence, haste, and even punishment in some cases – can instill a rebellious attitude or a refusal to go to the bathroom.
- Too little time spent in the toilet when the impulse or desire to defecate arises.
- Nerves, stress, a traumatic event in the family, such as a death, moving house or town, the arrival of a new member, etc.
- An erratic eating schedule. Many constipated children eat more between meals than at meal times.

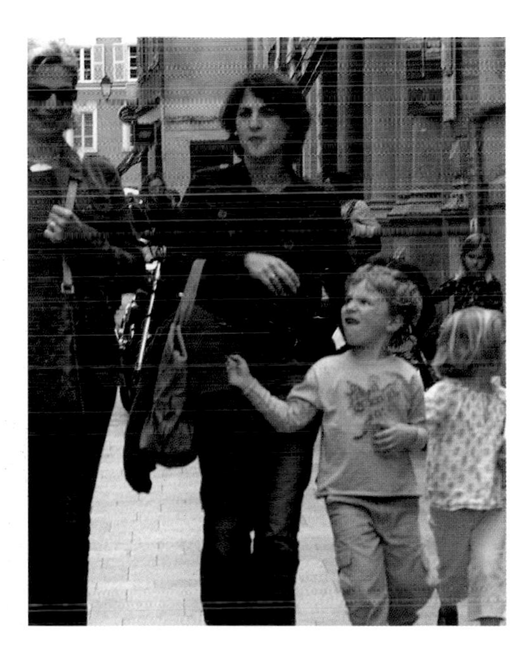

A small baby's rate of defecation depends on her diet, (breast-fed babies tend to have greater regularity of bowel movements, and greater liquid content than formula-fed babies). A baby under 6 months old should generally defecate at least once a day; after 6 months, she should do so at least 3 times a week. From the age of 2, children tend to defecate once or twice a day.

Any increase in fiber intake should be introduced gradually, as a diet with a high fiber content can cause a child to suffer from wind, distension of the abdomen, and colic, as well as interfering with the absorption of other nutrients she needs in order to grow.

Signs of constipation in a child

- The feces are hard and dry.
- Less than 2 bowel movements per day in babies fed with mother's milk.
- Less than 3 bowel movements per week in babies fed on formula.
- Less than 2 or 3 bowel movements per week in children and adolescents.
- Bowel movements are painful or incomplete.

Treatment

Here are some ways of treating constipation in children, although these should never be put into practice without first consulting a doctor:

• Phosphate enemas, combined with either mineral oil or laxatives, to obtain immediate relief.

• Intestinal re-education: encourage the child to sit on the toilet for 20 minutes after meals and make sure she never holds back the urge to defecate.

• The use of feces softeners like mineral oil, paraffin, glycerin suppositories, etc. They can be used for a maximum of 3 months, until the intestinal habit is regularized. The use of other laxatives and enemas should be avoided.

• Dietary changes: increase the quantity of fiber, liquids, fruits, and vegetables, with an emphasis on foods particularly rich in fiber such as wheat bran and pulses. Popcorn is a snack with a particularly high fiber content.

• Temporarily eliminate or reduce the intake of foodstuffs that worsen constipation, such as bananas, potatoes, and carrots.

Most constipation is connected with diet and lifestyle. In the first instance, there should be an emphasis on food with fiber, such as fruit and vegetables; second, exercise and movement will help resolve the problem by preventing a sedentary lifestyle.

The surface of the anus can be torn during defecation (anal fissure), causing pain and possibly a small amount of bright-red blood in a baby's feces. Most anal fissures heal rapidly in babies without any treatment, but a gentle laxative can help the healing process.

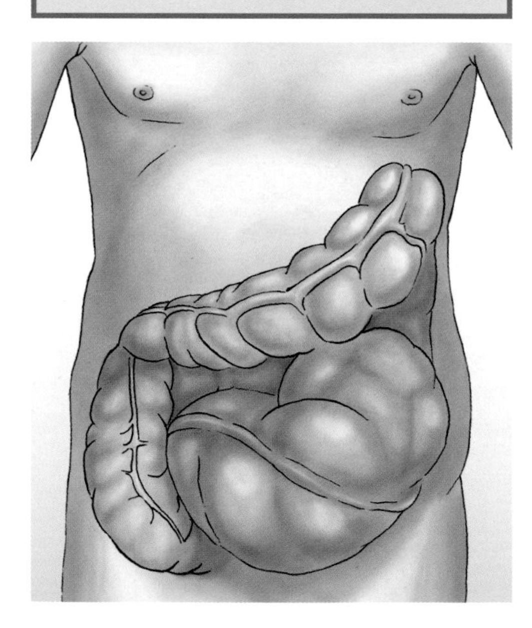

Intense and persistent constipation, especially in the first month of life, can be an indication of a serious problem, such as Hirschsprung's disease or congenital megacolon (dilation of the large intestine due to deficient nervous stimulation), or malfunctioning of the thyroid gland.

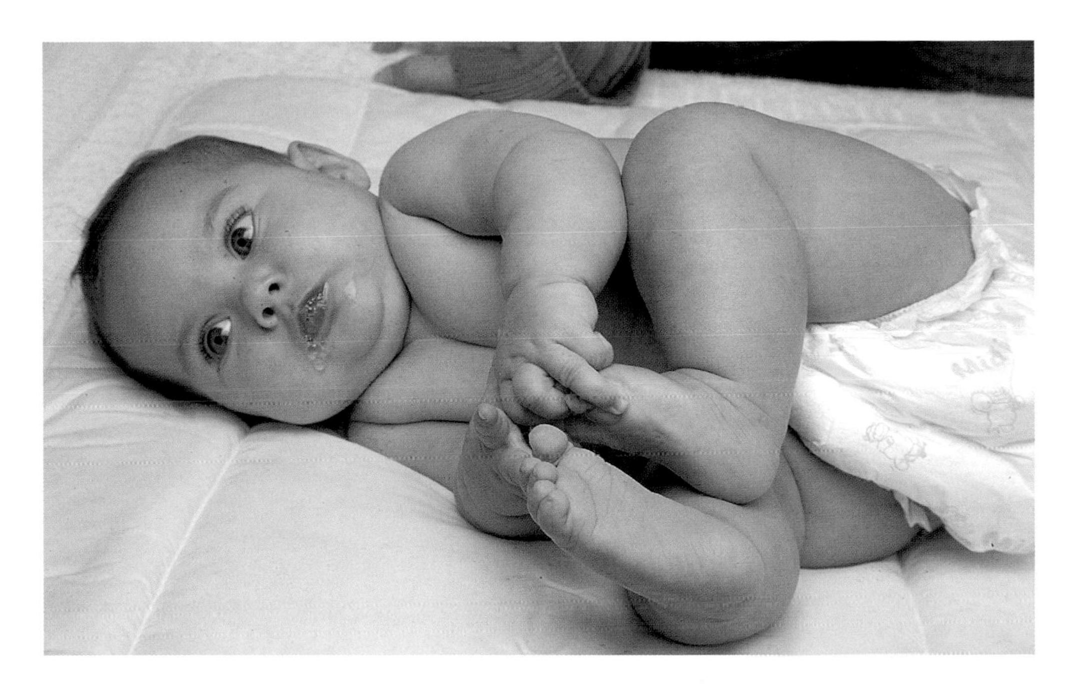

The anus of a baby aged less than 3 months can be narrow, and so defecation requires a real effort. A doctor can diagnose this problem by gently inserting a gloved finger into the anus. The discomfort is normally relieved by dilating the anus once or twice.

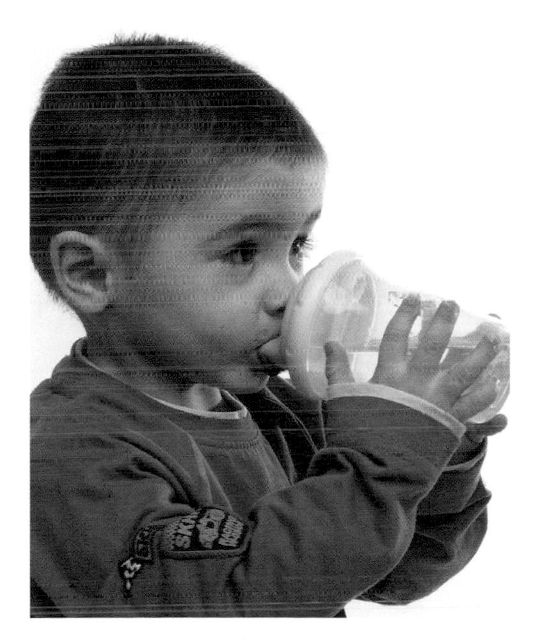

Educating or re-educating a child about intestinal habits involves devoting all the time necessary and, above all, not putting off any impulse to defecate.

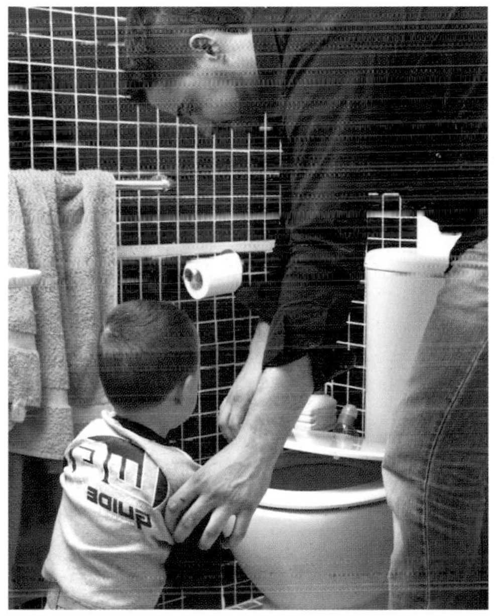

diarrhea

When the stool is abnormally frequent and liquid it is called diarrhea. As this is very common, its significance can be underestimated, but it can have serious consequences, such as dehydration, to which children are particularly vulnerable, especially in summer. The stools of a breast-fed baby are usually prolific and pasty, and this can make it difficult for parents to see whether their baby really is unwell, especially at the onset of diarrhea. It is important for parents to be aware of other symptoms associated with diarrhea in order to detect it in time, consult a doctor about the best solution, and avoid more serious complications.

Classification and causes of diarrhea

Classification of diarrhea according to its duration:

- Acute diarrhea. This is the most common type of diarrhea, lasting less than 2 weeks and can be of bacterial or viral origin. It can also be a reaction to medicines, especially antibiotics, which cause diarrhea by destroying the intestinal flora; in these cases, the flora will reform and the diarrhea will disappear once the treatment has been interrupted or completed.
- Chronic diarrhea. This lasts over 2 weeks. The basic causes in children are intolerance or poor absorption of certain nutrients (lactose, celiac sprue, etc.), or intestinal parasites (giardiasis).

Most frequent symptoms

- Stomach cramps
- Abdominal pain, similar to colic
- Feeling of heaviness in the stomach
- Nausea
- Strong urge to defecate
- Fever

Despite the relative simplicity and effectiveness of current treatments for diarrhea, it is a real problem that is responsible for the majority of infant hospital admissions in developed countries. Moreover, it is one of the main causes of infant mortality in developing countries.

In developed societies, this intestinal disorder is the result of poor hygiene or infection in play school or during a hospital stay.

In poorer countries, diarrhea can be related to lack of hygiene, cooking methods, shortage of drinking water, and an unbalanced diet.

The rotavirus is the most common cause of diarrhea of infectious origin, which, in its turn, is the main cause of diarrhea in childhood.

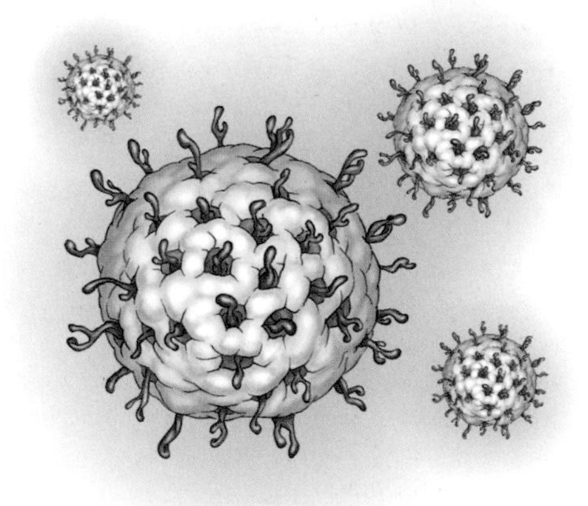

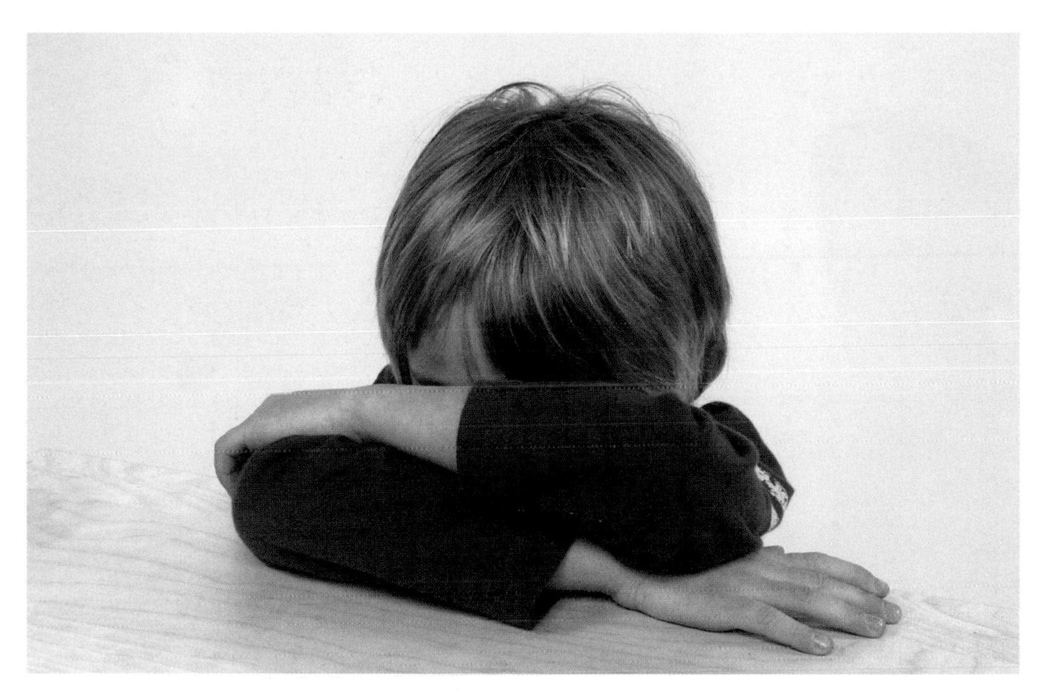

At the onset of diarrhea, a child is weak and listless, and also has difficulty in eating or drinking. If she is pale and has sunken eyes, along with blood in the stool, she must be treated immediately, as these are serious symptoms.

Infectious diarrhea

• Infections are the main cause of diarrhea in children. These can be caused by bacteria, parasites, or, most commonly, viruses. Over 70% of the micro-organisms that cause diarrhea have now been identified. The most common one, particularly in small children, is the human rotavirus, which is the cause of 50% of the cases of diarrhea that require hospital admission.

• The main cause of infection is the consumption of contaminated food or water. Micro-organisms manage to overcome the defensive barriers in the digestive tract and penetrate the intestine, where they can act in 2 ways:

Treatment

The aims of treatment are:

- To prevent dehydration, by restoring or maintaining the balance of water and salts in the intestine.
- To reverse any damage to the intestinal flora.
- To avoid any malnutrition and to maintain good health.

All types of diarrhea improve with the intake of liquids and salts: in most cases these can be taken orally, but, when this is not possible or in more serious cases, they can be administered intravenously.

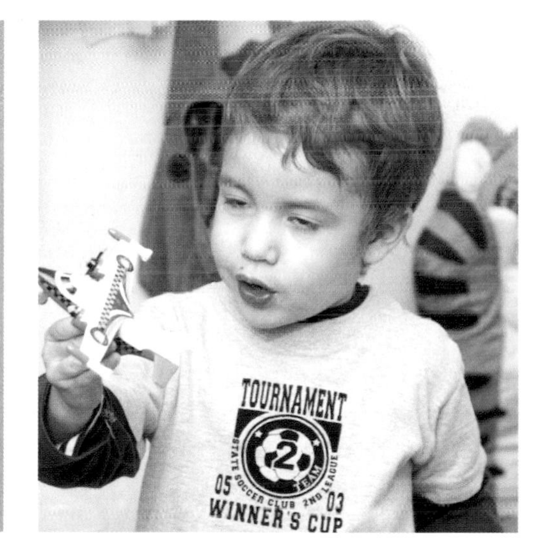

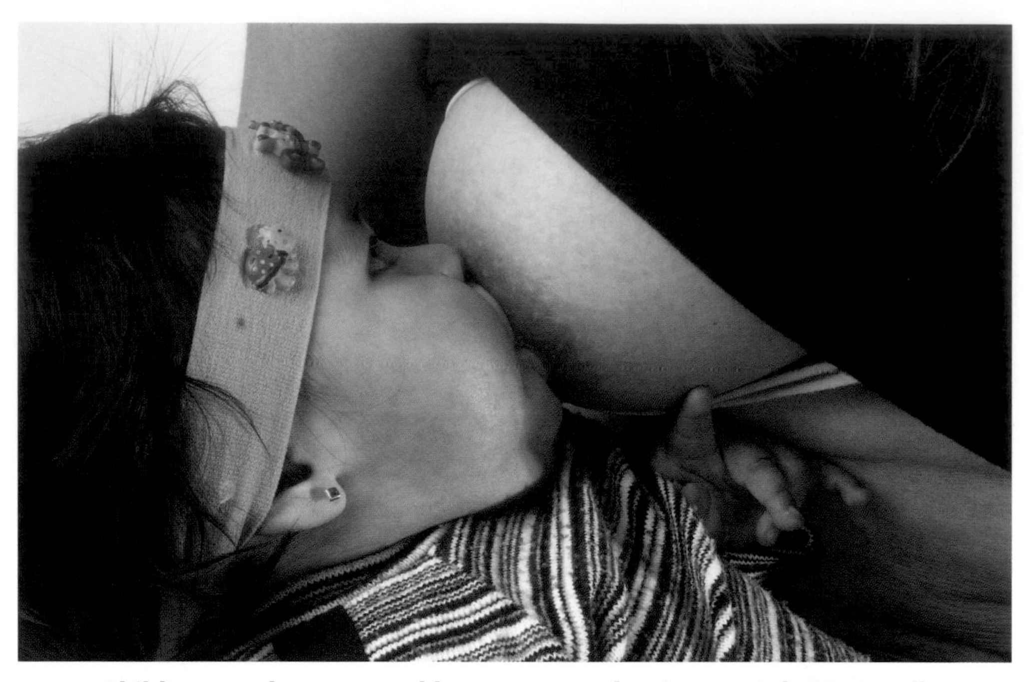

Children can be protected by measures that improve their overall diet and enhance their immunity against sickness–by being.

– By infecting and destroying cells, thereby producing inflammation. This phenomenon is known as invasive diarrhea.

– By producing toxins that stimulate the secretion of liquids and electrolytes (sodium, potassium, etc.) from the intestinal cells into the intestinal tract and blocking their reabsorption. This is known as secretory diarrhea.

• It is vital to give the child the appropriate oral solution as soon as possible. She should also be offered frequently, small amounts of liquid 1–2 tablespoons (15–30 ml), even if she throws it up. If the vomiting does not stop or if it grows worse, wait for around 15 minutes and then try to give her liquid once again. The quantity of liquid and the duration of the child's special diet will depend on the doctor's recommendation and will vary according to the seriousness of the diarrhea and the degree of dehydration.

A child with diarrhea usually loses her appetite and finds it difficult to eat at first. It is advisable to offer her small amounts of food, however, to encourage her to eat, as this will help the diarrhea to abate and speed her recovery. If her food intake is reduced or truncated, this can cause nutritional deficiency. A child who has suffered from diarrhea needs to eat an extra meal every day during the recovery period, for at least 2 weeks.

• If a child is suffering from severe dehydration or a significant deterioration in her general health, or if she cannot tolerate oral rehydration solutions, she will need to be admitted to hospital for intravenous rehydration.

• After an episode of acute diarrhea, it is advisable for a child to follow a balanced diet immediately to recover her nutritional equilibrium, and to try and eat basic foodstuffs.

• If your baby is being breast-fed, rehydration with liquids should be complemented by mother's milk, in an increased number of feeding sessions.

• If your baby is being fed on powdered milk, this should be withdrawn for a short period

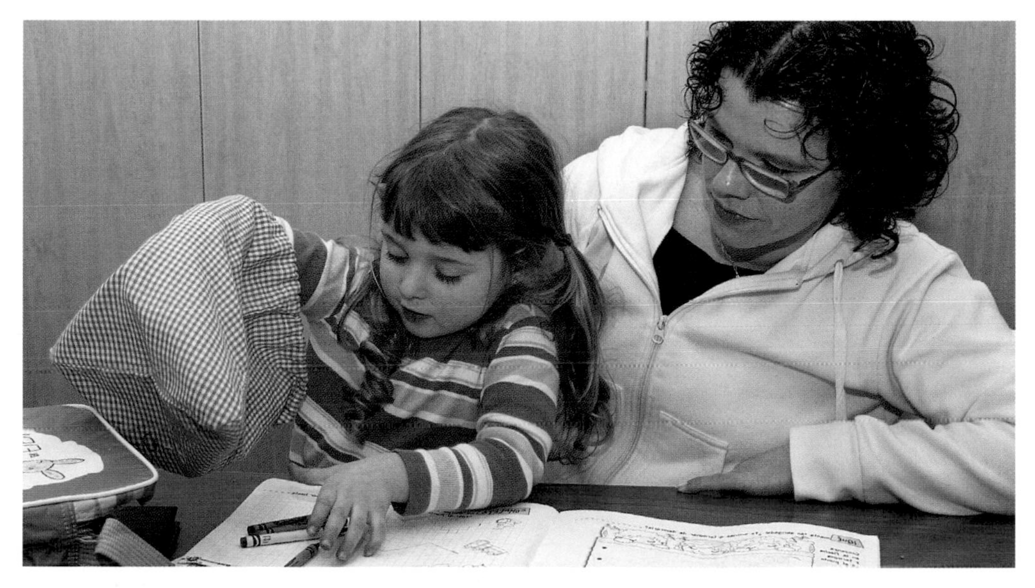

Hydration and a normal diet are the recommended measures for preventing dehydration in a child.

(usually 12–14 hours), during which time only the rehydration solution should be offered; after this, your baby can continue with the formula milk once again. Some studies, however, have concluded that

Symptoms indicating a serious problem

- Acute abdominal pain
- Blood in the stools
- Frequent vomiting
- High fever
- Dry, sticky mouth
- Weight loss
- Infrequent urination (less than 6 wet diapers per day)
- Frequent diarrhea
- Extreme thirst
- Lack of tears when crying
- No desire to eat or drink

Oral rehydration solutions are the most important advance in the treatment of diarrhea. These solutions contain the quantities of sugar and salts needed to restore the normal balance of the digestive tract. They are sold ready prepared, or in the form of sachets of dried salts that are mixed with cooled, pre-boiled water or mineral water. Some brands are even flavored, to make them more appetizing for children.

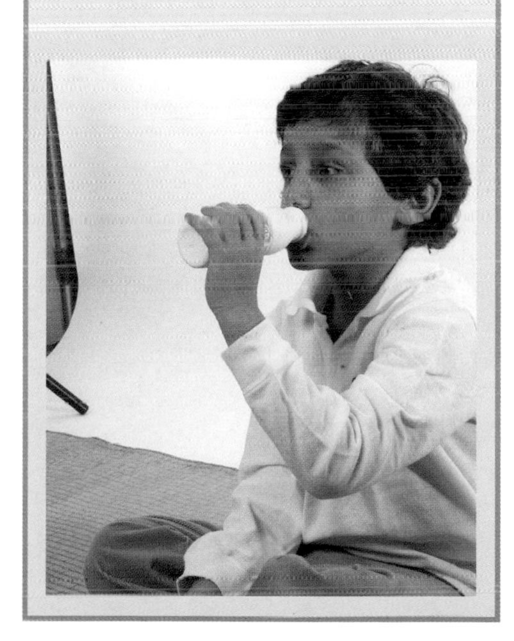

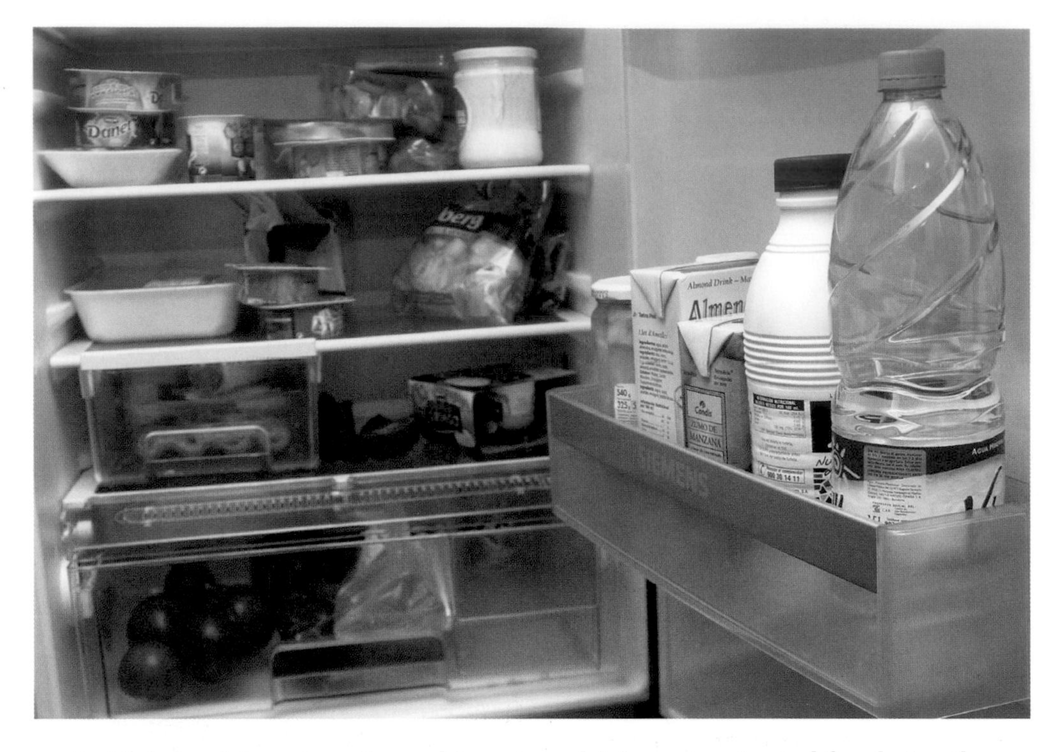

A child should not be allowed to eat or drink contaminated food. Another possible source of micro-organisms is stagnant water, rivers, or ponds. Children should avoid playing in such places, as it is very easy for them to swallow water in the process.

it is better to start feeding the baby again straight away, without giving her intestine time to rest. There is similar controversy about giving a baby formula milk during the episode of diarrhea itself; it has been argued that the milk's protein and sugar (lactose) content could act aggressively on the intestinal mucosa during a bout of diarrhea. Another subject of debate is the use of formula milk with no lactose, or with proteins of vegetable origin. It is generally agreed that they should be given only in proven cases of intolerance or in protracted episodes of diarrhea.

• The reintroduction of the food that your child used to eat before having diarrhea should be a gradual process, starting on the second day. Babies can be given rice flour or an astringent fruit puree (banana, apple), while an older child's solid diet would include pureed rice and carrots, boiled white meat or white fish, and natural yoghurt. Other foodstuffs can be introduced little by little, while avoiding any that might have a laxative effect for a few days, at least. An inadequate diet in the early stages of a bout of diarrhea will certainly increase the probability of it being prolonged.

• Medicines are rarely required, as both anti-diarrhea drugs and antibiotics are only prescribed in very specific cases. Antibiotics are prescribed only for very small children at risk of a possible generalization of the infection, in children with an immune deficiency, or in cases of persistent infection, after identification of the micro-organism responsible and the specific antibiotic that can elimi-

It is important to begin appropriate treatment for diarrhea from the very first symptoms. Effective vaccines are becoming available to treat some of the main micro-organisms responsible for diarrhea, such as the rotavirus.

nate the infection. This course of action alleviates the symptoms and reduces the possibility of passing on the infection to other children.

- No medicines are currently available to combat diarrhea of viral origin. The classic anti-diarrhea medicines are usually ineffective, expensive, and even counterproductive, especially in children.

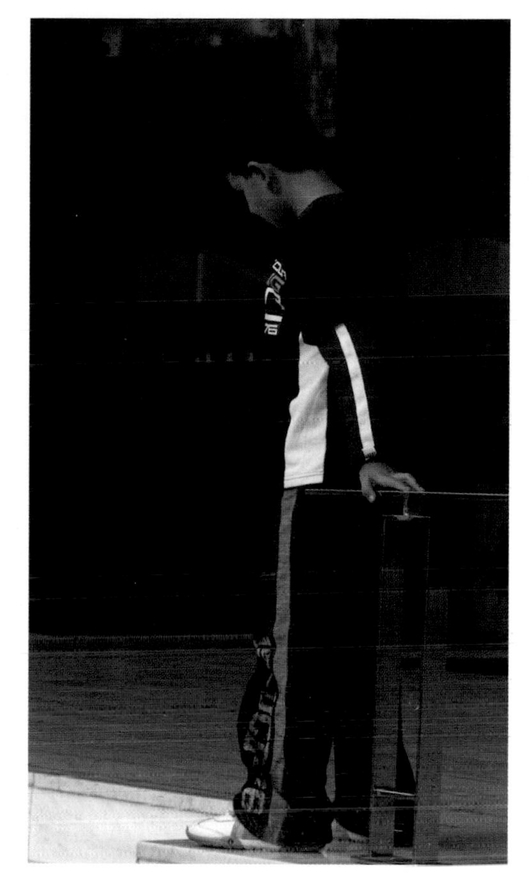

In mild cases of dehydration a child becomes irritable, with sunken eyes, a dry mouth and tongue, extreme thirst, weight loss, and dry skin. Children with severe dehydration are very listless, with dry, sunken eyes; they are incapable of drinking and have lost over 10% of their body weight.

FOODSTUFFS AND MEDICINES THAT CAN CAUSE DIARRHEA	
Food and medicine	**Ingredient that causes the diarrhea**
Apple juice, pear juice, sugar-free chewing gum, mint.	Hexitols, sorbitol, manitol
Apple juice, pear juice, grapes, honey, dates, walnuts, figs, soda pops (especially with a fruit flavor).	Fructose
Sugar.	Sucrose
Milk, ice cream, yoghurt, soft cheese, chocolate.	Lactose
Antacids containing magnesium.	Magnesium
Coffee, tea, cola drinks, over-the-counter analgesics for headaches.	Caffeine

food allergies

There has been a notable increase in the number of cases of food allergies in recent years, caused not only by genetic factors but also by environmental and nutritional agents. The introduction of new elements into the diet at an increasingly early age has much to do with this. Another reason is the growing tendency to stop breast-feeding sooner in favor of a feeding bottle and cereals, which have a great capacity for creating allergies. Infant food allergies mainly appear during the first 2 years of life: milk, eggs, and fish are responsible for 90 percent of the cases in children under a year old, while eggs are the main culprit in children between 1 and 2 years of age.

Act from the start

• Prevention of food allergy needs to start in infancy, shortly after birth. According to the World Health Organization (WHO), breast-feeding increases immunity – especially in newborn babies

The World Health Organization (WHO) considers breast-feeding to be a preventive mechanism against food allergy.

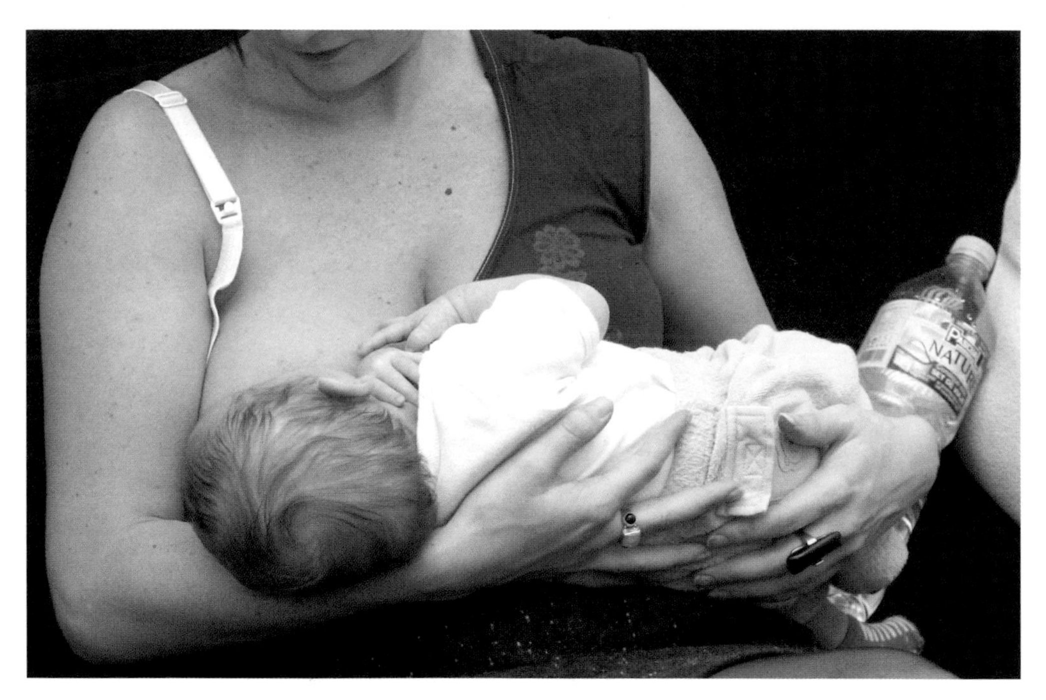

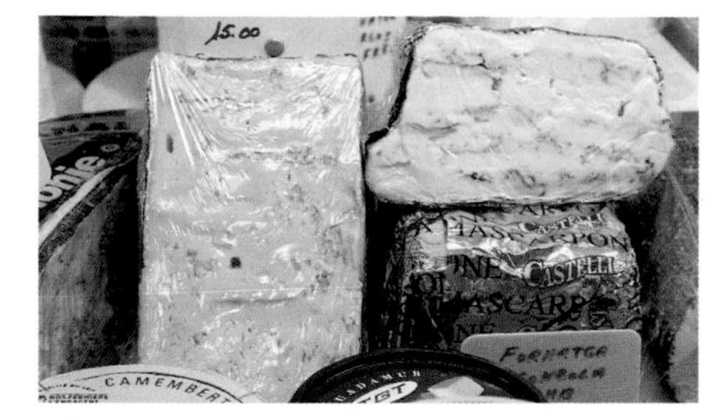

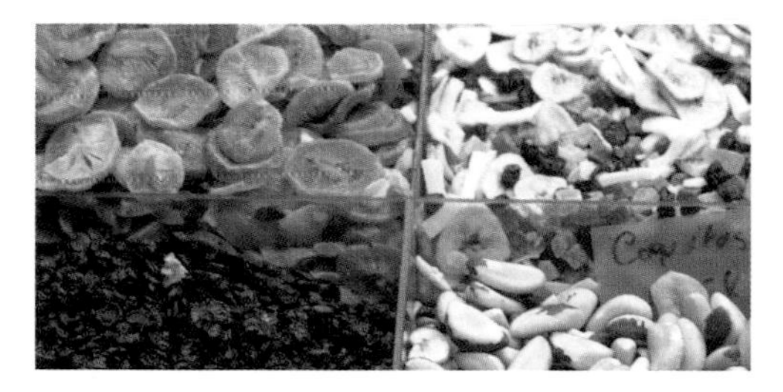

weighing under 5½ lb (2.5 kg) – as does the delayed introduction of eggs, fish, and dried fruit into the child's diet, along with a zinc supplement of 1mg/kg of body weight per day for 6 months.

• The prognosis for children with food allergies is usually hopeful. Children allergic to milk or eggs usually end up tolerating them once they reach the age of 2 or 3. From the age of 2, however, the list of potentially allergic foods gets longer; the most common are fish, pulses, nuts, fruit (dried and fresh), and seafood.

Food allergens

Around 170 foodstuffs have been reported as being responsible for allergic reactions. It is obviously impossible to detect them all and, for practical reasons, monitoring is concentrated on the most common and serious allergens, the so-called big eight: cow's milk, eggs, peanuts, dried fruits, fish, seafood, soya, and wheat. This group is responsible for 90 percent of food allergies. Other items that often cause allergies are pulses, fruit, and seeds (sunflower, sesame), not forgetting additives and preservatives.

Allergies are a result of the immune system's erroneous identification of a food item as harmful. Once the immune system has decided that a particular foodstuff is harmful, it generates specific antibodies (see box on the following page: sensitization phase). The next time the item in question is eaten, the immune system responds by releasing massive amounts of chemical substances (see box), including

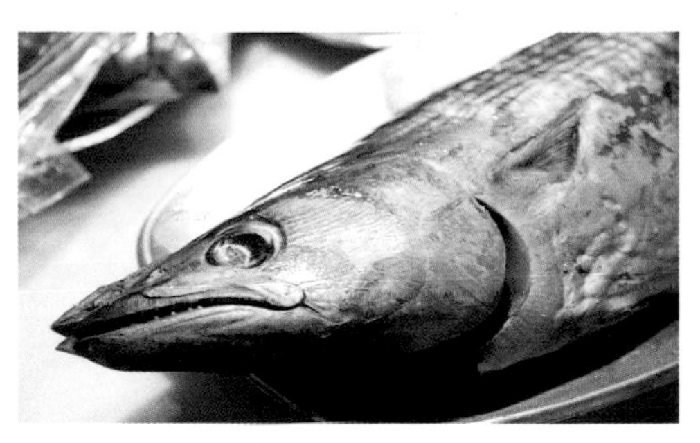

histamine, to protect the body. These substances give rise to a series of allergic symptoms that may affect the respiratory system, the gastro-intestinal tract, the skin, or the cardiovascular system.

A true allergic reaction to food has 3 main components:

• The allergen, i.e. a substance (almost invariably a protein) within the foodstuff that triggers the allergic reaction.

• The immunoglobulin (IgE in this type of allergy), which is the molecule in the immune system that reacts to the allergen.

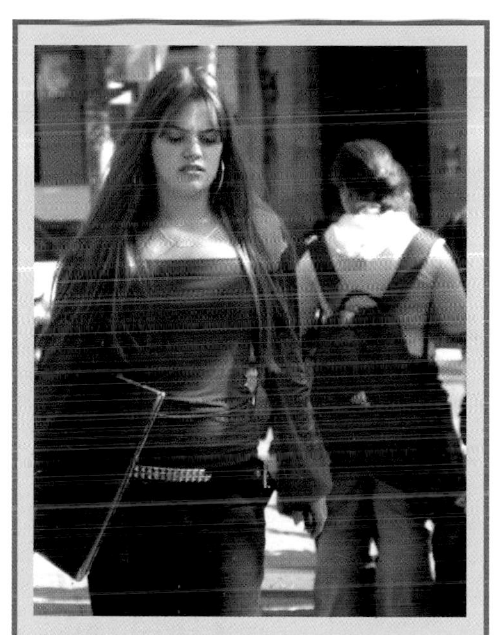

It has been estimated that 8% of children and 3% of adults suffer from a food allergy. In Spain alone, around 600,000 people suffer from this problem. At the moment, there is no curative treatment for this type of allergy: the only way to prevent an allergic reaction is to avoid the allergen.

> It is worth remembering that allergy is not the same as food intolerance. Food intolerance does not affect the immune system, although some of the symptoms can be identical to those of a food allergy.

• Mastocytes (tissue cells) and basophylls (blood cells) that, on coming into contact with IgE antibodies, release histamine and other chemical substances that cause allergic symptoms.

Many allergic reactions to food are mild. A small percentage of people, however, undergo a serious reaction, known as anaphylaxis. This is potentially dangerous, as various parts of the body experience allergic reactions simultaneously, and this can cause urticaria, obstruction in the throat, and breathing difficulty.

The treatment of food allergy requires the elimination of the item responsible from the diet. No effective preventive medicines or desensitizing treatment are available (in contrast to other types of allergy). Hypoallergenic diets offer good results, but they are very strict and cannot be maintained for much time (although some less demanding diets can be followed for several months).

Most common symptoms of food allergy

Although they can vary greatly from one child to another, some of the most frequent manifestations are:

- Vomiting.
- Diarrhea.
- Cramp.
- Rash.
- Inflammation.
- Eczema.
- Itching or swelling of the lips, tongue, or mouth.
- Breathing difficulties.
- Wheezing.
- Low blood pressure.

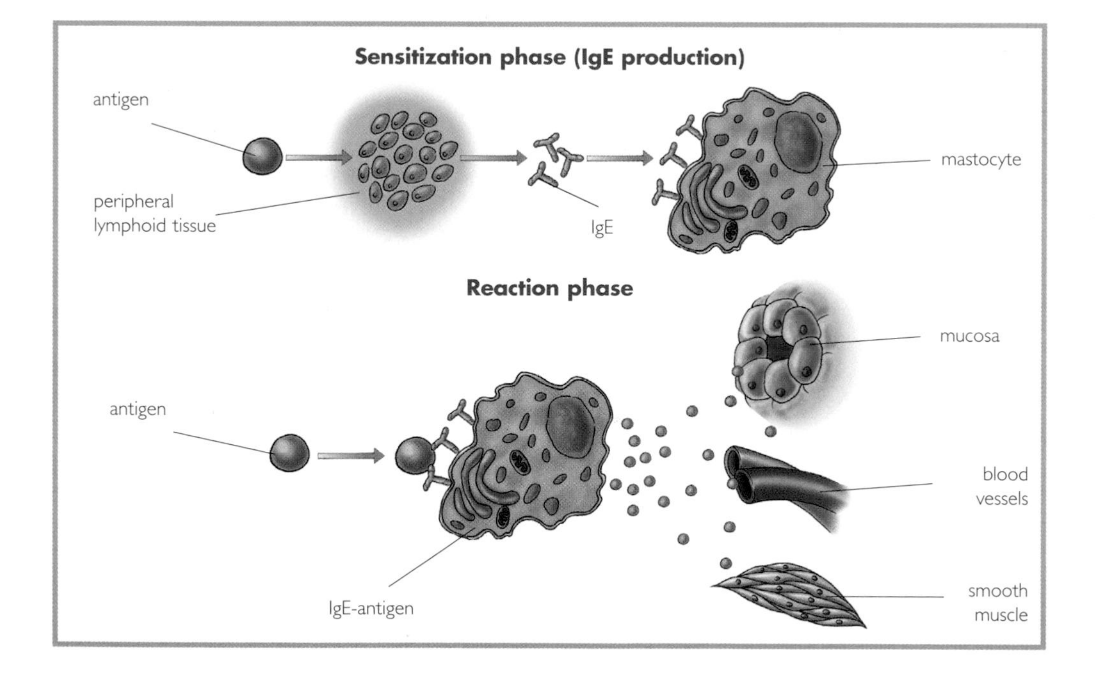

the child who refuses to eat

Lack of appetite or the systematic rejection of food is a common problem in young children – and one that often leads parents to consult a doctor. In most cases, the root of the problem is not of a medical nature, but rather a behavioral issue: the child tries to control the situation at mealtimes (as she does in other aspects of everyday life) by being bossy. This attitude is often the result of over-protectiveness on the part of her parents, or her family's own approach to eating.

Reasons for rejecting food

Satiation

Although it is generally a child's parents who decide how much food their child requires, she knows her own needs better than anybody else.

• Although children need more energy than adults – in proportion to their body weight – they eat less.

• Being fat is not a sign of good health. There are plenty of thin children with a small appetite who are fit and strong.

• A child who tends to be sedentary will have less appetite and energy requirements than one who is physically active.

• A child's stomach is much smaller than that of an adult and therefore needs less food to fill it.

• Some children lose their appetite because they are overfed.

Lack of interest

• A change in mealtime schedule, or in the place where a child normally eats, can alter her habits and cause her to lose interest in food.

• A child's faddish reaction to certain foodstuffs can be a response to her parents' attitude. Some parents, fearful that their child is not eating properly, react to her rejection of one dish by preparing another. This merely encourages her to complain even more often, in the hope of obtaining only what she wants to eat.

Psychological disorders

• Many families expect their children to eat large amounts of food to make them fat to show that they are good parents with healthy children. In these cases, a range of techniques is normally used to make the child eat: pleading and threats, games,

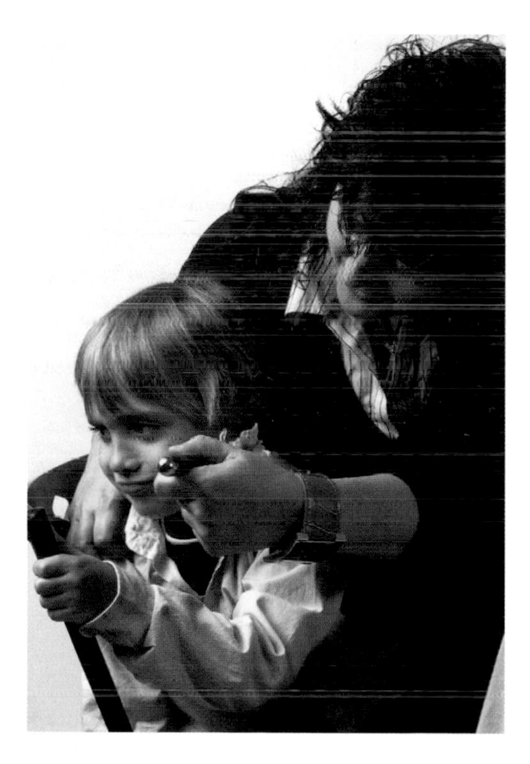

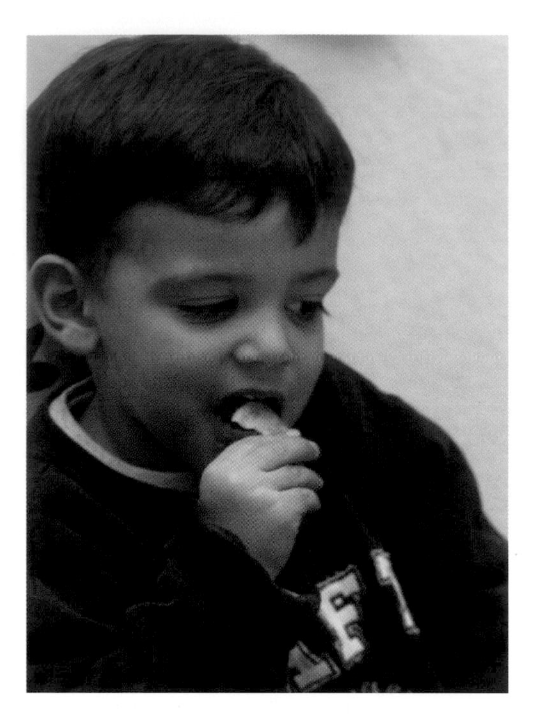

It is sometimes a child's parents who cause her to be disobedient and react negatively. In the face of excitable behavior, some parents will use any strategy, including bribery, to quell a tantrum, thereby only encouraging their child's unruly behavior. The message that a child unconsciously receives from this approach is that, if she goes on this way, she will obtain everything she wants, particularly the attention of her parents. A child can end up dominating the situation, and even her own parents, with her negative attitude.

Food eaten between meals (candies, pastries, sandwiches, etc.) provides calories and a feeling of satiation, and this often leads to a child having no appetite at meal times.

A child's refusal to eat is often caused by permissiveness and lack of control – or stress and impositions – at the meal table, as well as an inability to negotiate with the child.

distractions, bribes, force, or even violence – all of which will only make her more rebellious and more reluctant to eat.

• At times, loss of appetite is related to the memory of a disagreeable experience during a meal. Children are sometimes obliged to eat in situations where they have no appetite – sickness, a dish that disagrees with them, or simply lack of hunger – and recalling this incident causes them to reject food.

• Lack of appetite can also be a symptom of sadness, anxiety, or depression. It is important to speak to a child and find out what is worrying her.

Symptom of disease

Loss of appetite is one of the unspecific symptoms that can accompany any sickness, however minor. Infections, which are often frequent and repetitive in children under 6 years, can lead to rejection of food. This is, however, the least common reason for loss of appetite in children.

Children should not be given drugs or stimulants to increase their appetite. They will eat more than they need after taking these supplements and, furthermore, parents run the risk of having to give them for very long periods.

Most children are more interested in playing and exploring than eating. They consider meals a waste of time.

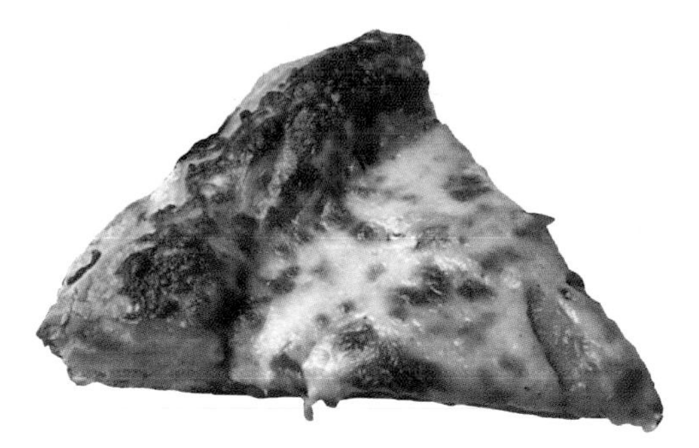

Helping a child eat properly

The first requirement is a different approach to meals on both sides. A child and her parents should see mealtimes as occasions to share and an opportunity for everybody to talk about how their day has gone, so that eating together becomes a relaxing and enjoyable experience.

- Do not respond to remarks your child may make about her food with pressure, arguments, or shouting. Meal time should be harmonious, with little intervention, and care should be taken to praise a child when she eats properly. Encourage dialogue and learn how to negotiate with your child, otherwise she will always get her own way.
- It is not up to a child to regulate her own diet. Children do not all eat in the same way; some need larger quantities than others. Do not place too great an emphasis on what is left over on a child's plate, but make sure she has eaten at least some of all the elements of a meal.
- It is better to serve small portions and then, if she wants more, give her further helpings.
- Avoid comparisons with siblings or other children.

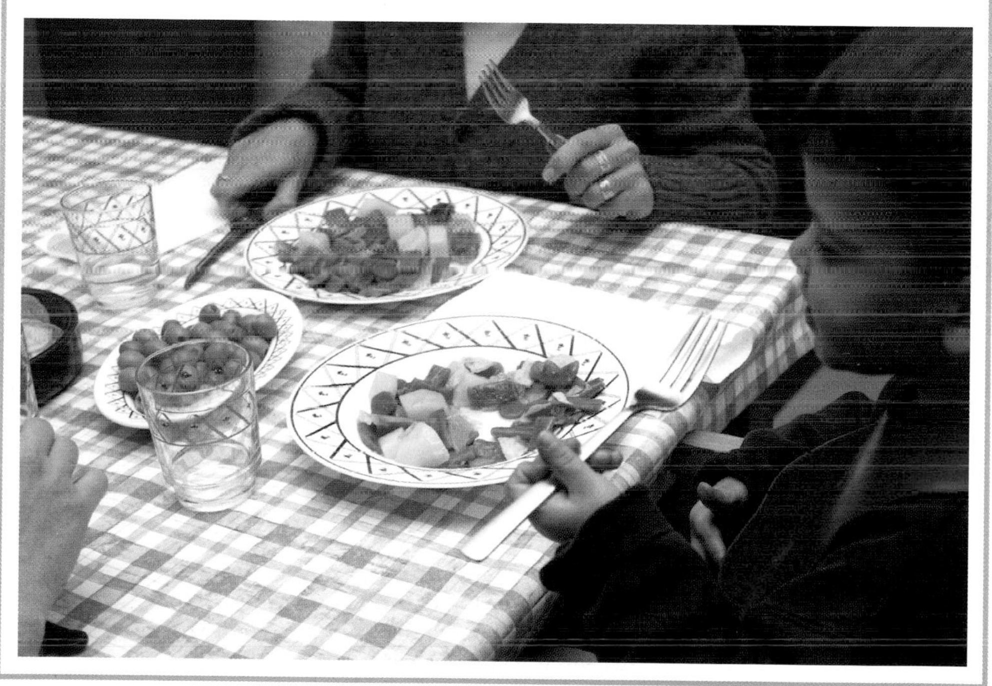

obesity

Obesity is generally defined as an excessive accumulation of fat or adipose tissue in the body, resulting in a surplus of over 20 percent, compared to the weight considered ideal for a particular stature and age. The last 20 years have seen an alarming increase in the number of obese children, to such an extent that it is now possible to talk of a worldwide epidemic. Obesity involves not only excess weight but also a series of physical and physiological disorders, making it a serious problem. The prevention and early treatment of obesity is therefore of utmost importance.

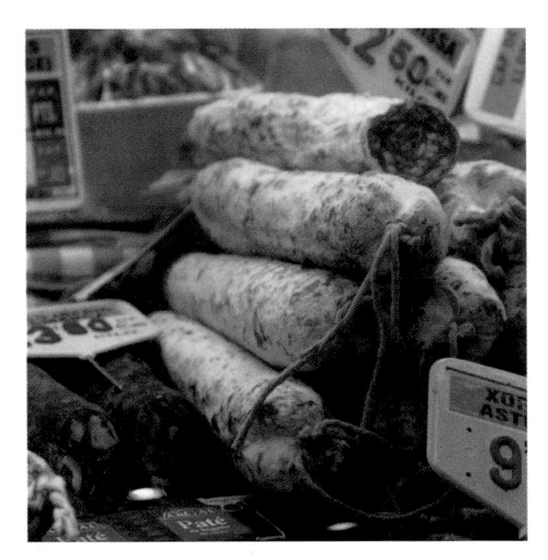

Some causes of obesity

• **Genes.** Obesity is often found in various members of the same family.

• **Environment.** Lifestyle (diet and exercise) has a considerable effect on the incidence of obesity.

Obesity is becoming increasingly common in our world, especially in industrialized countries, and above all the United States, where it is estimated that 34% of adults and 22% of children are obese. Obesity can be seen as a modern epidemic, a by-product of the excessive consumption of food with a high calorie content in developed societies.

• **Cushing's syndrome.** This is a change in the suprarenal gland that triggers an increased production of cortisol, which leads to obesity.

• **Hypothyroidism.** Reduced levels in the thyroid hormone can cause obesity. This pathology must always be ruled out, even though it is uncommon.

• **Insulinoma.** This is a tumor in the pancreas that triggers obesity; it is very rare, however.

• **Hypothalamic alterations.** Some tumors, swellings, and lesions in the central nervous system can cause changes to the nerve centers that regulate hunger, resulting in obesity.

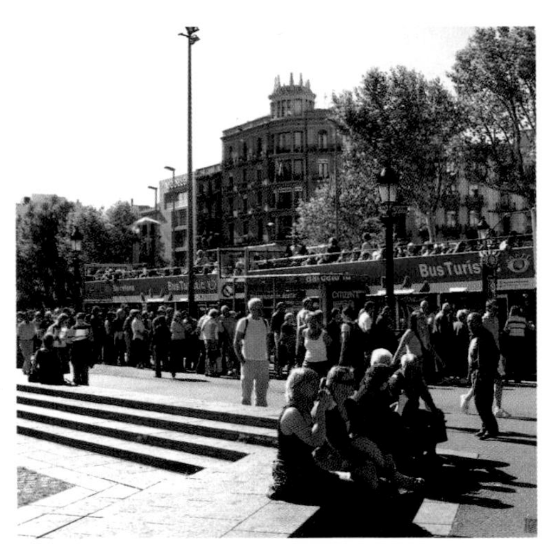

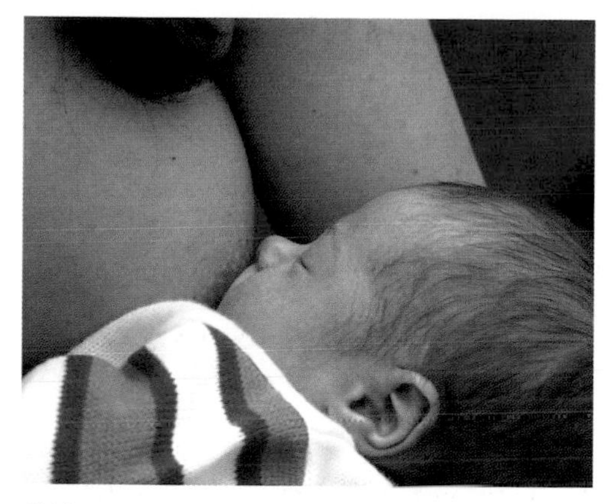

Children who become obese between the ages of 6 months and 7 years have a 40% probability of still being obese in adult life; this figure rises to 70%, however, in children who start to suffer from this problem between the ages of 10 and 13, as the cells that store fat (adipocytes) multiply in this period.

• **Polcystic ovary syndrome.** This is the most common cause of obesity in young women. It is associated with menstrual irregularities, acne, excessive body hair, and pancreatic disorders.

• **Hypogonadism.** A drop in the levels of testosterone in men enlarges the adipose tissues and leads to obesity.

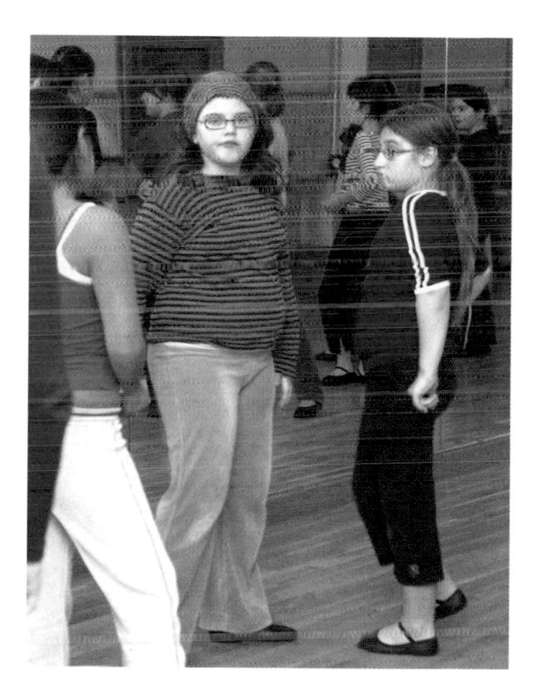

Consequences of infant obesity

The most important consequences involve the obese child's psyche and the increased risk of falling sick in adulthood.

• Psychological consequences:

- Low self-esteem.
- Poor results at school.
- A change in self-perception, particularly in adolescence.
- Introversion, often followed by social rejection.

• Risk of falling sick:

A greater number of conditions can appear at an earlier age than normal in obese children. These include:

- High blood pressure.
- High cholesterol levels.
- Diabetes.
- Heart disease.
- Respiratory disorders.
- Skin complaints.
- Sleep disorders (sleep apnea).
- Joint and bone problems.

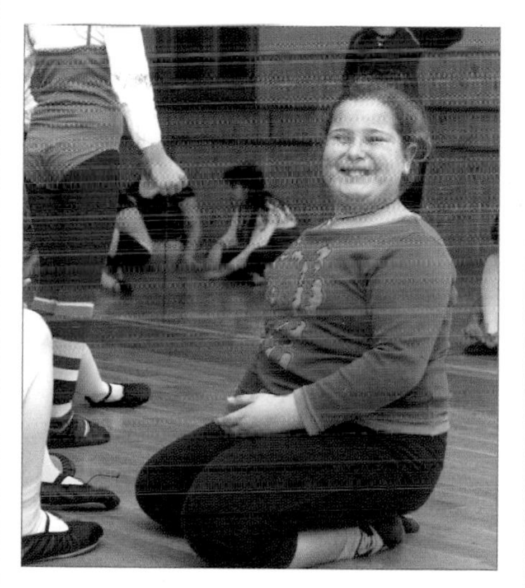

The greatest risk associated with infant obesity is an increased tendency to develop health problems in later life. The younger an obese child, the more likely she is to develop health problems at a younger age than normal.

Obese children can display a tendency, in both infancy and adolescence, toward introspection, as well as experiencing rejection from their peers. The low self-esteem that can sometimes contribute to obesity is made worse by mockery and social rejection.

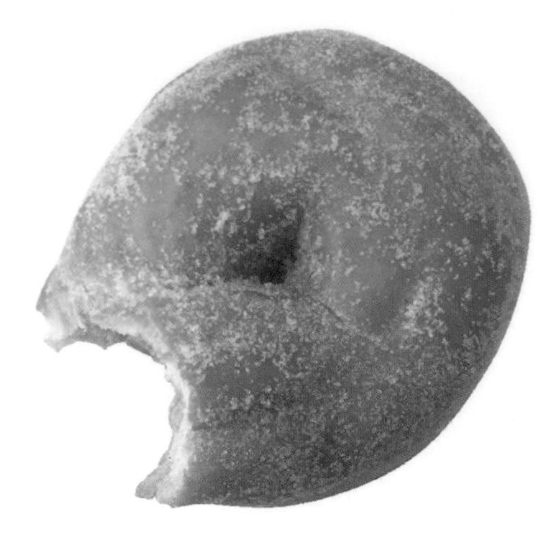

Treatment of childhood obesity

• The basic elements of therapy for obese children are diet and exercise, as these are both essential for good results.

• In growing children, the aim of weight control is often to maintain the status quo, i.e., to keep the weight constant while a child grows in stature.

• When monitoring a child's calorie intake, it is advisable to consult a nutritionist, who will tell you how to calculate the size of food portions and decide on the appropriate options for menus and diets. Remember that an obese child is not an adult and is growing fast. The consumption of certain foods should be restricted, but it is very important that she follows a balanced and varied diet.

• Exercise should consist of 30 minutes of aerobic activity every day (playing sport, running, walking energetically, swimming, or cycling).

• Behavior therapies are also useful in the treatment of obesity. The best technique is to encourage the child to monitor herself by keeping a record of the exercise she does and the food she eats.

• Changes in lifestyle are also important: sitting down to eat at a table, instead of in front of the television; meals served according to a regular schedule, so that the child grows accustomed to her eating times and cuts down on snacks; and enhancement of self-esteem by encouraging the child to take a positive approach to weight control.

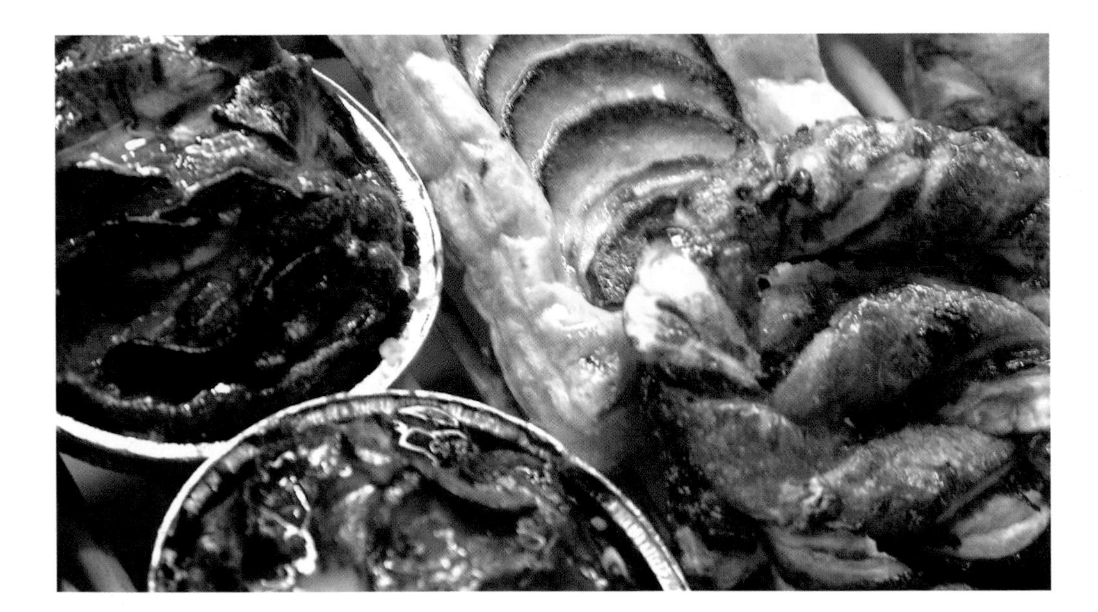

anorexia and bulimia

As in the case of obesity, in the last few decades, eating disorders, particularly anorexia and bulimia, have taken on epidemic proportions in developed countries. The root of this phenomenon is the increasingly evident cult of the body; this gives rise to a variety of emotional conflicts and psychological problems that manifest themselves through eating disorders. They are associated with an obsession with the appearance of the body and a refusal to believe the reality reflected in the mirror; eating disorders are starting to acquire alarming characteristics, especially among adolescent girls _ of whom, at least one in every thousand suffers from an eating disorder.

Anorexia is a mental disorder that creates a distorted image of the body. It is a syndrome characterized by a drastic reduction in food intake motivated by an obsessive fear of becoming fat. There are 2 types of anorexia:

- Restrictive. Weight is lost quickly, due to a self-imposed diet.
- Bulimic. Periods of restricted diet alternate with episodes of overeating followed by vomiting, the use of laxatives and/or diuretics, or intense physical exercise, all intended to keep the body thin.

Clinical manifestations of anorexia

- Precise starting point. The start of anorexia can be identified as the moment at which the adolescent decides to slim. Sometimes the resolution to lose weight can follow a significant event that acts as a trigger: the loss of a loved one, academic failure, or a family conflict.
- Uncontrollable desire to be thin.
- Mealtime rituals. Apart from cutting down on food, anorexics might play endlessly with food or cut it into tiny pieces. They may also store food in their mouth and later spit it out in secret; most avoid eating with their family or in public.
- Exaggerated interest in food. Although a typical anorexic eats less and opts for low-calorie dishes, she is thinking about food all day long, collecting recipes and cooking for others, even though she herself contents herself with watching the results.
- Amenorrhea. All women who suffer from anorexia stop menstruating, and in 25% of cases this change precedes any weight loss. Men experience a loss of interest in sex.
- Increased physical activity. As the weight goes down, so the physical activity becomes more intense. Anorexic patients do not keep still; they may walk around ceaselessly, for example, or do countless sit-ups.

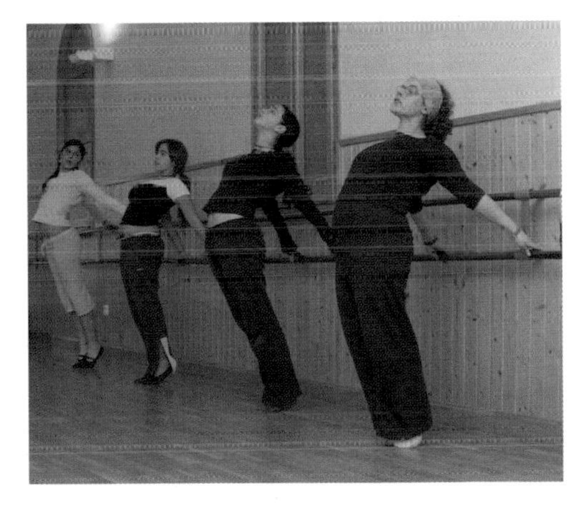

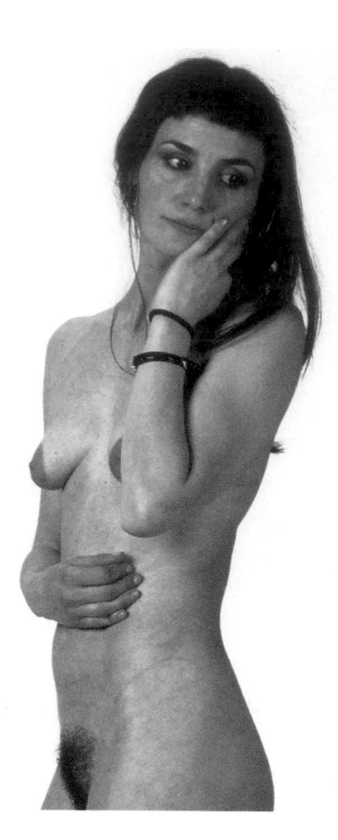

An increasing number of people are experiencing the desire to "have a different body." According to specialists, wishing for a perfect, or near-perfect body does not necessarily indicate mental illness, although it does increase the chances of it occurring. This type of obsession can turn into a nightmare in adolescence, as the combination of a still unformed personality and a society constantly displaying models of perfection and beauty makes adolescents feel obliged to have a slim figure, even at the cost of their health.

Clinical manifestations of bulimia.

- Recurring blow-outs, associated with a loss of control over food intake. These usually occur after personal efforts or external pressure to lose weight.
- Low self-esteem or depression.
- Appearance of compensatory behavior, such as vomiting, abuse of laxatives or diuretics, and/or exaggerated exercise.
- At first, the blow-outs and vomiting episodes are sporadic, but over time they increase in frequency and occur every day, or even several times a day.
- Blow-outs usually take place after a period of dieting.

- Vomiting and use of laxatives. Some anorexic patients make themselves vomit and take laxatives and/or diuretics.
- Academic results. Anorexic patients generally have average or above-average results at school and are considered to be highly motivated students.
- Contact with peers. Anorexics usually distance themselves from their companions. This enables them to avoid any confrontation over food and weight; it can also be a manifestation of low self-esteem.
- Apathy. Progressive weight loss is normally complemented by apathy about the ever-deteriorating state of the body.
- Food as a battlefield. Persistent weight loss turns food into a pressing issue in family conversations and discussions. This situation becomes increasingly difficult, as the anorexic's parents become frustrated and worried about their child's physical state, while she herself becomes more and more intransigent at mealtimes.

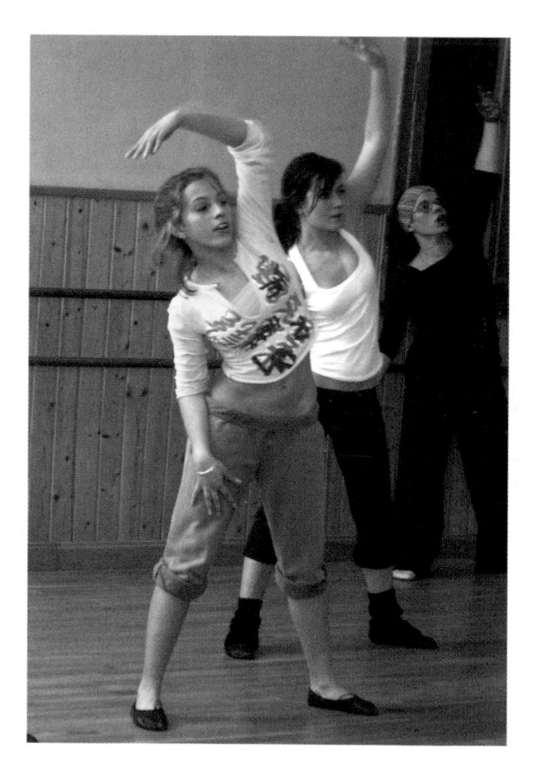

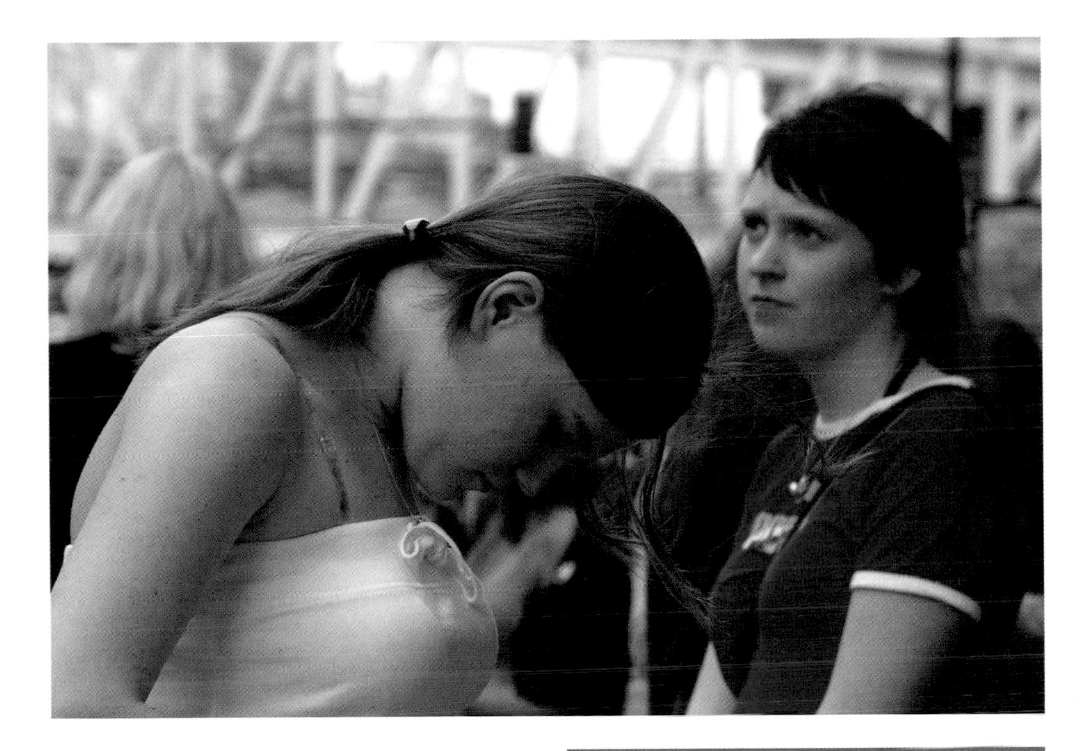

Blow-outs are generally followed by purgative measures, such as self-induced vomiting or the use of laxatives or diuretics.

Statistical data

- The incidence of cases of anorexia in adolescents and young women has been estimated as being between 0.5 and 3%. These figures are doubled if we take into account "healthy" adolescents with abnormal eating behavior or exaggerated concern about their weight.
- Models, ballerinas, athletes, and gymnasts are particularly susceptible to eating disorders.
- In the last few decades, a significant increase has been detected in the number of new cases of anorexia in the adolescent population.
- Eating disorders are most frequent in industrialized Western societies and in middle and upper socioeconomic classes, although they can be found in all strata of society.
- Women are most affected by eating disorders, although there has also been a notable increase in cases among men in recent years.
- The incidence of cases of bulimia in adolescents and young women is 1–3%. It generally appears in late adolescence or at the start of adulthood. Ninety percent of those affected are women. It is most common in developed countries with high socioeconomic levels.

medical checkups and vaccination schedule

Apart from consultations when a child is ill, periodic visits to the doctor are intended to detect and treat any possible health problems at an early stage, ensure that growth and development are normal, establish an appropriate vaccination schedule, and advise parents about issues such as diet and the prevention of accidents and sickness. The frequency of these checkups varies according to the age of the child and they are usually more spaced out after the first year.

Consultation as the basis of prevention

It is advisable for parents to be well informed about the main phases of growth and maturing. They also need appropriate advice about the attention a child requires at each stage, but not all the information they hear will necessarily be valid. Even if it were, and despite the relevance of certain general guidelines, remember that every child is a special case, with her own particular characteristics and needs, which cannot be applied to others.

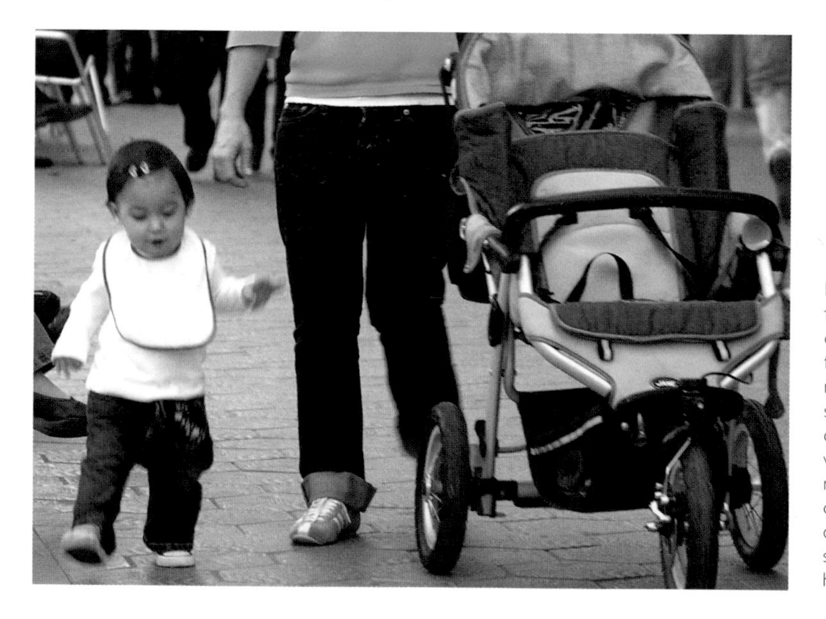

Preventive medicine is of the utmost importance during infancy: it is good for a child's health and reduces the risk of disease in later life. Routine checkups provide parents with advice and information about the development of their child, her vaccination schedule, and general healthcare measures.

SCHEDULE FOR PERIODIC MEDICAL CHECKUPS
Two weeks after birth
1 month
2 months
3 months
4 months
5 months
6 months
9 months
1 year
18 months
2 years
2 1/2 years
3 years
Thereafter, every year throughout childhood

ABBREVIATED SCHEDULE
Two weeks after birth
6 weeks
3 months
6 months
9 months
1 year
18 months
2 years
2 1/2 years
3 years
Thereafter, every year throughout childhood

Generic tables for children's growth can serve as guidelines, but it is important for a doctor to place each child within her own specificity. A child's own growth pattern indicates her normal path of development and will call attention to any major or abrupt changes that may be a sign of a disorder or an inadequate diet.

In the first years of a child's life, the doctor is responsible for supervising her healthcare, by following her development step by step and becoming acquainted with both her medical history and that of her family. Doctors provide parents with support and advice, and parents need to feel comfortable about confiding their doubts and anxieties to them, and able to follow any recommendations about the treatment and prevention of any disorders that may affect the child.

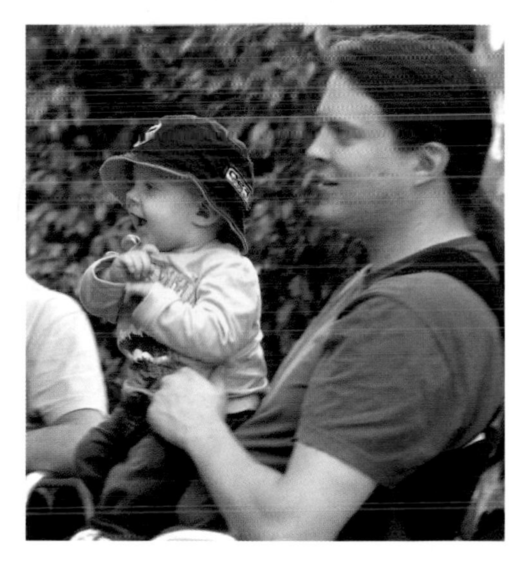

Recording weight and height

These are some of the most important registers involved in the monitoring of healthy children. On the basis of a child's weight and height, and their evolution over time, the doctor can trace her growth curve and compare it with the general parameters for children, in order to ascertain whether she is growing normally.

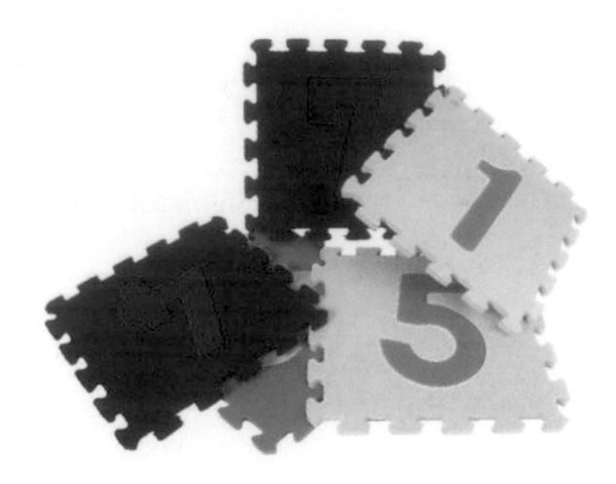

A child's most effective monitors are her parents. Even a doctor's knowledge of her health problems is largely based on information provided by her parents. This information should be as clear and as complete as possible, so there needs to be a relationship of trust and communicativeness between doctor and family. Parents' observations and opinions can be just as revealing as any physical examination.

TABLE FOR GROWTH IN BOYS

Age	Weight (lb/kg)			Height (in/cm)		
	low (3)	medium (50)	High (97)	low (3)	medium (50)	high (97)
36 weeks	4.17/1.89	2.95	3.82	17.32/44.00	18.66/47.40	20/50.80
37 weeks	4.89/2.22	6.86/3.11	8.80/3.99	17.83/45.30	19.13/48.60	20.43/51.90
38 weeks	5.14/2.33	7.12/3.23	9.11/4.13	18.14/46.10	19.60/49.80	20.94/53.20
39 weeks	5.3_ .41	7.34/3.33	9.39/4.26	18.50/47.00	19.80/50.30	21.06/53.50
40 weeks	6.06/2.75	7.74/3.51	9.88/4.48	18.32/46.54	19.74/50.16	21.17/53.78
1 month	7.94/3.60	9.70/4.40	12.57/5.70	19.76/50.20	21.25/54.00	22.60/57.60
2 months	9.68/4.39	11.86/5.38	14.66/6.65	20.96/53.25	22.47/57.09	23.98/60.92
3 months	11.24/5.10	13.67/6.20	16.98/7.70	22.20/56.40	23.77/60.40	25.35/64.40
4 months	12.35/5.60	15.17/6.88	18.63/8.45	23.01/58.45	24.50/62.25	26.16/66.45
5 months	13.45/6.10	16.76/7.60	20.28/9.20	23.85/60.60	25.59/65.00	27.12/68.90
6 months	14.44/6.55	17.61/7.99	21.47/9.74	24.70/62.75	26.27/66.74	27.85/70.74
7 months	15.06/6.83	18.63/8.45	22.88/10.38	25.11/63.80	26.77/68.01	28.38/72.10
8 months	15.83/7.18	19.47/8.83	24.07/10.92	25.63/65.11	27.40/69.60	29.09/73.90
9 months	16.58/7.52	20.37/9.24	25.04/11.36	26.25/66.70	27.99/71.11	29.73/75.53
10 months	17.09/7.75	21.12/9.58	25.90/11.75	26.74/67.92	28.46/72.30	30.32/77.02
11 months	17.64/8.00	21.56/9.78	26.63/12.08	27.15/68.98	28.99/73.65	30.82/78.30
12 months	18.21/8.26	22.38/10.15	27.49/12.47	27.71/70.39	29.53/75.01	31.35/79.63

TABLE FOR GROWTH IN GIRLS

Age	Weight (lb/kg)			Height (in/cm)		
	low (3)	medium (50)	high (97)	low (3)	medium (50)	high (97)
36 weeks	4.25/1.93	6.22/2.82	8.16/3.70	17.32/44.00	18.66/47.40	19.99/50.80
37 weeks	4.67/2.12	6.61/3.00	8.58/3.89	17.83/45.30	19.13/48.60	20.43/51.90
38 weeks	4.98/2.26	6.94/3.15	8.93/4.05	16.62/45.70	19.33/49.10	20.66/52.50
39 weeks	5.20/2.36	7.19/3.26	9.19/4.17	18.26/46.40	19.52/49.60	20.78/52.80
40 weeks	5.73/2.60	7.28/3.30	9.26/4.20	17.95/45.60	19.33/49.10	20.62/52.40
1 month	7.05/3.20	9.48/4.30	11.46/5.20	19.48/49.50	20.90/53.10	22.44/57.00
2 months	9.04/4.10	11.02/5.00	13.45/6.10	20.82/52.90	22.24/56.50	23.62/60.00
3 months	10.58/4.80	12.57/5.70	15.21/6.90	21.92/55.70	23.18/58.90	24.48/62.20
4 months	11.24/5.10	13.67/6.20	17.20/7.80	22.83/58.00	24.40/62.00	25.78/65.50
5 months	12.57/5.70	15.43/7.00	18.74/8.50	23.54/59.80	25.15/63.90	26.57/67.50
6 months	13.45/6.10	16.31/7.40	20.06/9.10	24.25/61.60	25.70/65.30	27.08/68.80
7 months	14.11/6.40	17.64/8.00	21.61/9.80	24.80/63.00	26.37/67.00	27.95/71.00
8 months	14.77/6.70	18.08/8.20	22.49/10.20	25.23/64.10	26.81/68.10	28.58/72.60
9 months	14.99/6.80	18.96/8.60	23.81/10.80	25.74/65.40	27.32/69.40	28.89/73.40
10 months	15.65/7.10	19.62/8.90	24.47/11.10	26.18/66.50	27.95/71.00	29.64/75.30
11 months	16.53/7.50	20.06/9.10	25.57/11.60	26.69/67.80	28.38/72.10	30.27/76.90
12 months	16.98/7.70	21.16/9.60	26.23/11.90	27.12/68.90	28.85/73.30	30.62/77.80

In the first years of a child's life, the doctor advises parents how to stimulate her overall development. Later on, when she is at school or in adolescence, the doctor will encourage her to lead a healthy and active life, in accordance with her capacities, so that she can fulfill her potential.

Psychomotor development

At each checkup, the doctor evaluates the child's psychomotor development, i.e., her capacity to perform certain physical and neurological tasks.

Key markers that can be accurately assessed in accordance with a child's age are used to monitor this process; they include the ability to open and close the hands, focus the eyes, and respond to specific stimuli.

The objectives of regular checkups

- To educate and encourage healthy lifestyles. This involves establishing a relationship of trust with parents in order to guide them about healthcare, in both physical and emotional terms, while also allowing the doctor to assess whether there are any family problems that could affect the child's development and require outside assistance.
- To monitor the child's growth and weight, and to promptly prevent or correct any possible problems.
- To assess how the child is developing.
- To promptly prevent or detect any abnormalities that parents would be unable to spot.
- To compile the child's medical history. This allows for the most appropriate decisions to be made in an emergency, or where there are clinical complications.
- To establish a feeding schedule appropriate to the particular child and evaluate the need for vitamin supplements.

Vaccination schedule

It is worth bearing in mind the following points:

- Children need most of their vaccinations during the first 2 years of their life, starting soon after birth. Further booster vaccinations should be given before they go to school.

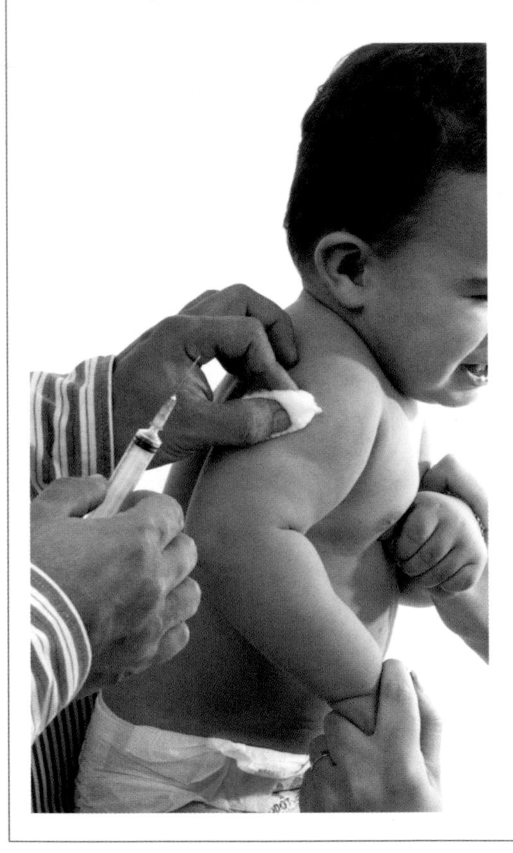

- Older children and adolescents also need vaccinations. Ask your doctor for the recommended vaccination schedule, so that you know when your child has to be vaccinated.
- Keep a written record of all your child's vaccinations. Ask the doctor to help you fill this in after every dose. This will help you to be certain about what vaccinations have been given and whether they are up to date. Sometimes several vaccines are combined in a single injection, so be sure to ask exactly which ones have been used.
- A child with a minor sickness can be vaccinated without any problem. Included in this category would be slight fever, ear infection, a cough, a runny nose, or mild diarrhea, in an otherwise perfectly healthy child. Children with serious health problems may have to avoid certain vaccinations, however, or receive them at a later stage than usual. Consult your doctor.
- Some vaccinations may trigger a reaction, but these are generally mild. It is unusual to see a stronger reaction, such as a high fever, a widespread rash, or a large inflammation on the site of the injection.
- If a child does have a side effect after a vaccination, ask the doctor whether it is wise for her to receive another dose of this particular vaccine.

Preparing a child to go to the doctor

Explain the purpose of visiting the doctor

- If a child's next consultation is a checkup, explain to her that it is merely a routine examination.
- Stress that all children go to the doctor for this type of checkup.
- If a consultation is intended to diagnose and treat an illness or disorder, explain to your child that the doctor needs to examine her in order to improve her health.
- If your child needs to see a doctor because of an illness or disorder, she may have unexpressed feelings of guilt. Talk openly to her.
- Talk to her about the illness or disorder affecting her in neutral language that is easy to understand. Reassure her that it is not her fault or the result of something bad that she has done.
- If you or any relatives or friends have suffered, or are suffering from the same sickness or health problem as your child, share this information with her. The knowledge that other people have gone through the same experience will reassure her.
- If your child needs medical attention on account of a condition that gives rise to rejection or mockery from other children (or even adults), you should make a special effort to reassure her and dispel her feelings of shame and guilt.
- If your child has been injured in an accident after disobeying safety instructions, you must stress, as naturally as possible, the cause–effect relationship between the action and the injury. You should try to relieve any sense of guilt.
- If your child repeatedly disobeys rules and hurts herself, talk to the doctor. This behavior requires closer analysis. In any case, always be sure to explain, especially to small children, that visiting the doctor is not a punishment.

Anticipating what will happen at the doctor's

- In the case of a routine checkup, you can use a doll or stuffed toy to show your child how she will be weighed and measured. Show her how the doctor will look inside her mouth, eyes, and ears, as well as listening to her chest or back with a stethoscope. Explain that the doctor may gently strike and press down on her stomach to feel what is inside, lightly tap her knee, and look at her feet.
- If it is not a routine consultation – for example, a visit to a specialist, or if the child is going to have some kind of test – it is advisable to give her the relevant information in simple language appropriate to her age. Build up her confidence by reassuring her that you will remain by her side at all times.

(*) In a high-risk situation, a dose should be given at the age of 9 months or earlier.
(**) A booster is recommended every 10 years.
(***) For children who did not receive a second dose before the age of 6.

VACCINATIONS RECOMMENDED BY THE INTERNATIONAL COUNCIL OF THE SNS - 2003

	Months						Years							
Vaccinations	2	4	6	12	15	18	3	4	6	10	11	13	14	16
Poliomyelitis	OPV1	OPV2	OPV3		OPV4			OPV5					Td (**)	
Diphtheria, tetanus, whooping cough	DTaP1	DTaP2	DTaP3		DTaP4			DTaP5 (or DT)						
H flu b	Hib1	Hib2	Hib3		Hib4 (optional)									
Measles, German measles, mumps				MMR1 (*)			MMR2				MMR (***)			
Hepatitis B	HB 3 doses 0, 1–2 and 6 months; or 2, 4, 6 months									HB 3 doses				
Meningitis B	1	2	3											

Involving the child in the process

• Except in the case of an emergency, allow your child to participate in the description of the symptoms to the doctor. Mention all the symptoms you have noticed, even those that appear to be unrelated to the problem in question. Also prepare a clinical history, in the form of a list of previous sicknesses and medical disorders.

• Ask your child to think of the questions she would like to ask the doctor. Write them down and hand them over in the consultation, or allow her to write them down, if she is capable, and ask them herself.

Choosing a doctor who relates to children

Apart from a doctor's training and professional expertise, it is worth remembering that your doctor must always be your greatest ally, particularly in the case of children, and so it is important to choose very carefully.

Immunization, or vaccination, is a process by which a person acquires protection against a disease. It plays an important role in infant healthcare. Most vaccines should be administered before a child's second birthday, to protect her from fatal but preventable diseases like whooping cough and measles. So, a child should be vaccinated in good time and keep her vaccination card up to date.

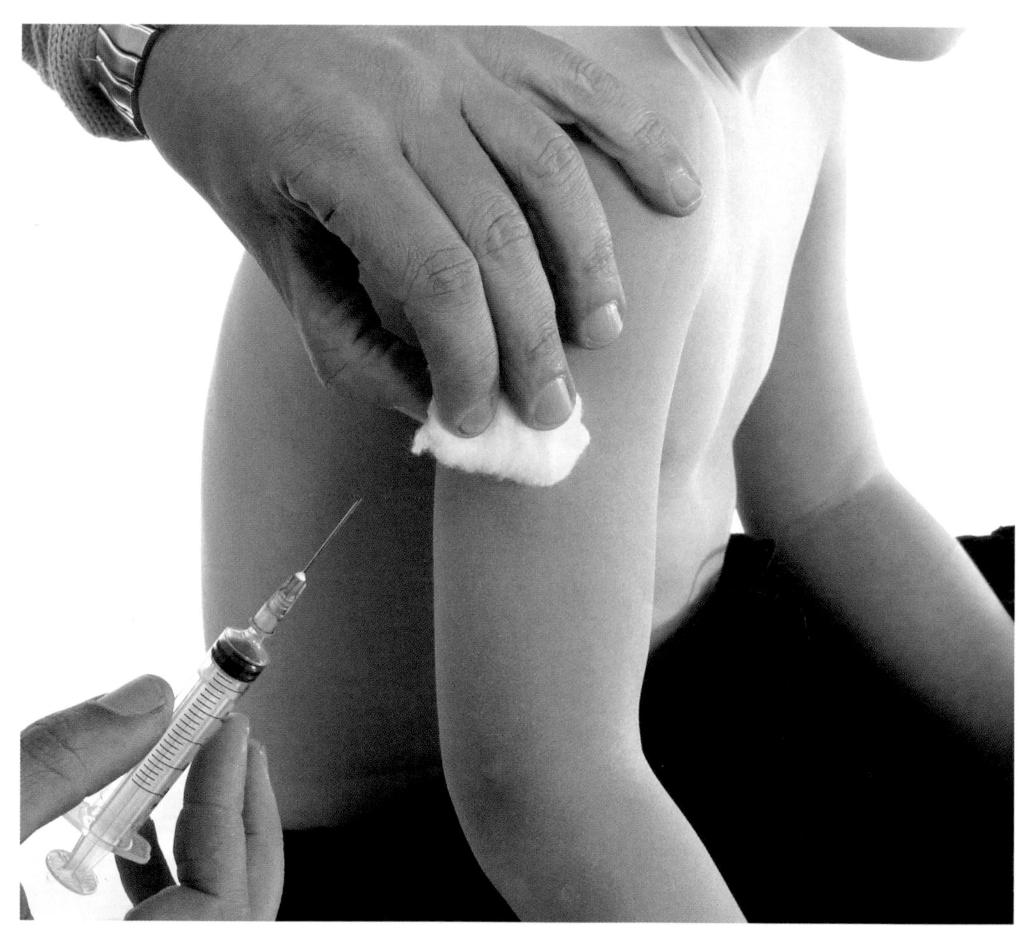

teeth

Teeth start to emerge in the sixth month of life, going on to constitute the 20 milk teeth. These start to be replaced by permanent teeth at the age of 6, in a process that culminates in the appearance of the third molar or wisdom tooth, which normally comes through between the ages of 18 and 30 (although in some people it never emerges at all).

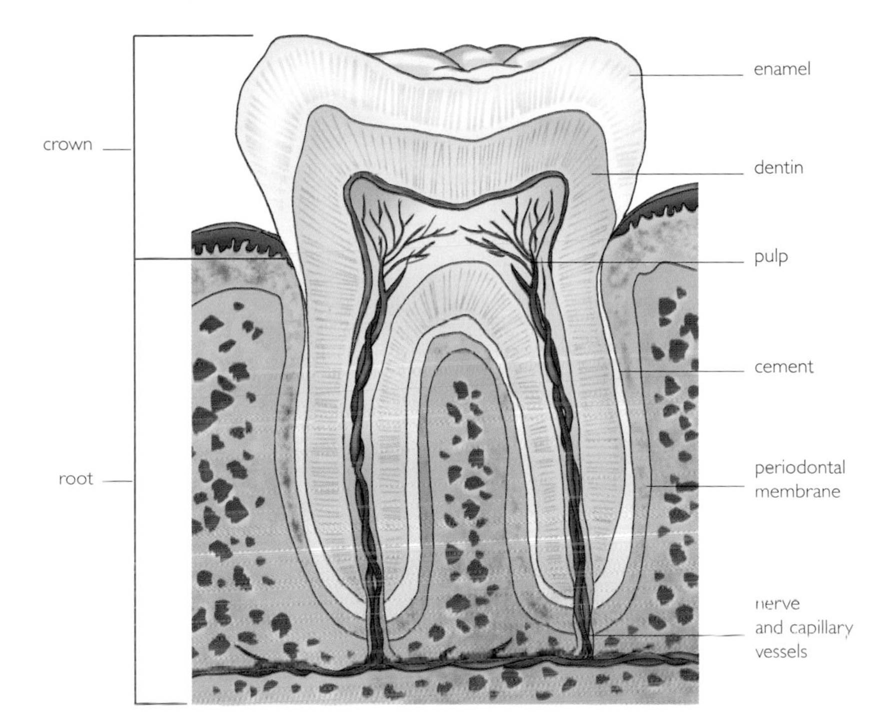

Teeth

The tooth and its structure

- Teeth are hard anatomical structures embedded in the jaw bones that participate in the digestive process, by cutting and grinding food, as well contributing to vocalization and speech, along with other elements in the mouth.
- The periodontium is a unit made up of the tooth itself and the area around it, which comprises the alveolar bone, the periodontal ligament, and the gum.

Dentition phases

Until the age of 8 or 9, children only possesses 20 teeth, known as the *first dentition* or, more popularly, *milk teeth*. These are later substituted by a total of 32 teeth, which make up the permanent dentition. The teeth are divided into 4 groups, each with specific functions: the incisors, the canines, the premolars, and the molars.

• The tooth itself is made up of 3 mineralized elements (enamel, dentin, and cement), along with a nucleus of fibrous tissue (the pulp).

• The tooth is divided into the following sections:

– The crown is the free part of the tooth visible in the oral cavity, while the layer covering it is enamel.

– The neck is level with the gum and links the crown to the root.

– The root is embedded in the dental alveolus, inside the bone, and the layer covering it is dentin.

Milk teeth

In most children, the first teeth appear around the age of 6–7 months, although there can be great variations. Some babies are born with a tooth, while others have to wait a year for this milestone. The early or late appearance of teeth tends to follow the same pattern among members of the same family. There are no hard-and-fast schedules with respect to the appearance and loss of the various different teeth. The timetable detailed here shows the most common parameters.

It is not unusual for the emergence of teeth to be accompanied by symptoms like fever, uncha-

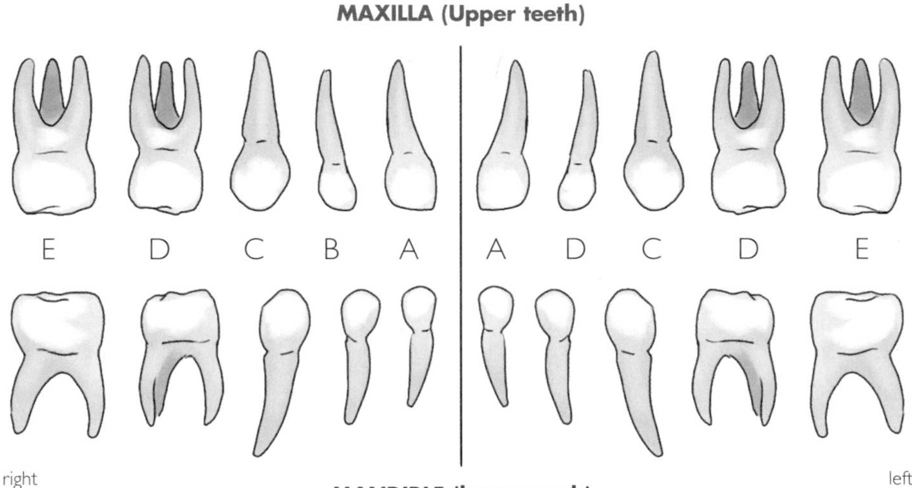

	Upper teeth	Timetable of emergence and loss
A	central incisor	7–8 months; falls out at 7–8 years
B	lateral incisor	9 months; falls out at 8–9 years
C	canine	18 months; falls out at 11–12 years
D	first premolar	14 months; falls out at 10–11 years
E	second premolar	24 months; falls out at 10–12 years
	Lower teeth	
A	central incisor	6 months; falls out at 11–13 years
B	lateral incisor	6 months; falls out at 10–12 years
C	canine	16 months; falls out at 9–11 years
D	first premolar	12 months; falls out at 7–8 years
E	second premolar	20 months; falls out at 6–7 years

How to soothe teething pains

- Use soft plastic teethers with water inside; these can be frozen or chilled in the fridge.
- With cold foods (liquid or jelly).
- With cold gel for the gums, free of alcohol, sugar, or anesthetics (consult your doctor).

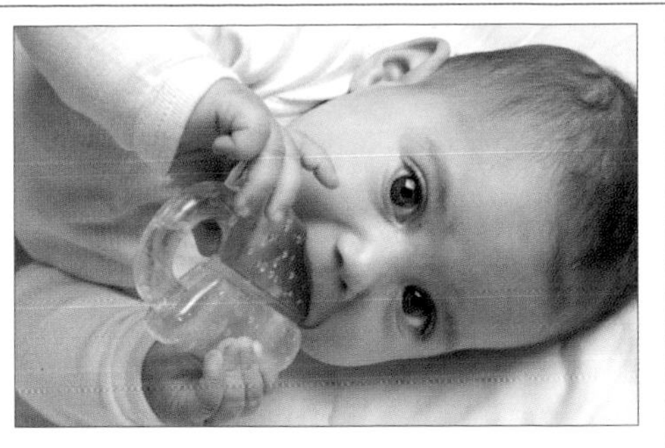

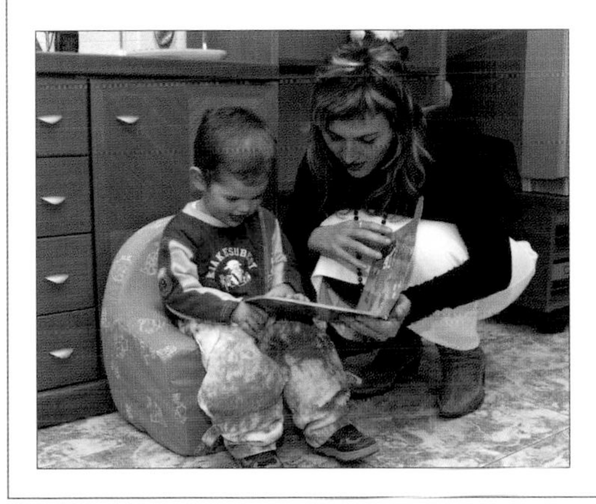

- Analgesics, antipyretics, and anti-inflammatory drugs can help, following your doctor's advice.
- Keep the baby company and reassure her, as she does not understand what is happening.
- Dentists and pediatricians usually recommend the use of fluoride from the age of 6–8 months to prevent tooth decay. Fluoride is only effective, however, if it is complemented by adequate dental hygiene.

racteristic irritability, sleep disorders, and dribbling. These symptoms can also appear for other reasons, which should be ruled out with the help of a doctor.

Permanent teeth

The permanent teeth appear during the period known as the second infancy. The first to emerge is the first molar, situated behind the 2 molars that

Although a feeding bottle is a good option for mothers who cannot, or do not want to, nurse their baby, it can give rise to dental problems.

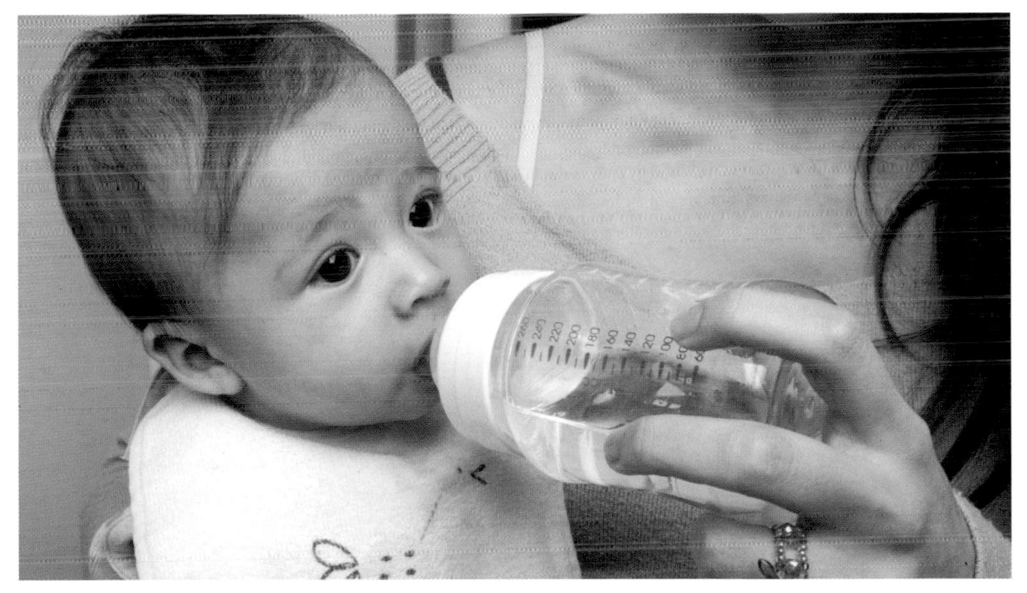

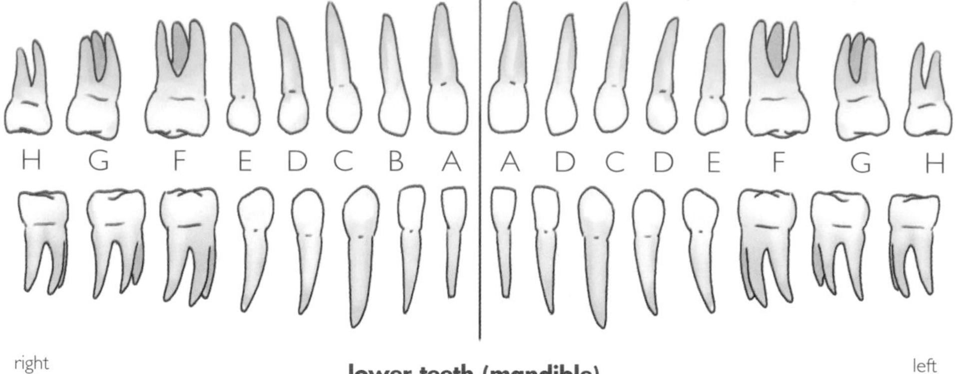

form part of the milk teeth. It normally arrives at about the age of 6.

In contrast to milk teeth, the emergence of the permanent teeth does not occasion any significant discomfort. Furthermore, the child is now aware of what is happening to her and knows how to express her complaints and requirements. The cutting of the third molars (commonly known as the wisdom teeth) may be very painful, however, and their evolution should be monitored by a dentist.

	Upper teeth	**Timetable of emergence (in years)**
A	central incisor	7–8
B	lateral incisor	8–9
C	canine	11–12
D	first premolar	10–11
E	second premolar	10–12
F	first molar	6–7
G	second molar	12–13
H	third molar	17–21
	Lower teeth	
A	central incisor	6–7
B	lateral incisor	7–8
C	canine	9–10
D	first premolar	10–12
E	second premolar	11–12
F	first molar	6–7
G	second molar	11–13
H	third molar	17–21

Dental problems

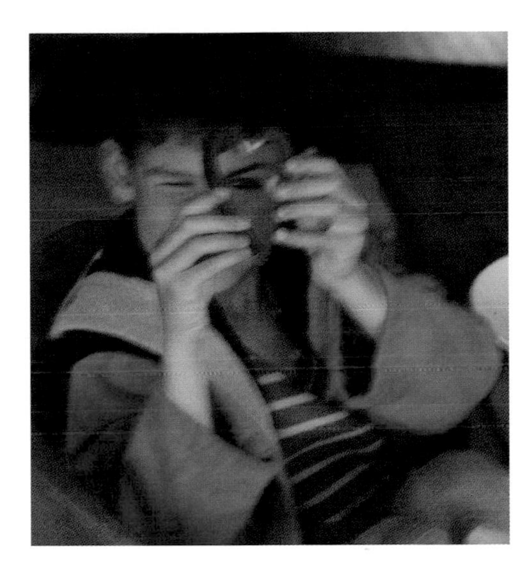

Deterioration of the teeth after using a feeding bottle

• This is a problem that occurs in the first 2 years of life, due to the teeth's exposure, for a prolonged period, to liquids with a high sugar content, such as milk and juices,.

• This problem can also affect babies who breast-feed for a long time – for example, after the mother falls asleep while she is still nursing.

• The bacterial plaque that appears on teeth uses this sugar as a source of energy to form acids that attack the teeth's enamel.

Prevention of tooth decay

- Never leave a child in bed with a feeding bottle.
- Avoid prolonged use of pacifiers.
- Rinse a baby's teeth and gums after every meal with a clean sponge or cloth, to remove the plaque.
- Start to use dental floss between the teeth as soon as the first milk teeth appear.
- Do not put sweetened drinks in a child's feeding bottle.
- Make sure that your child takes fluoride in some form or other, especially if the water supply is not fluoridated.
- Examine your child's teeth frequently and take her to the dentist regularly as soon as the milk teeth appear.

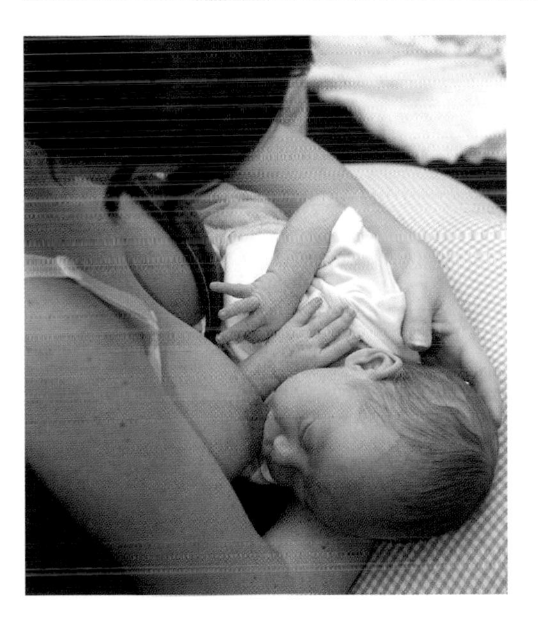

Preventing tooth decay

• Do not sweeten a baby's pacifier with honey or other sweetened products.

• Do not allow a baby to sleep with her feeding bottle or mother's breast in her mouth.

• Depending on the fluoride content in the local water supply the doctor may recommend the use of a supplement.

• Start brushing your child's teeth when she reaches the age of 2 (without toothpaste at first). Before that, the teeth should be cleaned with a soft sponge or cloth.

A mother should not sweeten her nipple with sugar, honey, or any other delicacies before offering her breast to a baby, as this can cause tooth decay.

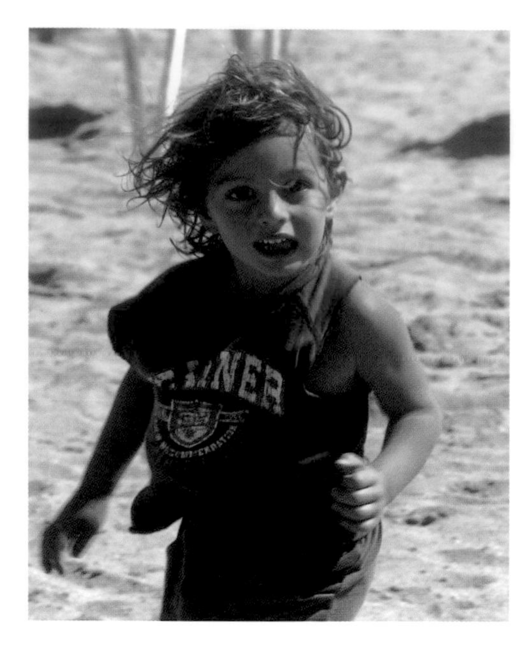

• Avoid food that can cause tooth decay. Sucrose, which is abundant in candies, is the most damaging sugar in this respect. Starch, present in cereals and pulses, is the least harmful food component.

• Between the ages of 3 and 6, it is advisable to use toothpastes containing less than 0.25% of fluoride; between 6 and 10, those with 1–1.5%, and, from then on, those with over 2.5%.

• Make sure you know how to brush teeth correctly and instil this habit in your child in the first years of her life.

• Take your child regularly to the dentist from an early age; also consult the dentist at the appearance of any unusual changes in the teeth, or if your doctor recommends a visit.

The most important way of guaranteeing that your child's teeth are in good condition is, quite simply, by taking her to the dentist regularly. This does not mean going only if you notice something unusual in the form of visible decay or toothache. It is essential to see a dentist before any such problem arises, precisely to prevent them or correct any factors that make them more likely.

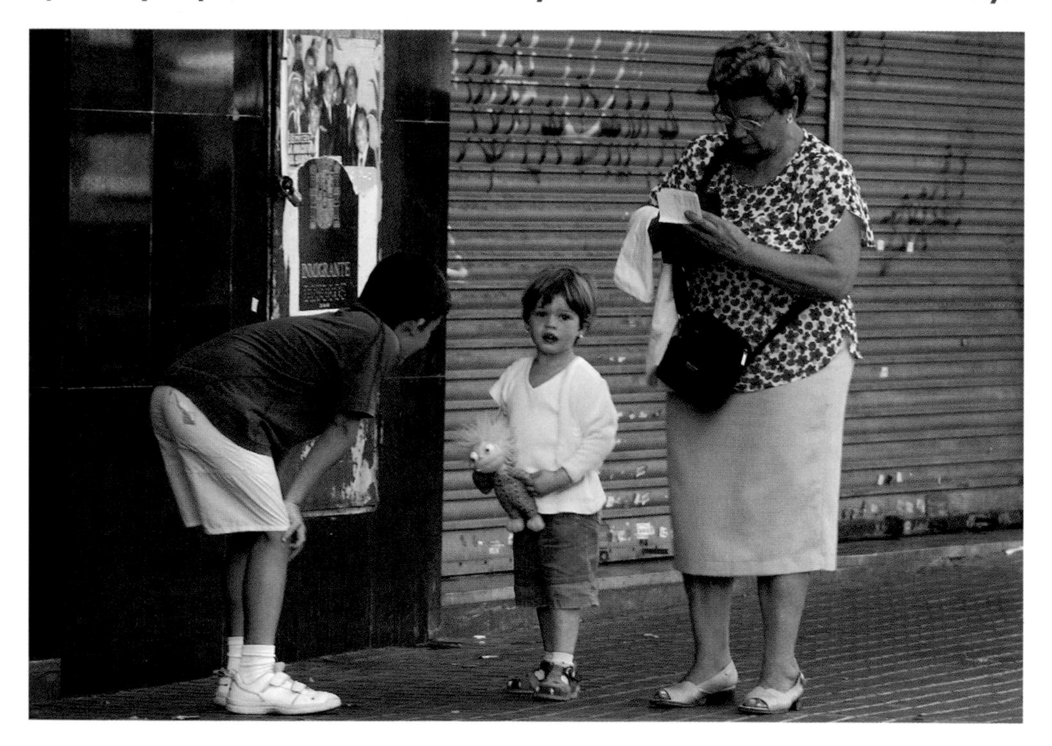

Why do teeth grow crooked?

Irregular alignment of the teeth can have a number of causes:

- Childhood habits like sucking the thumb or a pacifier, which impedes the appropriate molding action of the tongue and lips.
- Premature loss of teeth.
- Milk teeth that remain in place for too long, preventing the permanent teeth from coming through in the right place.
- Breathing with the mouth open, because of repeated inflammation of the tonsils and adenoids or certain allergies.
- Genetic inheritance.
- Overly large teeth.
- Gum diseases that make the teeth move out of position.

Orthodontistry

Children should start visiting the dentist regularly as soon as their first teeth appear. Childhood checkups make it possible to monitor the progress of the dentition and to prevent any complications that could lead to unsightliness or other problems in later years if not treated in time, such as crooked teeth, as a result of anomalies in the teeth themselves or during the growth of the jaw. In these cases, the dentist may recommend a visit to an orthodontist who will assess the need for braces.

Parents should try to ensure that their child has trust and confidence in the dentist before visiting the dentist. It is worth establishing a good relationship between your child and dentist to prevent the fears that are so common in adulthood. For this reason, it can be useful to go to a children's dentist who decorates and adapts the surgery to the needs and tastes of youngsters.

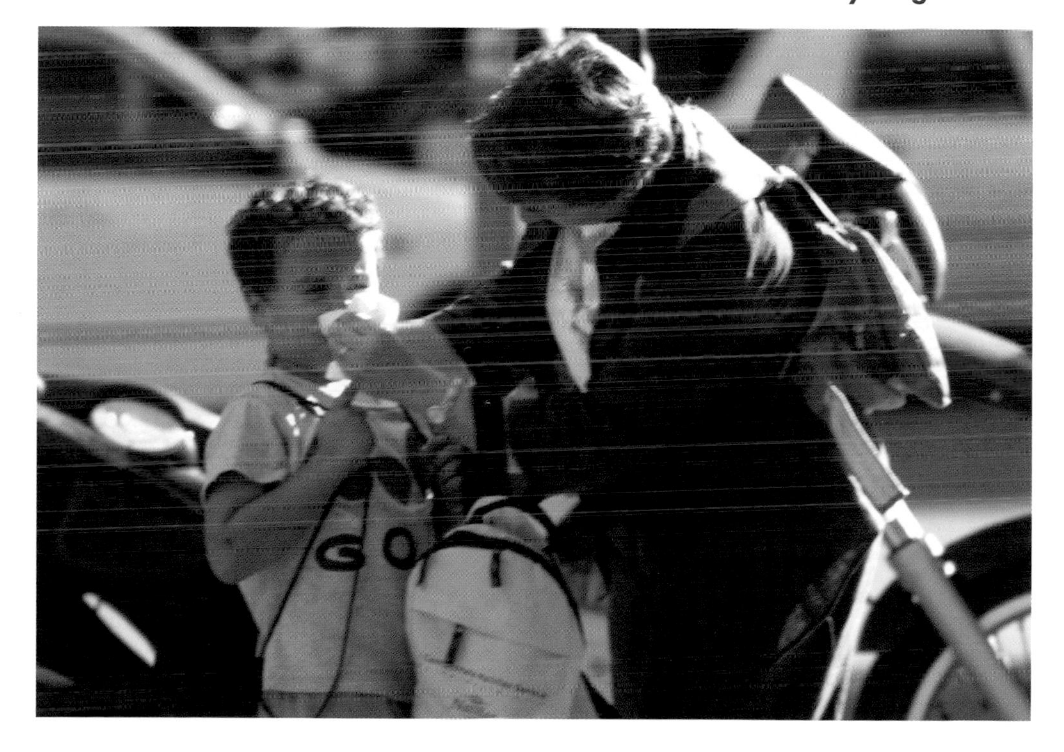

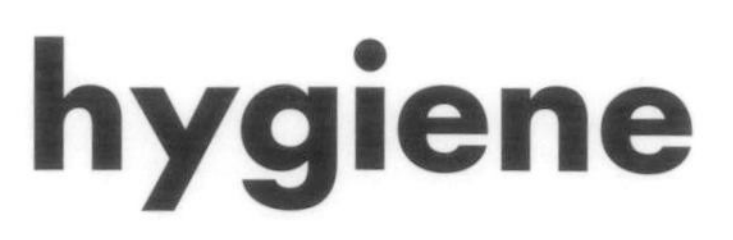

hygiene

Hygiene provides another means of staying healthy and feeling good. Maintaining hygiene is important not only for preventing infection and disease, but also for boosting confidence, as it facilitates integration into social life. During the first stages of a child's life, parents must take responsibility for their child's hygiene while also instilling good hygiene-related habits and rules as he grows up.

Hygiene in a baby

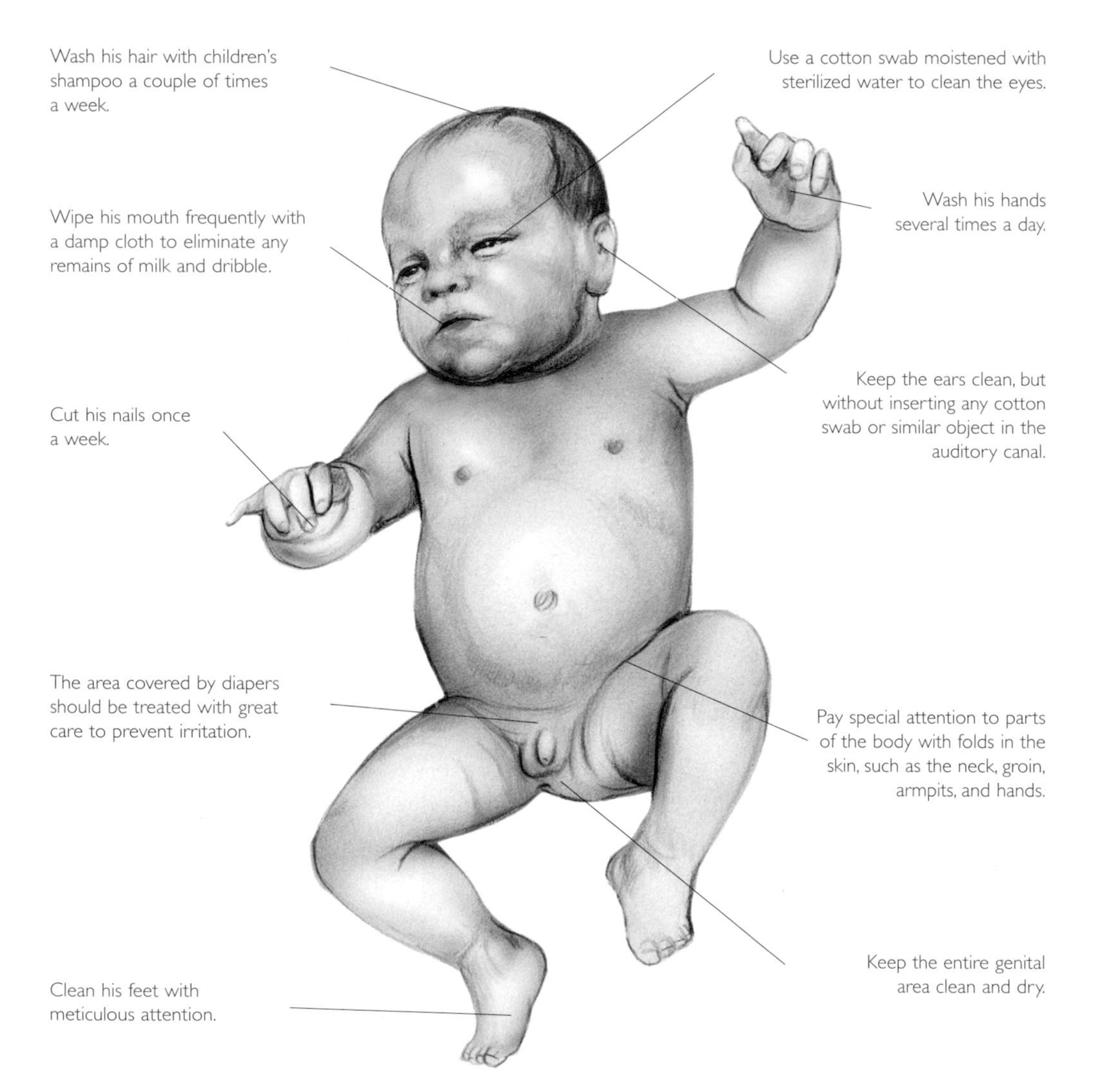

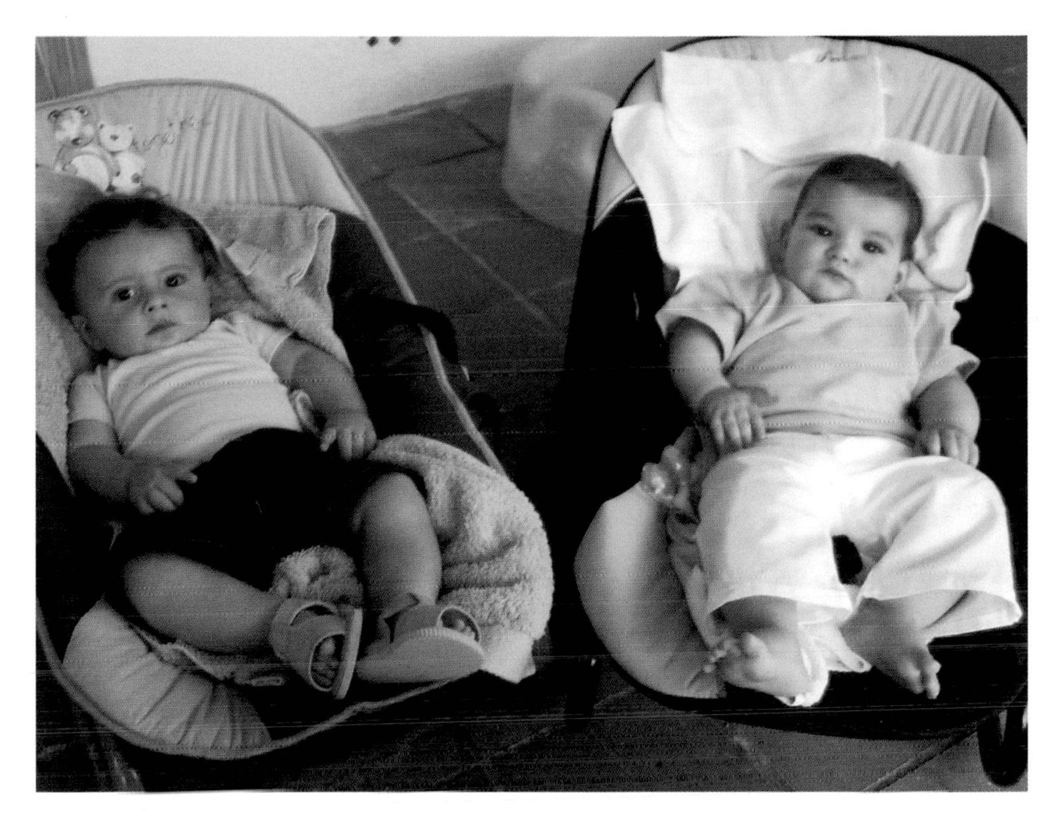

Changing diapers

• Changing diapers is one of the first tasks facing the parents of a newborn baby (8 times a day, on average). Bowel movements are frequent in the first few months, and the baby should be washed regularly to prevent any irritation of the skin from contact with feces and urine.

• Consult a doctor if the skin does become irritated, or at any signs of a dermatological problem.

• It is normally advisable to change a baby's diaper first thing in the morning, just before bedtime, after every feeding session, when he is restless and, obviously, whenever you are sure the diaper is wet or soiled.

• The use of talcum powder is not recommended.

• It is important to buy diapers that fit the baby properly.

• As the genitals of a boy and girl are different, so the method of washing them is also distinct:

• In girls, a damp cloth should be passed from front to back, to avoid the penetration of intestinal bacteria into the vagina and subsequent infections. Irritation can be avoided by thoroughly drying any folds in the skin. Do not apply any powder to the vulva region.

• In boys, the folds in the thighs and the base of the genitals should be washed carefully, followed by the penis. Do not try to pull back the foreskin, because this could damage the skin; excessive rubbing can also lead to irritation.

• Take advantage of diaper changing to play and talk with the baby, as well as caressing and tickling him, etc. This turns a chore into a pleasant interlude, enjoyed by both the baby and his parents. As he grows older, it becomes more difficult to keep him still. In order to distract him, it is a good idea to have a few toys at hand (rattles, soft toys or empty pots of cream or gel, cleaned and tightly closed or free of their lid). It is advisable to lay him on a high changing table with a waterproof cover that can be cleaned after every session.

• In wintertime, it is better to cover the plastic cover with a towel, to prevent the baby from catching cold. After washing and drying him thoroughly, allow him to exercise his legs for a few minutes without the diaper.

• Basic equipment:

– Small, clean bowl with warm water mixed with a small amount of neutral liquid soap.

– Disposable wipes.

– Diapers of the appropriate size.

– Protective cream (consult the doctor). This is not essential, but can help avoid irritation.

– High changing table for the home, and a folding one for outings.

– A soft, absorbent and not particularly large towel.

Bath time

• It is not usually advisable to give a baby his first bath until the incision of the umbilical cord (navel) has healed. As always, you should follow your doctor's advice.

• Before putting your baby in the bath, make sure that you have all the necessary equipment readily available, and use a thermometer to check the temperature of the room (71.6–77 °F/22–25 °C) and the water (95–98.6 °F/ 35–37 °C).

• A baby's first bath should be a celebration for both the baby and all his family.

• The frequency of bath sessions depends on the amount of free time available to his parents. If he is not suffering from any skin disorder, the normal schedule is once a day, but if he relaxes and enjoys it, he can take a bath more often.

• You should use neutral or glycerin soaps specially made for a baby's delicate skins.

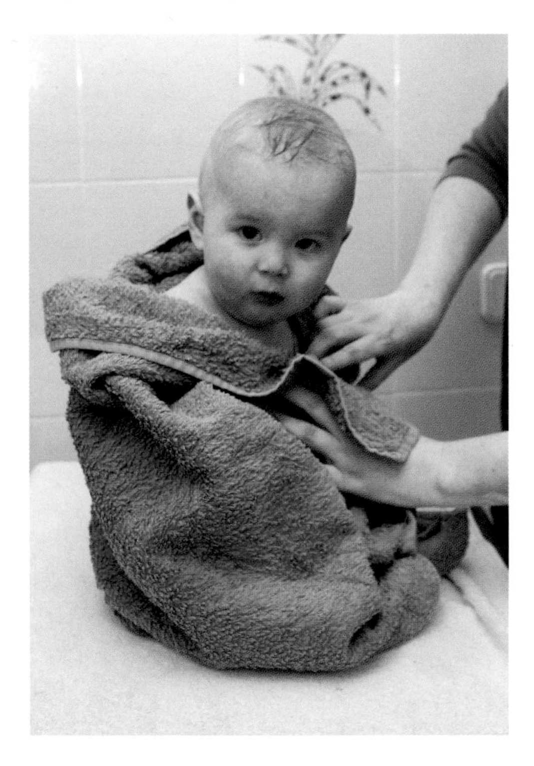

• A folding bath is very practical and comfortable. This consists of a metal support and a stiff plastic tub with its own drainpipe and a padded wooden lid that can be used to dress the baby. You can also use a plastic tub of any size, or even the kitchen or bathroom sink. If you are thinking of using a freestanding tub, it is worth placing it on a high table, so that the person in charge of washing the baby can be more comfortable.

• When you take your baby out of the water, wrap him in a soft, absorbent towel that covers him up to his head and start to dry him gently, taking special care with the folds in his skin. Do not rub him dry, to avoid causing any irritation.

• After the bath, it is a good idea to moisten his skin with a lotion or oil. Choose the most natural brand you can find, free of any cologne or alcohol. Talcum powder is not recommended nowadays, as it dries and irritates the skin. Toilet water is also to be avoided, unless it is put on the baby's clothes and not his skin.

Useful tips

A dirty child with body odor will be subject to mockery and humiliation. This not only endangers his health but is also an affront to his dignity, making him feel vulnerable and severely undermining his self-esteem.

• **Oral hygiene.** Hygienic habits, including those associated with dental hygiene, need to be instilled in children at an early age; this is a complicated process that requires great patience on the part of parents, who should set an example. As role models for a child, parents should try to keep their home spick and span. They might also teach their child how to brush their teeth by calling him to the bathroom, explaining the purpose of the brush and toothpaste, and giving him a demonstration. Another important factor in the reduction of tooth decay in children has been the fluoridization of water.

• **Good habits need to be learnt in infancy.** A child will always understand more than he can express; this is why his parents need to constantly explain why hygiene is important and what benefits it brings to his health. For example, you can say to a 6–month old baby, "Let's change your diapers so that your bottom is not sore."

• **Regularity.** Habits need to be followed on a daily basis and be incorporated into all aspects of a child's life. It is important to keep the instructions you give a child as simple as possible.

Washing special parts of the body

Scalp
Special brushes for washing the scalp are available. It is generally advisable to use shampoo only once or twice a week. Choose a neutral shampoo, with no alcohol or perfume.

Eyes
The eyes do not usually require any special care, but they can be washed with cotton soaked in boiled water, going from the outside to the tear duct. Use a separate piece of cotton for each eye.

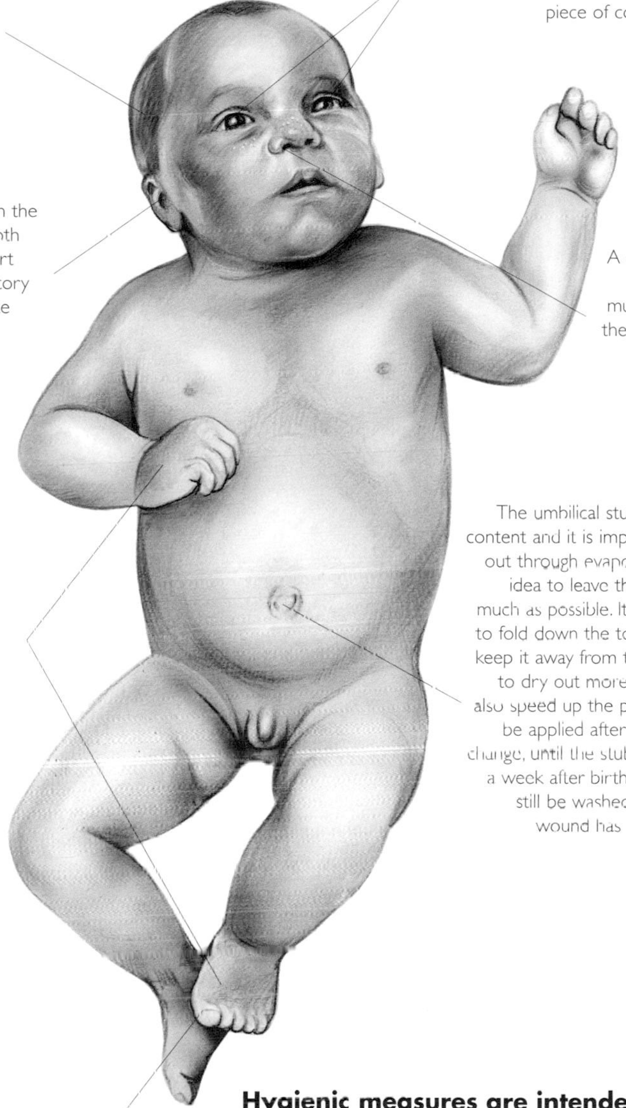

Ears
Clean behind the ear and in the outer folds with a damp cloth or cotton swab. Never insert cotton swabs into the auditory canal, as you could perforate the ear drum.

Nose
A damp cloth can be used to remove mucus, or to moisten the nostrils if they are excessively dry.

Umbilical stub
The umbilical stub has a high water content and it is important that it dries out through evaporation. It is a good idea to leave the stub exposed as much as possible. It may be necessary to fold down the top of the diaper, to keep it away from the stub, allowing it to dry out more quickly. Iodine can also speed up the process. This should be applied after a bath or a diaper change, until the stub falls off (normally a week after birth). The navel should still be washed regularly until the wound has completely healed.

Hands and feet
Wipe both sides of the hands and feet (including the lines on the palm and soles) with a damp cloth. Separate the fingers and toes to remove any accumulated dirt.

Nails
As a baby cannot control his movements, he can scratch himself if he has long nails, so these should be cut regularly (even if he does not like it). It is easier to perform this task while he is fast asleep.

Hygienic measures are intended to keep a baby clean at all times, but his skin should be washed only with water and special soap designed for babies. All other products, such as alcohol, eau de cologne, and talcum powder, are to be avoided. If you want to make your baby smell attractive, you should always apply toilet water to nothing but his clothes or sheets.

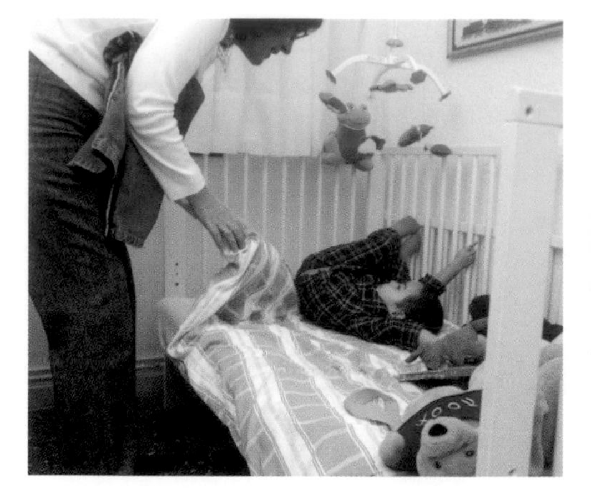

The biggest problem associated with hygiene, apart from social factors, is the passing on of disease. The home itself can become the primary source of infections in a baby. Windows closed all day long, overcrowding, cigarette smoke, and atmospheric pollution all allow the viruses present in the environment to propagate and give rise to colds or pneumonias. Furthermore, hygiene should also be scrupulously maintained in the kitchen.

• **A child should be able to find everything he needs.** A child's wash things should be kept within his reach. Toothpaste cannot be locked away, toilet paper needs to be readily available, etc. If a child does not have conditions that enable him to maintain his hygiene, he will grow discouraged. If he has his own wash bag he can look after his own creams and soaps, and always know where they are.

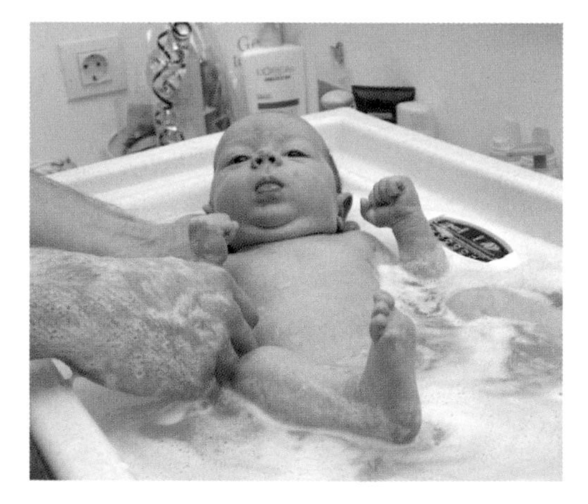

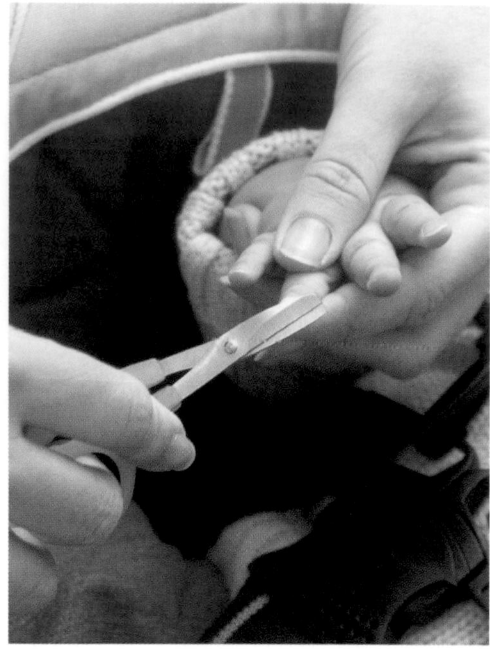

• **Time devoted to personal hygiene should be fun.** Avoid threats and punishments. On the contrary, it is better to emphasize positive aspects, by saying, for example, "How nice it is to have clean hair!" The example of parents plays a key role here, too: when they groom themselves, they should demonstrate the pleasure it gives them so that their child associates such habits with happiness.

• **The importance of creativity.** If you feel you are getting nowhere in your attempts to teach your child good habits, do not despair, and above all avoid scolding him. It is always better to try another approach. An approach that worked with one child will not necessarily work with another. Parents should have the capacity, and above all the patience, to experiment with new methods.

sexuality

For over a century psychoanalysts, prompted by Sigmund Freud, have been discussing infant sexuality but, nevertheless, it remains a taboo subject and a great source of doubt and anxiety for many parents. Perhaps the best starting point is the notion that a child is just as sexual a being as any adult, despite their differences and specificities. If we accept this premise and leave aside our own fears and seek the appropriate information, it is possible to educate a child about sex and sexual behavior.

Infant sexuality

When a child is born, he has no dominant cultural and educational guidelines, nor does he know about the concepts of good and evil. He is therefore not repressed, and he does not assume his sexual desires to be something bad or perverted, let alone a reason for guilt. He knows nothing of taboos or prohibitions. On the contrary, he uses his sexuality as a source of pleasure, but also as a source of knowledge. It provides a means for understanding the world and having fun, for finding out about both himself and other people.

If parents react overdramatically to their child's sexual behavior and apply repressive or even violent educational methods, they can induce traumas that can manifest themselves in great frustration and difficulties in sexual and emotional relationships in adult life. Parents need to understand that sexuality is just another characteristic of their child. Everybody is born with their own sexual identity and this develops as the child grows. A healthy

Infant sexual development

Typification. This refers to the development of sexual identity, along with those of the masculine and feminine roles. The basis of sexual typification is acquired at home, although teachers and classmates act as moderators and, to a certain extent, strengthen a child's attitude. The influence of the media should also be taken into account.

Sexual orientation. This corresponds to the learning of behavior that leads a child to discover pleasure. It embraces experimentation with respect to sexual behavior and eroticism, on the basis of trial and error.

Complementation. This describes the discovery of love and intimacy, and the capacity for communication that is opened up by interpersonal relationships, and also relates to how sexuality enriches these relationships. In short it describes how boys and girls learn about the dynamics of affection, attraction, and falling in love.

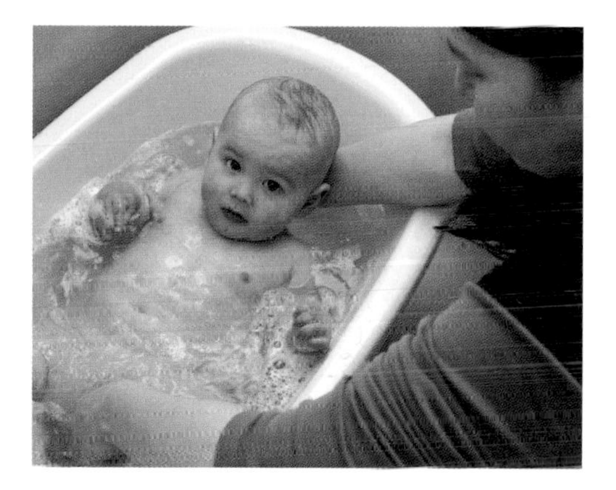

An adult male does not have phymosis if his foreskin descends freely and does not experience pressure with an erection – an excess of skin is not phymosis.

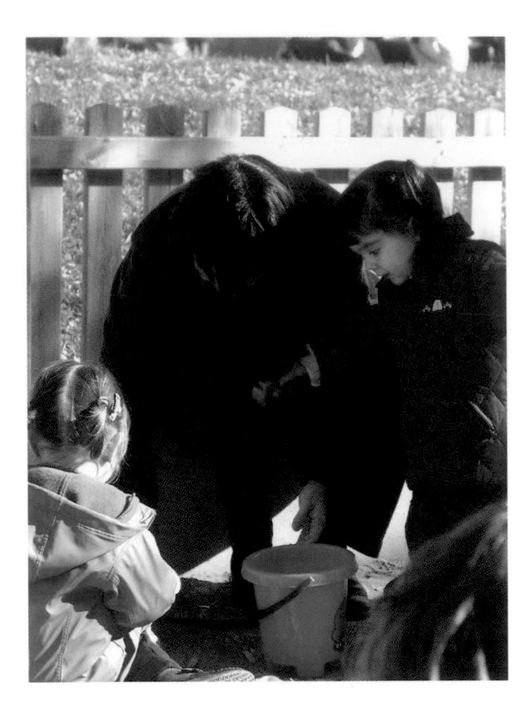

It is entirely normal for children to explore their own body and genitals from the age of 2, or even earlier. Even masturbation can occur at a very early age. Exploration of the genitals is linked to the discovery of pleasure, a desire for relaxation, and simple curiosity, so young children sometimes masturbate as part of their natural inquisitiveness about their own body.

sexual development – guided by education but free of guilt, abuse, or extreme behavior – is essential to the development of a well-rounded human being.

Phases of infant sexual development

- Birth to 2 years

Various studies have demonstrated that the reflex mechanisms of the sexual response (male and female erections) are present from early infancy.

Self-exploration is an experience basic to healthy sexuality. Parents' attitudes should be as relaxed and natural as possible in these situations. If a child is scolded or punished for masturbating, he will see sexuality as being something bad, to be prohibited, and he may feel guilty about this practice.

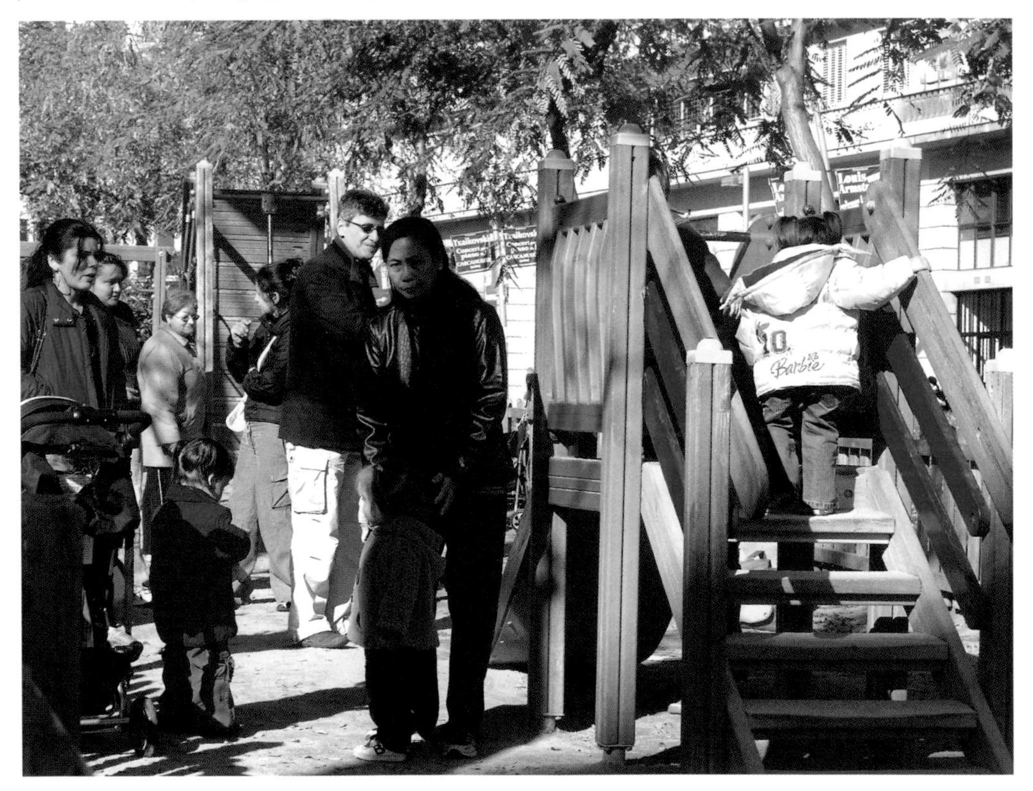

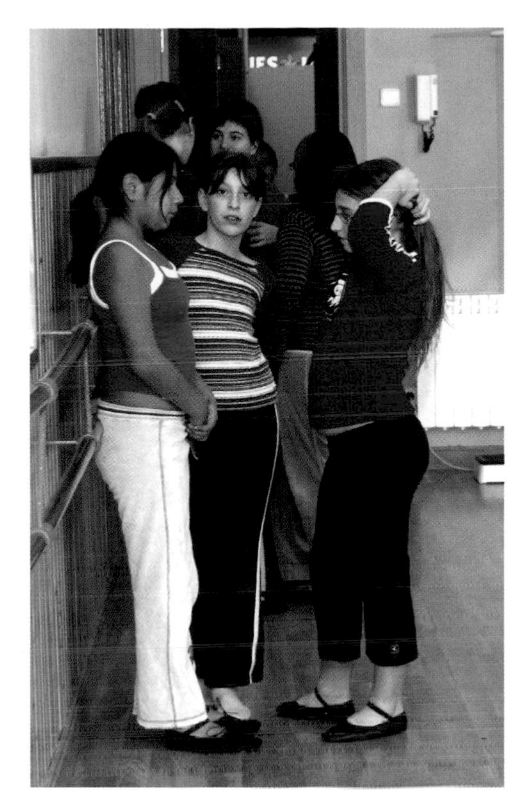

Children display signs of sexual excitement after contact with various physical stimuli, including breast-feeding, having a bath, diaper changing, and caressing. These reactions should not be repressed or punished. On the contrary, a relationship of relaxed intimacy between a baby and his parents will help him to learn about feelings and affection. A baby deprived of this atmosphere may have sexual problems in the future.

When a child is 1 year old, he may play with his genitals when he is in the bath or otherwise naked, and he can display irritation at any attempts to stop him doing so.

• Between the ages of 2 and 5

Between the ages of 2 and 3, a baby establishes a clear sexual identity and starts learning about gender roles.

This is a phase marked by great curiosity about the sexual organs and the feelings of pleasure derived from them.

During this stage, children ask about reproduction, play at doctors, observe sexual relationships between adults (at home and on the television) and animals, and can even experiment with homo- and heterosexual relationships with older children (ages 6–9).

• From 6 to puberty (primary school age)

This phase is characterized by games that permit sexual exploration, from pastimes involving visual inspection to touching, kisses, rubbing, inserting objects into the rectum or vagina, and even attempts at oral sex or coitus (either hetero- or homosexual).

Almost all children experiment with their sexuality by privately indulging in hetero- and homosexual games, maybe even with siblings.

This is a period of sexual fantasies and falling in love. These contacts generally teach a child to relate to other people and play an important part in the establishment of psychosexual equilibrium in adulthood.

It is important to realize that homosexual games do not determine the future identity of a child. Similarly, sexual contact between siblings at this age should not be interpreted as incestuous behavior, but merely as erotic play. In these cases, any hostile reaction from parents is not positive; it is much more effective and healthy to take a realistic, comprehensive attitude and pursue sexual education appropriate to the child's age.

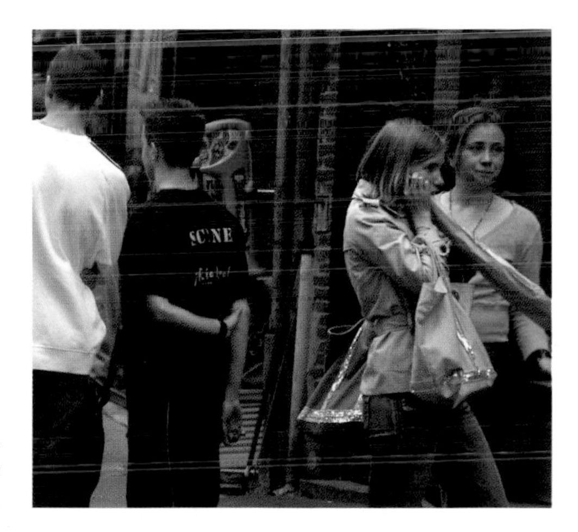

In pre-adolescence, boys mainly stick with members of their own sex and generally behave aggressively toward girls of their own age.

Sexuality in pre-adolescence (age 10–12)

- The impulsiveness of this phase leads to a reappearance of behavior typical of the age of 2 or 3 (rebelliousness, stubbornness and contrariness, exhibitionism, a liking for dirt and disorder, etc.). A child becomes more inaccessible and difficult to control at this age.
- There is a notable concern about the working and protection of their sexual organs, but they do not associate their own genitals with amorous situations or personal satisfaction.
- They express their sexual curiosity by means of jokes, giggling, and secrets.
- An interest in collecting objects and forming groups is common at this age.
- Transitory symptoms appear as a release of tension: phobias, nervous tics, head and stomach ache, nail biting, stammering, playing with the hair, and constantly touching every object in sight.
- Children gradually start to experiment with new forms of behavior in order to appear more grown-up; their emotions are unstable, although this volatility can vary from one child to another (and even fluctuate within the same child).
- The stimulation of the genitals is an activity that occurs naturally from birth. At this age, children do this in private, as a way of experiencing pleasure, channeling anxiety, and learning about their body. Masturbation does not, however, play the all important role that it will later take on in adolescence.
- Boys mix almost exclusively with other boys. They show aggression toward girls by attacking and snubbing them, as well as acting haughtily and contemptuously. They express their pre-genital impulses through restlessness, voracity, sadistic attitudes, obscene language and onomatopoeia, and exhibitionist, phallic displays. They also spurn cleanliness and are not concerned about smelling unattractive.
- By this age, girls have already strongly repressed their pre-genitality, so they address the opposite sex more openly, becoming aggressive and seductive in games of love. Their greatest conflict is with their mother, as they need to free themselves from her. They take decisive steps toward adapting to reality, accepting rules and behaving as expected of them.

Girls show themselves to be more open toward the opposite sex, behaving aggressively and seductively in games of love.

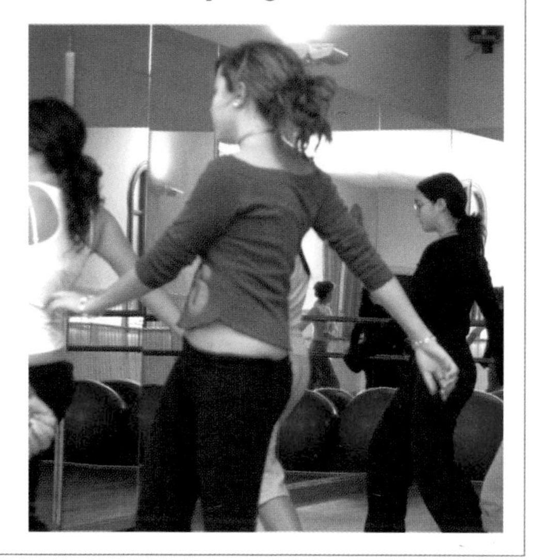

Sexuality in adolescence

Genitality and sentimentality can and should be dominated and channeled, but they first need to be understood. This need for understanding is what sparks the curiosity so typical of an adolescent – a curiosity that is satisfied by an exploration of their own bodies and those of others, or by reading (books, magazines and publications of all kinds), by conversations with their companions and with people who they trust, or even through more impersonal, anonymous, and up-to-date means, such as Internet forums and chatrooms.

Boys tend at first to focus on a friend of the same sex, with whom they establish an idealized and mutually fulfilling relationship. Such friendships gradually fade away as they move toward heterosexuality.

In this phase of transitory homosexuality, adolescent boys learn about their male identity from sexual games or intimate chats that allow them to identify with their own sex.

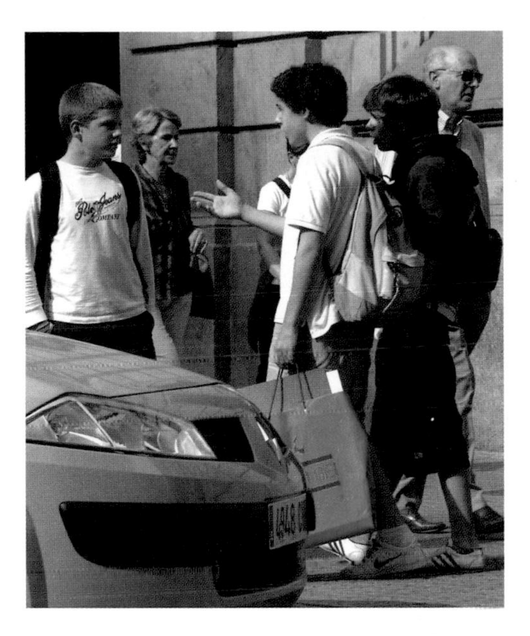

Girls also place great emphasis on friendships, but with both sexes. This attitude springs from normal bisexual tendencies that will, for the most part, give way to heterosexual choices. The tendency to bisexuality marks the entrance into adolescence, properly speaking.

The construction of a personal form of sensuality is a basic undertaking for girls, as this is the way they enjoy their sexuality, while also allowing them to find out whether or not they are attractive to boys.

The assertion of virility follows a similar path. Certain parts of their body cause them particular concern: the size and external characteristics of the genitals occupy a central place in the fears and fantasies of adolescent boys. This leads to comparisons with each other, in the belief that true masculinity – bursting with power and a guarantee of sexual success – is directly related to the size of the penis.

Not only do the conditions of adolescence itself exert an influence, the demands and pressures of the environment also play a role. If modern society and the media present sex as the most human way of expressing love, adolescents feel impelled, to some degree, to seal a relationship with sex, which can have negative psychological repercussions at such an early age. Youngsters are in fact starting to have sex at an increasingly early age.

In most cases, adolescent sexual relationships surge spontaneously, i.e. they occur without the planning that is usually characteristic of adult relationships. This pattern can be seen as an enrichment of tenderness and love, but it can also have dramatic consequences, as it may give rise to undesired pregnancies and a lack of precautions against sexually transmitted diseases.

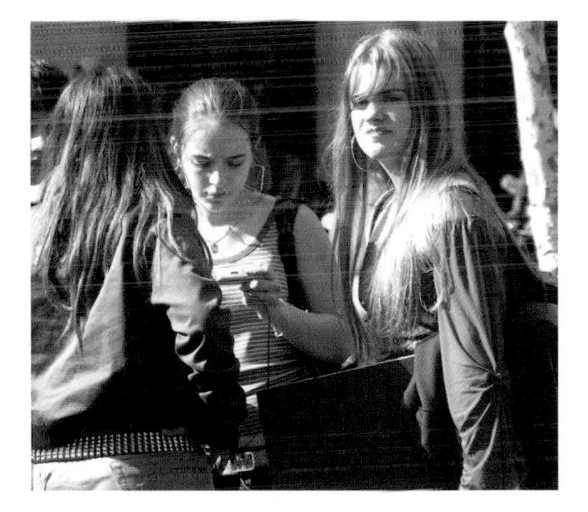

The risk at this age is that the need to search for an identity can propel an adolescent into premature sexual relationships. Friendships, studies, sport, activities with companions, and dialogue with parents and teachers protect an adolescent from impulsive sexual behavior.

alarming symptoms

Although a child may display many symptoms that are cause for concern to his parents, some are particularly worthy of mention on account of their frequency and seriousness – especially vomiting, fever, and feverish convulsions. The first two are very common during childhood, but feverish convulsions are found in only 3–5 percent of children aged between 6 months and 6 years. When a child with a high body temperature does start to tremble, however, other pathologies like epilepsy need to be ruled out.

Vomiting

This is the expulsion through the mouth of the contents of the stomach; these may be partially digested or simply consist of digestive juices with no traces of food. It must be stressed that the occasional presence of blood may be caused by the effort of the vomiting itself and not have any special significance or importance. Nevertheless, it is wise to consult a doctor in such cases.

Vomiting: what to do before consulting a doctor

- Dehydration can be avoided by giving your child small amounts of liquid (water or natural juices), at a rate of about a tablespoonful every 5–10 minutes.
- If the vomiting is accompanied by diarrhea, it is preferable to use the rehydration solutions on sale in pharmacies. Homemade solutions should not be used.
- Observe your child; if he tolerates liquid, gradually increase the frequency.
- If he keeps on vomiting, stop giving him liquid for an hour _ or even longer in older children _ and then start again with spoonfuls every 10 minutes.
- Once he is taking liquid without any problem, offer him food, in small quantities (and without ever obliging him to eat).

Causes

- **Fever.** Fever can itself cause vomiting. The presence of both fever and vomiting requires observation, in order to rule out serious problems like pneumonia, meningitis, and urinary infection.

Vomiting: when to consult a doctor straightaway

- If your child is less than 3 months old and has vomited after 2 or 3 feeding sessions.
- If the vomiting is persistent.
- If the vomit contains bile or blood, or looks like coffee grounds.
- If your child is listless, sleepy, and very thirsty, with sunken eyes, and cries without tears and produces little urine.
- If he has very strong abdominal pains or headaches.

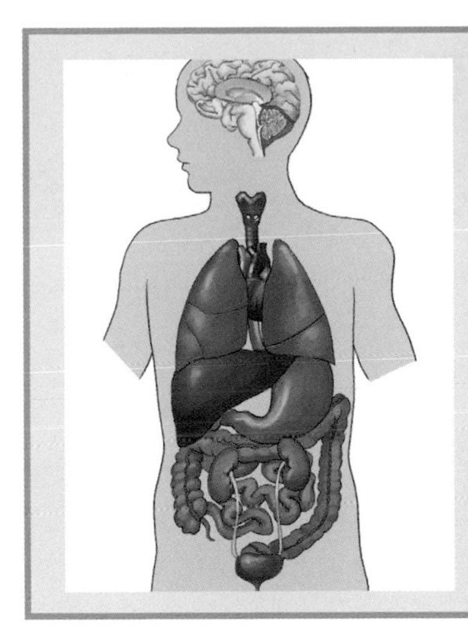

Possible reasons for vomiting

- Abdominal disorders:
  appendicitis, cholecystitis, intestinal obstruction, gastroenteritis, liver or pancreas disorders, infections, etc.
- Disorders of the nervous system:
  encephalitis, vertigo, migraines, meningitis, etc.
- Psychological disorders: anorexia or bulimia, emotional stress, etc.
- Lung disorders:
  Infections such as pneumonia or very severe coughing fits, etc.
  Consumption of certain medicines.

- **Diarrhea.** The combination of vomiting, fever, and diarrhea is very common in cases of acute gastroenteritis.
- **Abdominal pain.** This can be a transitory complaint or a more serious disorder, such as acute appendicitis, so it is advisable to consult a doctor.
- **Headache.** A headache complemented by vomiting and fever may be a sign of meningitis, so once again a medical examination is in order.
- **Medication.** If a child is taking medicine, it must be taken into account that any medication can cause digestive disorders. Your doctor will decide whether the treatment needs to be interrupted.
- **Acetone breath.** In cases of fever, vomiting, or lack of food intake, the body reacts by creating acetone, which can in itself bring on more vomiting, thereby creating a vicious circle.
- **Listlessness, pallor, and cold sweat.** These symptoms can signal the onset of a more serious intestinal disorder, so your child needs to be seen by your doctor.

Fever

This is an increase in the body temperature above normal levels. Body temperature varies according to where it is measured (armpit, mouth, rectum, or ear) and the age of the child. The thermometer has to remain in place for 1 or 2 minutes in the rectum or ear, and for 5 minutes in the armpit or fold of the groin.

Causes

Although the most common cause of fever is an infection, there are other disorders that a doctor has to take into account when establishing a diagnosis and the cause of fever.

- **Sunstroke or heatstroke:** when the environmental temperature is excessive, the body does not evaporate heat properly and the body temperature rises.

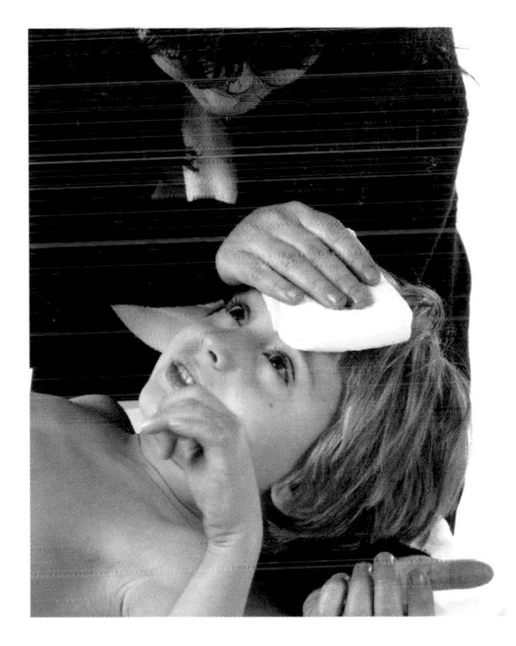

In cases of fever, rehydration and the use of cold cloths and baths are basic measures to be taken while waiting for the doctor to prescribe more specific treatment.

NORMAL VARIATIONS IN TEMPERATURE	
Age	**Temperature (ºF /ºC)**
3 months	99.32 +/- 32.72 (37.4 +/-0.4)
6 months	99.5+/- 32.72 (37.5 +/-0.3)
1 year	99.68 +/- 32.36 (37.6 +/-0.2)
3 years	98.96 +/- 32.36 (37.2 +/-0.2)
5 years	98.6 +/- 32.36 (37 +/-0.2)
7 years	98.24 +/- 32.36 (36.8 +/-0.2)
9 years	98.06 +/- 32.36 (36.7 +/-0.2)
11 years	98.06 +/- 32.36 (36.7 +/-0.2)
13 years	97.7 +/- 32.36 (36.5 +/-0.2)

• **Hormonal disorders:** hyperthyroidism, thyrotoxicosis, pheochromocytoma.

• **Muscular effort:** the temperature can be raised by physical exercise, playing sport, an epileptic fit, a tetanus crisis, etc.

• **Malignant hyperthermia.**

• **Some medicines** trigger a fever, as do some vaccinations.

• **Others,** such as the recent consumption of very hot or very cold food, the presence of bruising, stress, etc.

Febrile convulsions

This is a crisis that can also include unconsciousness; convulsions can occur in children with a high fever aged between 6 months and 5 years.

The child's body can stiffen and start to shudder or become completely flaccid; the mouth is often purple and closed tight.

The convulsions usually stop after less than 5 minutes; after this, the child may urinate or defecate, and then the tendency is to fall asleep. Convulsions almost invariably occur during the first day of a fever – sometimes even before the child's parents have noticed that he has a high temperature at all.

Fever: what to do before consulting a doctor

- Keep the room temperature at a comfortable level. Do not wrap your child up excessively.
- A child with fever needs to drink a lot of fluids. Offer him drinks, but without being over-insistent.
- Monitor your child's temperature and treat the fever (if he is disturbed by it) with antipyretic (fever-reducing) drugs at the normal dosage, respecting the recommended intervals between the doses.
- Baths or compresses with cool water reduce a fever only for a very short time. Never use compresses with alcohol or very cold water.
- Turn your child on his side, to help him breathe more easily, and keep him away from any objects that could cause him damage.
- Do not put anything in his mouth.
- Take off his clothes to help lower the temperature.
- If he has not received any medicine for fever in the last two hours, you can administer a suppository.
- It is advisable to have the child examined by a doctor at once. Take him to the nearest health center or hospital.

Fever: when to consult a doctor straightaway

- If your child is less than 3 months old.
- If your child is sleepy, listless or, in contrast, very irritable.
- If he has suffered a convulsion.
- If he is complaining of a headache and vomiting.
- If he is having difficulty in breathing.
- If the armpit temperature is over 104.9 ºF (40.5 ºC).
- If marks appear on his skin.

the asthmatic child

Asthma is a chronic disorder of the respiratory canals that causes a suffocating feeling of being unable to breathe. It affects between 5 and 10 percent of the infant population in developed countries. There has been an alarming increase in the incidence of asthma in recent years, which could be related to environmental factors. A clear diagnosis and regular monitoring, even during asymptomatic periods, are essential to the prevention of long-term lung complications.

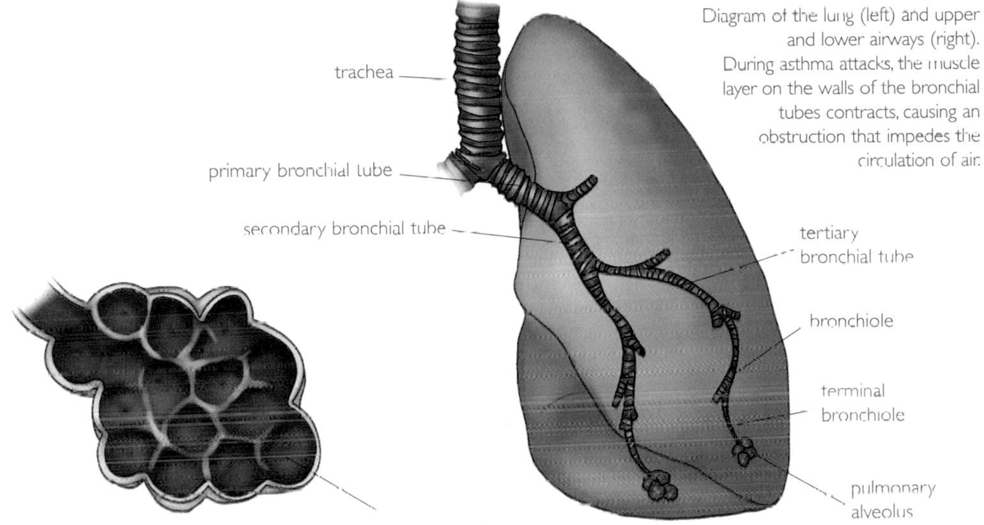

Diagram of the lung (left) and upper and lower airways (right). During asthma attacks, the muscle layer on the walls of the bronchial tubes contracts, causing an obstruction that impedes the circulation of air.

Asthma

Asthma is a chronic disorder of the respiratory canals that causes a suffocating feeling of being unable to breathe. It affects between 5 and 10 percent of the infant population in developed countries. There has been an alarming increase in the incidence of asthma in recent years, which could be related to environmental factors. A clear diagnosis and regular monitoring, even during asymptomatic periods, are essential to the prevention of long-term complications in the lungs.

Asthma is an inflammatory disease of the air ways that restricts the amount of air flowing in and out of the lungs. When an asthma attack occurs, the muscles of the bronchial tree tense up and the

Asthma is found in 3% to 55% of adults and 7% to 10% of children. The majority of asthmatics develop the disease before the age of 30, and half of them do so before the age of 10. Asthma symptoms can become less severe over time, especially in children.

Physical exercise in an asthmatic child

Exercise and play are necessary for all children, and asthmatic children do not have to be an exception, even though 80 percent of them find their participation in sports impaired (except when they take the appropriate measures). It is a great mistake, however, to overprotect an asthmatic child and deny him a normal level of physical exercise, particularly in view of the psycho-emotional and social benefits of sport. Everybody becomes tired and breathless after trying a demanding physical activity for the first time. An asthmatic child who has never played the sport before will experience these reactions with a particular intensity. An asthmatic child therefore needs to be introduced to sporting activity very gradually, so that he can learn to distinguish between the breathlessness normally associated with vigorous exercise and that associated with an asthma attack. An asthmatic child can play any sport (apart from diving with oxygen bottles), but some are more suitable than others:

- Athletics, football, and basketball are the sports that can give rise to most bronchospasms.
- In contrast, sports such as swimming in an air-conditioned indoor pool (warm, damp air), gymnastics, golf, hiking, and cycling on flat land are much less asthmogenic. Tennis and ball games, although requiring plenty of running, tend to demand intense but intermittent effort, and so they are also recommendable, as are martial arts (judo, karate, taekwondo), fencing, etc.
- Diving with air bottles is not a good idea, because of the changes in pressure involved and the impossibility of handling an asthma attack underwater; it would be very difficult to perform the decompression maneuvers required for returning safely to the surface when overcome by breathing difficulties.
- Mountain sports like rock climbing and skiing, etc. pose the problem of breathing in cold, dry air, although this can be mitigated by the use of masks or helmets.

lining of the airways swells up, reducing the flow of air and producing a distinctive whistling sound. Asthma is also marked by an increased production of mucus.

Most people with asthma have periodic wheezing attacks interspersed with asymptomatic periods. These attacks can last anything from a few minutes to several days, and they can be dangerous if the airflow is drastically reduced.

An asthma attack can be unleashed in susceptible children by:

- **Inhaled allergens** (triggers of allergies), such as fur from a toy, dust mites, insects, mold, or pollen.
- **Respiratory infections.**
- **Exercise.**
- **Cold air, tobacco smoke, and pollutants.**
- **Stress.**
- **Food or allergies to foods.**
- **Medicines**, such as anti-inflammatory drugs and aspirin.

Many asthmatics have a personal or family history of allergies, such as hay fever (allergic rhinitis) or eczema, while others have no such precedents and no problems with allergies.

Symptoms

- Wheezing:

– This starts suddenly, is usually episodic, and disappears spontaneously.

– It can worsen during the night or in the early hours of the morning, and after exercise or exposure to cold.

– It improves with bronchodilators (medicines that dilate the airways).

- Cough, with or without sputum (phlegm).

– Difficulty in breathing, aggravated by exercise.

– Breathing accompanied by retraction of the skin between the ribs.

Symptoms indicating an emergency

- Extreme difficulty in breathing.
- Intense anxiety brought on by breathing difficulties.
- Blue face and lips.
- Rapid pulse, sweating.

Asthma is generally classified as either mild, moderate, or severe. Children and adolescents usually suffer from the mild and moderate forms where the attacks alternate with asymptomatic periods. In their more serious form, asthmatic symptoms are almost constantly present. Asthma can also be classified according to its cause, distinguishing between extrinsic asthma, where it is possible to demonstrate allergic sensitization (80% of cases in children), and intrinsic asthma, where no allergic cause can be demonstrated.

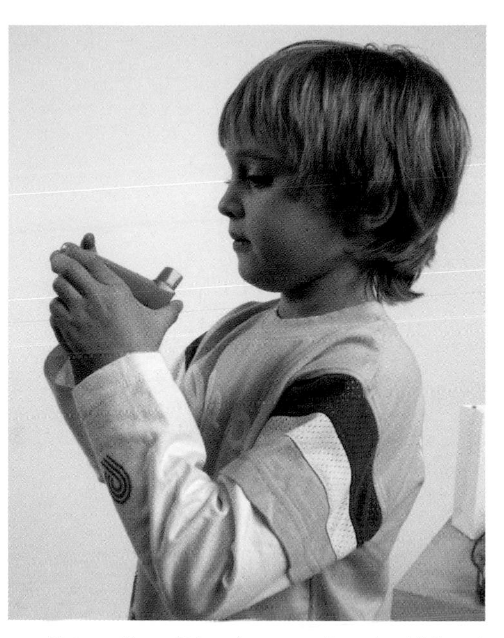

• Sleepiness or confusion during an asthma attack.

Other symptoms that can complement asthma:

• Nasal flaring.
• Chest pain.
• A feeling of tightness in the chest.
• Abnormal breathing pattern, with delays in exhalation.
• Temporary respiratory arrest.
• Sensation of being suffocated.

A diagnosis of asthma is established primarily on the basis of the child's clinical history and the presence of the abovementioned symptoms. It is also necessary to ascertain the characteristics of attacks, such as their form and the intervals between them, what triggers them and their relationship to seasonal changes, and the general evolution of the disease. A more general investigation into the child's medical history is also necessary to rule out other respiratory diseases that share symptoms with asthma.

A functional diagnosis will be made to assess the extent of the obstruction of the airflow; this involves a test of the respiratory function (spirometry). This has the disadvantage of requiring the child's collaboration, and is therefore only suitable for patients aged over 6.

Treating asthma

The 3 basic pillars of treatment are:

• **Prevention.** This means avoiding any elements that have been identified as triggers for attacks.

• **Education.** Educating an asthmatic child and his parents is a cornerstone of preventive treatment. It is essential that they understand his sickness, along with its triggers and symptoms, as well as how to administer medicines and approach sport and exercise, etc.

• **Pharmacological treatment.** There are 3 types of drugs: those that impede the release of substances that cause the allergic reaction; those that block the action of these substances; and those that reduce inflammation and bronchial obstruction, such as derivatives of cortisone and bronchodilators.

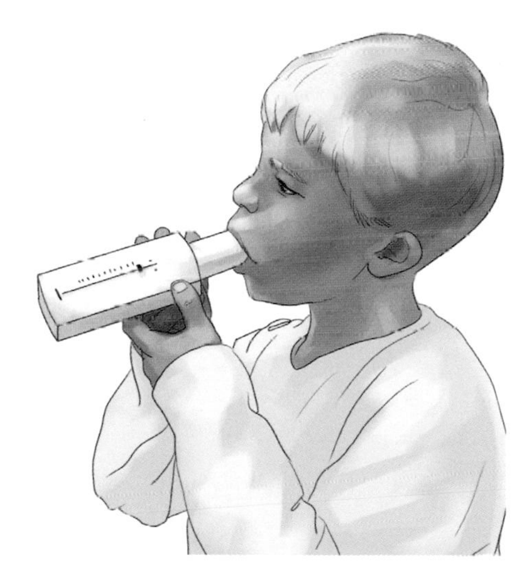

If a child is suspected of suffering from bronchial asthma, he will be given a spirometry. This is a painless test of the volume and rhythm of the airflow in the lungs.

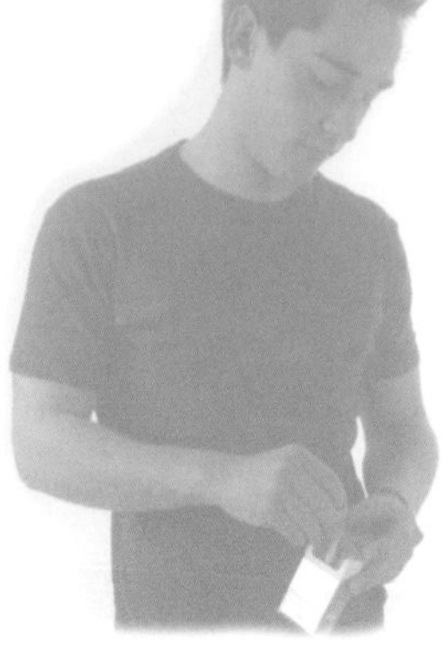

allergies

Allergy can be defined as an exaggerated response on the part of the immune system to contact with a substance, known as an allergen, which is capable of triggering a series of mechanisms that release chemical mediators, including histamine, that are responsible for the appearance of symptoms. It is estimated that allergies affect approximately 20 percent of the population, particularly in the summer months; the rapid growth in the number of new cases, however, leads us to believe that this figure may rise to 50 percent in a couple of decades.

The immune system and allergic reaction

Under normal conditions, the immune system responds to aggressive external agents, such as bacteria, viruses, and toxins, by producing substances known as antibodies (immunoglobulins), which neutralize the threat and destroy it, and thus protect the organism. For some reason, in certain circumstances the immune system reacts in this way to substances that are normally harmless (allergens), giving rise to the various symptoms of allergies.

Four components are required to trigger an allergic reaction:

- **Allergen:** the substance that causes an allergy.
- **Immunoglobulin (IgE):** antibody produced by the immune system in response to the allergen.

Immunological mechanism of the allergic reaction. If an allergic reaction, the immune system reacts to substances that are normally inoffensive. In the first phase, contact is made with the allergenic substance, which gives rise to the formation of antibodies (particularly immunoglobulins) on the surface of certain cells (mastocytes) that circulate in the blood or in some tissues. In the second phase, the antibodies, confronted with the same allergen once again, recognize it and bind with it, triggering the release of a series of chemical mediators, particularly histamine, which are responsible for the appearance of allergic symptoms.

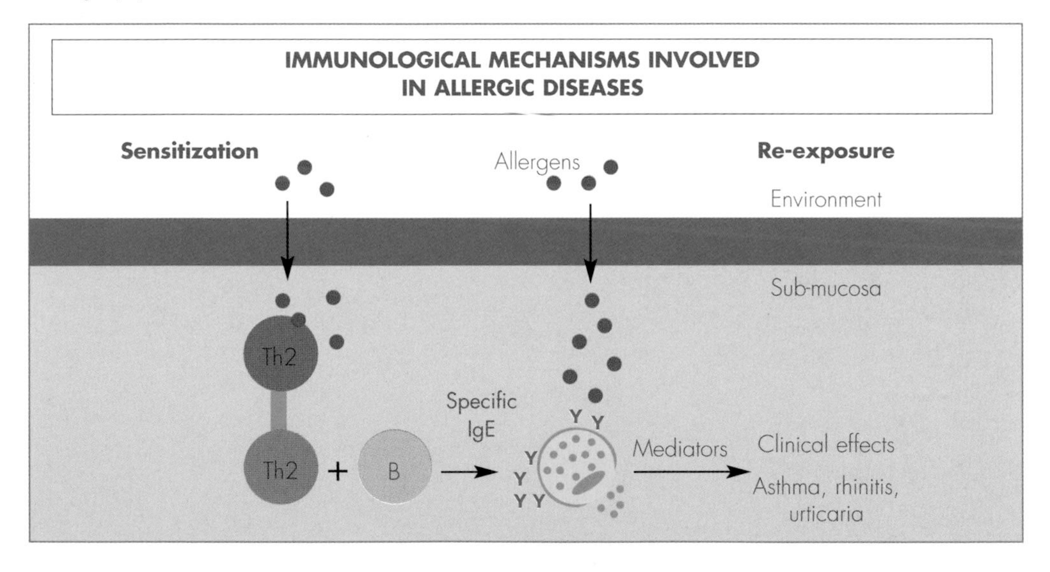

THE MAIN ALLERGENS INVOLVED IN ALLERGIC REACTIONS

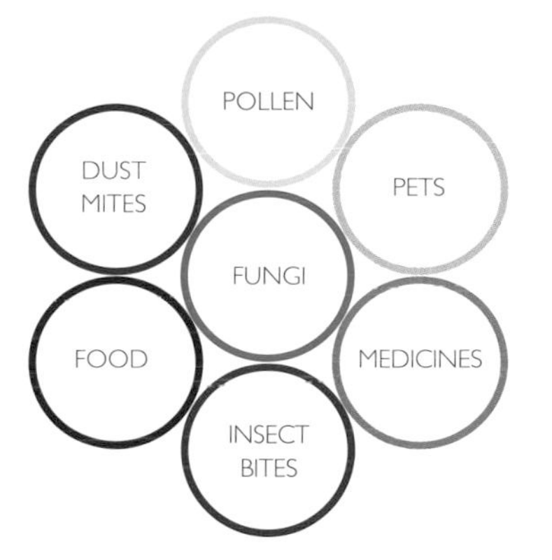

Around 30% of children suffer from some type of allergy. It is not a serious ailment but it can disrupt a child's life, especially if it is associated with other complications like asthma. A precise diagnosis and appropriate medical monitoring are required to enable an asthmatic child to lead a totally normal life.

- **Mastocytes:** special cells containing histamine granules, located in the skin and mucous membranes (nose, eyes, mouth).
- **Histamine:** substance released during the allergic process; it is responsible for the symptoms of the allergy.

There are a number of potential allergens that can make contact with the body via various means:

- Air: pollen from plants, house dust (mites), fungal spores, animal fur, etc.
- Food: fish, eggs, nuts, etc.
- Medicines: penicillin, aspirin, etc.
- Insect bites and stings.
- Contact with the skin: cosmetics, industrial products, etc.

Bites from mosquitoes, fleas, ticks, etc. can create localized skin reactions, distinguished by lesions similar to urticaria that are often painful. Bees and wasps can produce allergic reactions of an anaphylactic nature, involving obstruction of the airways and a circulatory collapse that endanger a child's life.

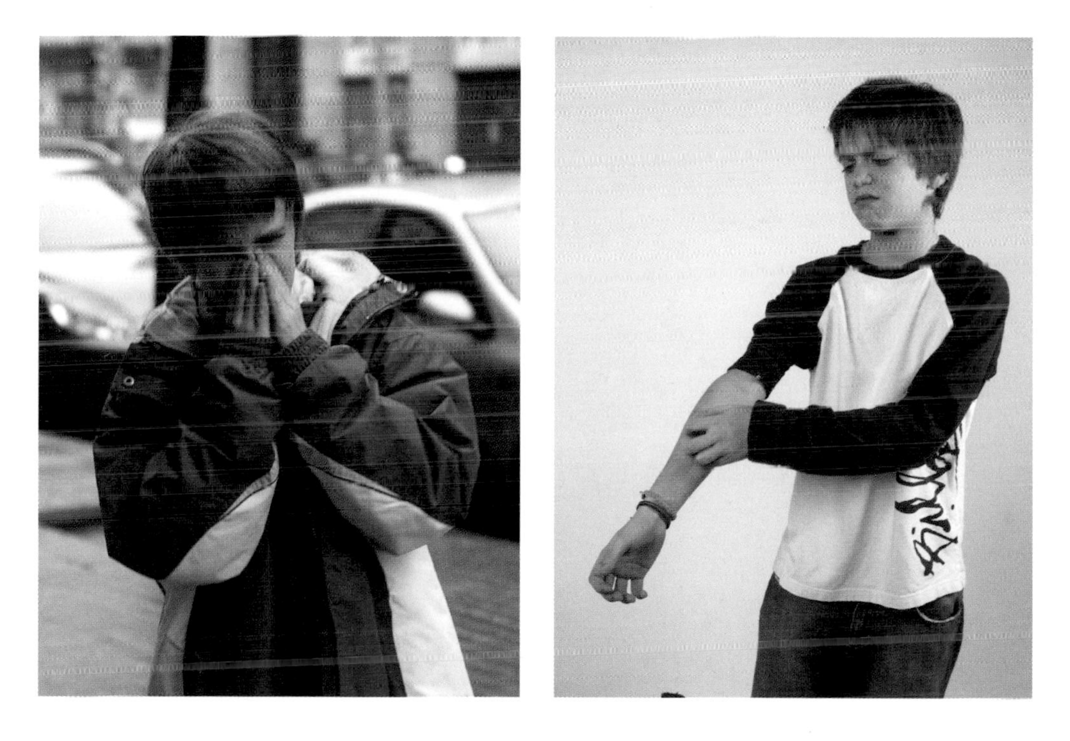

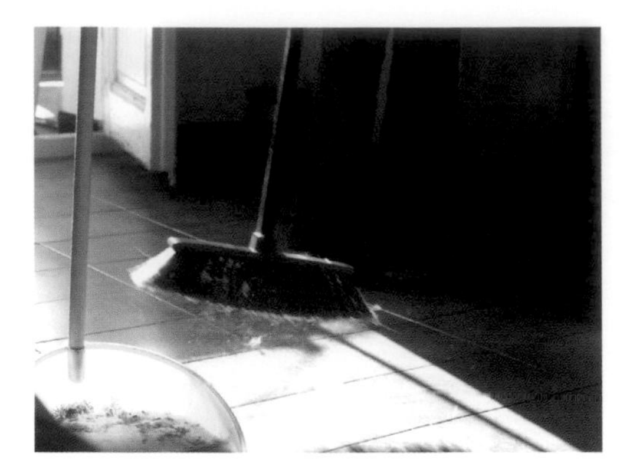

Urticaria

This is a common skin complaint, characterized by the sudden appearance of thick red rashes with sharp edges, in various sizes, which can be accompanied by itching. As urticaria gradually spreads over the body, parents often find it very alarming. It can be caused by eating certain foods (fish, seafood, walnuts, peanuts, or additives), contact with plants, medicines, animal saliva, insect bites, pollen, lacquers, viral infections, parasites, bacteria, or fungi, among others.

Allergic manifestations

Allergic rhinitis

Fur or feathers from pets and dust are the allergens most frequently associated with this complaint, although in many cases the reaction is triggered by the inhalation of pollen or fungal spores, or the consumption of certain foods. The symptoms of allergic rhinitis include sneezing, a constantly runny nose, and obstruction and itching in the nose. This last symptom makes children screw up their nose and rub it constantly.

Allergic conjunctivitis

The allergens responsible for this are the same ones that cause allergic rhinitis. It is characterized by red, itchy eyes with a watery discharge that can become purulent. Ocular cytology makes it possible to distinguish between allergic and infectious conjunctivitis.

Atopical dermatitis (Eczema)

This is an inflammatory skin complaint caused by a wide variety of foods, fabrics, chemical substances (such as detergents and soaps), and inhalants. It is characterized by extremely itchy, red skin, which may also be flaky and weepy and disfigured by crusts. Affected children tend to suffer from rhinitis or bronchial asthma at the same time. This allergic reaction starts in infancy, with small lesions on the face, which later extend to the neck, wrists, hands, and folds of the elbows and knees. Its onset frequently coincides with the introduction of new foods into a child's diet such as cow's milk, cereals, eggs, or citric fruit, although it is not always possible to establish a direct connection. This allergy tends to improve at the age of 5, thanks to the tendency of the skin to thicken and dry up.

Treating allergies

Prevention is the best cure, and this obviously involves avoiding the allergen to which a child is allergic, whenever it has been identified. This is not as easy as it sounds, however.

Anti-histamines. Anti-histamines block the histamine receptors, thereby preventing it from taking effect and preventing the main symptoms of allergies, such as sneezing, conjunctivitis, runny nose, etc. They have the additional advantage of acting against all types of allergies. The latest anti-histamines have no side-effects and are very effective; they are available in capsules, creams, nasal sprays, syrups, and eye drops. In short, anti-histamines are the most useful drugs on the market for treating the most troubling allergic symptoms.

Corticosteroids. Corticosteroids is also available in various forms: creams, lotions, nasal sprays, and eye drops. In the form of a nasal spray corticosteroids are recommended for the relief of symptoms of rhinitis. They are highly effective, but must be applied on a regular basis throughout the entire allergic period _ although they cannot be used for more than 3 consecutive months and should not be prescribed to children. Creams and lotions are prescribed for skin reactions.

Cromoglycates (cromolyn). Sodium cromoglycate and disodium cromoglycate are used prophylactically, so they need to be prescribed about a month before the allergy season. They do not prevent an allergic reaction once it has been triggered, but instead act against the degranulation of mastocytes and, therefore, the release of histamine.

Immunotherapy. In some very specific cases, an allergy specialist may consider immunotherapy appropriate. This is normally reserved for patients

Coping with allergens

- Use humidifiers and air-conditioning with anti-pollen filters.
- Avoid opening windows during car journeys.
- Keep windows closed in the early hours of the morning and the late afternoon, as these are the times of maximum pollination.
- Take a shower and change your clothes as soon as you arrive home (there may be pollen deposits on your hair and clothes).
- Take vacations in places and seasons in which the pollen count is low.
- Avoid irritants such as smoke, dust, aerosol sprays, and insecticides.
- Use a vacuum cleaner regularly (choose a model with an anti-mite filter).
- Air-conditioning systems must be enclosed or fitted with an air filter, which must be changed frequently (at least four times a year).
- To avoid breathing in the dust raised by cleaning, use a damp cloth, and also a damp cloth to protect your mouth and nose; you can even cover your entire head.
- Avoid any objects that gather dust, particularly in bedrooms, for example, carpets, curtains, rugs, upholstery, tablecloths, decorative items on walls, pictures, and books.
- Dispose of any mattresses, cushions, and covers containing material of animal or vegetable origin, such as wool, jute, hemp, vegetable fibers, hay, straw, or horsehair. These are all cozy nooks for mites.
- For the same reason, do not decorate a room with upholstered furniture or tapestries.
- Use latex or foam-rubber mattresses and cushions, and cover them with non-porous, synthetic materials that cannot be penetrated by mites.
- Use sheets and bedcovers that can be washed at more than 131 °F (55 °C); mites cannot survive this temperature.
- Do not allow pets to enter the sitting room or bedrooms.
- Groom pets regularly and make sure the places they use most are kept clean.

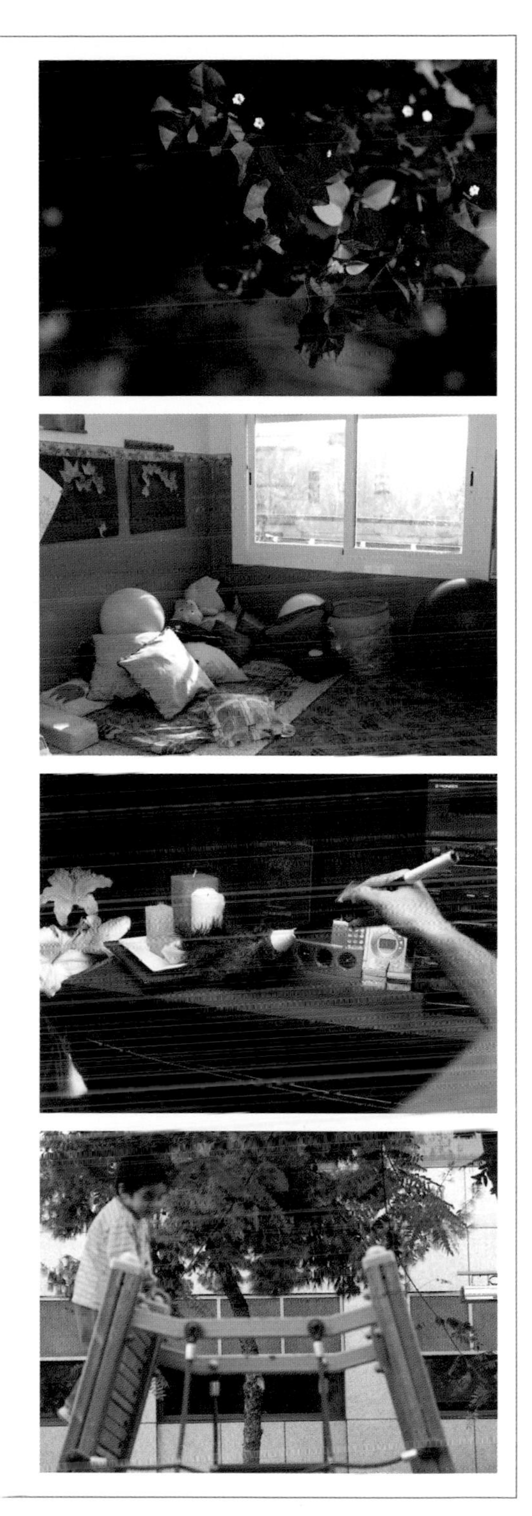

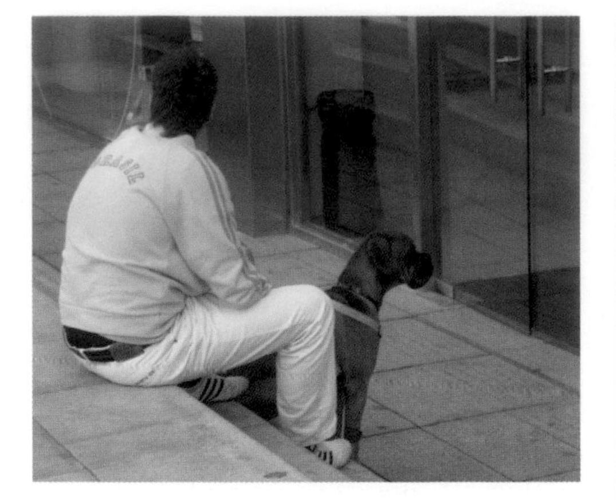

with severe allergies that do not respond to medication. It involves injecting increasingly greater amounts of the allergen to induce a degree of immunity against it. This is a long process with an inherent risk of anaphylaxis and bronchospasms immediately after the treatment.

Diagnosing an allergy

Two types of tests are used to determine whether a child has an allergy:

- **Skin tests.** Extracts of the substances to which the child is possibly allergic are applied to his skin in the form of drops, and then slight punctures are made on these points. This enables a tiny amount of the allergen to penetrate the skin, to see whether or not it produces a reaction. A reading is made after 15–20 minutes: those points where spots or marks have appeared correspond to substances to which the child is allergic.
- **Blood tests.** These are an essential complement to skin tests. They make it possible to not only confirm a diagnosis but also to quantify the intensity of the allergic sensitization.

A specific allergy is generally not hereditary, but the tendency to develop allergies often is. If both parents have allergies, it is probable that their children will also be affected by this tendency.

TYPE OF ALLERGY	POSSIBLE MANIFESTATIONS
To animals	Sneezing. Itchy, watery eyes. Asthma. Urticaria or localized erythema.
To a medicine	Erythema, urticaria, dizziness, breathing difficulties, anaphylactic shock.
To insect bites	Inflammation and reddening of the affected area, spots, itching, nausea, breathing difficulties, anaphylactic shock.
To dust mites	Rhinitis, asthma.
To food	Reddening of the skin, inflammation of the mucosa in the mouth, breathing difficulties, vomiting, anaphylactic shock.
To pollen	Sneezing, itching, burning skin, watery eyes, rhinitis, asthma.

respiratory diseases

The respiratory system is a complex network of hollow structures designed to transport atmospheric air, in appropriate conditions of humidity and temperature, to the alveolar sacs, where gases are dispersed on contact with the capillary vessels. In childhood, a host of (mainly infectious) disorders can affect any of these structures, including the ears, which can also be affected by a respiratory disease, on account of their relationship with the airways. Given the great frequency of such disorders, and their tendency to recur up to 6 or 8 times a year, it is worth understanding their main characteristics.

BREATHING

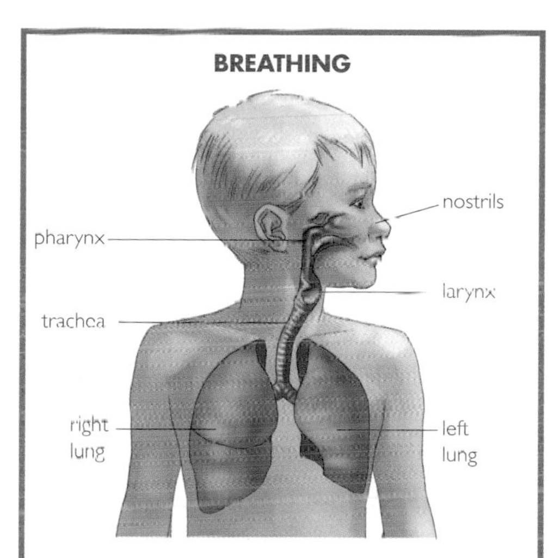

Breathing is an involuntary, automatic process that serves to extract oxygen from the air breathed in and expel waste gases through the air breathed out. Air is inhaled through the nose, where it is heated and moistened. It then goes on to the pharynx, continues through the larynx, and penetrates the trachea. Halfway up the chest, the trachea divides into two bronchial tubes which, in turn, divide first into secondary and tertiary bronchial tubes and, finally, into some 250,000 bronchioles. These lead to clusters of alveoli, small bags of air in which gases are dispersed in the blood.

Infection of the upper airways

Common cold

• This is one of the most common conditions found in children, and one that causes the most visits to the doctor and the most absences from school.

• It is triggered by a range of over 200 viruses (particularly the rhinovirus and the corona virus), which inflame the tissues or mucous membranes covering the upper airways.

• The symptoms of a cold appear two or 3 days after contact with the virus, and they can last for about one week.

• In babies, the symptoms are a blocked nose, fever, nervousness, insomnia, and occasionally vomiting and diarrhea.

• In older children, the symptoms are a blocked or runny nose, a sore throat, watery eyes, sneezing, a mild, dry cough, fever, generalized muscle pain, headache, and tiredness. The mucus is watery at first but then turns thick and yellowish.

The common cold is different from influenza, which is a more serious disease with a greater risk of complications.

As some of the symptoms can be similar, it is important to be able to differentiate the two illnesses:

Symptoms of a cold	Symptoms of flu
Low fever or normal temperature	**High fever**
Headache (on occasions)	Headache (invariably)
Blocked and runny nose	Nose blocked or unblocked
Sneezing	Sneezing (on occasions)
Mild, dry cough	Cough that often becomes severe
Mild pains and discomfort	Often severe pains and discomfort
Slight fatigue	Fatigue for several weeks
Sore throat	Sore throat (on occasions)
Normal level of energy	Extreme exhaustion

Some points of interest

- Most young children suffer from at least 6–8 colds a year – or even more, in the case of children who go to play school.
- After the age of 6, however, they occur less frequently.
- Adolescents catch around two to four colds a year.
- Colds occur most frequently in autumn and winter.

The increased incidence of colds in these seasons can be attributed to the fact that children spend more time in closed settings and in contact with other children and adults. Furthermore, many of the viruses responsible for colds flourish in chilly, dry environments, and cold snaps cause the nostrils to lose moisture, making them more vulnerable to infection.

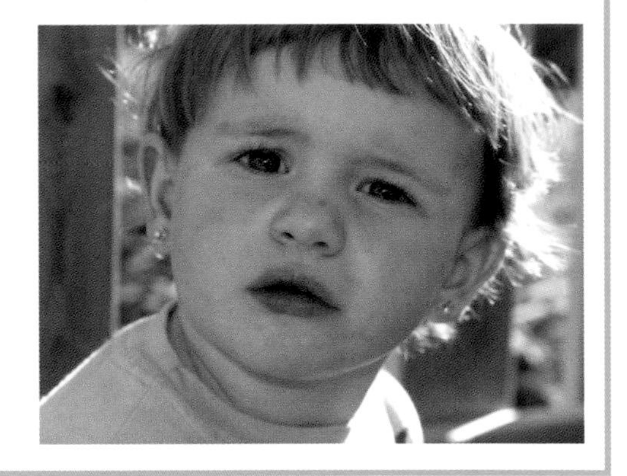

A nose wash with a saline solution and aspiration of nasal secretion are two of the most effective measures for treating a cold, even though they may cause a child discomfort.

Sinusitis

• This is an inflammatory process in the para nasal sinuses, a series of air cavities in the front of the head. These fill up with mucus, causing discomfort.

• Sinusitis is classified as acute, if it lasts for less than 3 weeks; sub-acute, if it lasts between 3 weeks and 3 months; or chronic, if it lasts for over 3 months.

• It is usually caused by a cold that has developed complications or failed to clear up properly.

• Sinusitis causes pain and local obstruction, catarrh, nasal congestion, fever, headache, and even dizziness and vertigo. The most sensitive diagnosis method is an X-ray of the para nasal sinuses.

Apart from treatment, it is important:

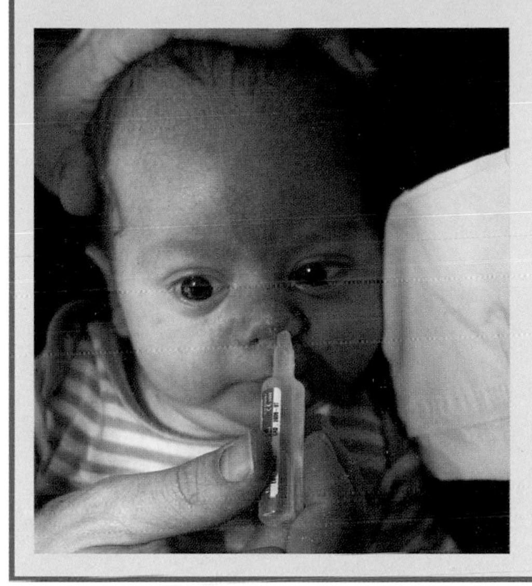

- To give your child plenty of fluids.
- To prevent him from coming into contact with tobacco smoke.
- To use a saline solution to moisten the nose.
- To aspirate the mucus in your child's noise to help him breathe.
- To use a cold-steam humidifier in his bedroom.
- The use of analgesics such as paracetamol and ibuprofen can be effective, but you should always consult your doctor before giving them. Because of its possible association with Reye's syndrome, a serious neurological disorder, your child must never be given aspirin without a doctor's prior approval.

Pharyngitis and tonsillitis

• Acute inflammation of the mucosa in the pharynx and/or tonsils, characterized by a sore throat that can be very painful. It is most commonly caused by a viral infection (45–60%), although it can also be of bacterial origin (15%) or have no known cause (25–40%).

SINUSITIS

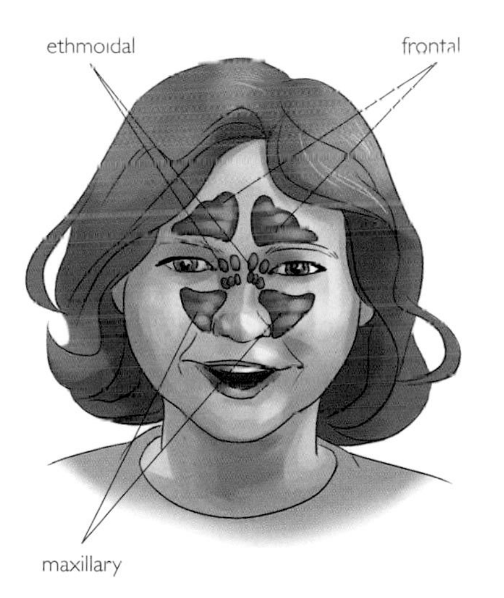

• Viral pharyngitis causes a sore throat, a dry, itchy cough, difficulty in swallowing, and, in some cases, fever with general discomfort. If the latter symptoms are intense or last for more than 3 days, they may be of bacterial origin, so you should consult a doctor to ascertain the cause of the infection and what specific antibiotic treatment is needed.

• Another possible diagnosis is infectious mononucleosis, a special variant of pharyngitis of viral origin. This requires much the same treatment as a common cold, but you should consult your doctor, who will decide whether antibiotics are required. As this is an infectious disease that is transmitted via nasal secretion and saliva, it may affect several members of the family.

• Bacterial pharyngitis, frequently caused by the hemolytic streptococcus, is characterized by an extremely sore throat, difficulty in swallowing, high fever, a layer of pus covering the tonsils and pharynx, and swollen neck glands (cervical adenopathy). The severity of its potential complications, which include rheumatic fever, kidney disorders, and scarlet fever, means that any suspicion of this disease calls for antibiotic treatment with penicillin (or its derivatives) or erythromycin (an alternative in cases of allergy to penicillin). It may be necessary to perform cultures of the pharyngeal secretions before starting antibiotic treatment, in order to identify the bacterium responsible for the outbreak.

Infectious mononucleosis

- This is a viral infection caused by the Epstein-Barr virus, characterized by fever, pharyngitis, swollen neck glands, and an enlarged spleen. It affects children, adolescents, and young adults.
- It is mainly passed on via saliva, which is why it is popularly known as kissing disease.
- Its incubation period (without symptoms) usually lasts between one and 2 weeks. The most noteworthy symptoms are fever, listlessness, a sore throat, muscle pains, and loss of appetite.
- The most intense symptoms (fever, swollen glands, and enlarged spleen) can last for around 10 days, but the listlessness and general feeling of being off-color can go on for 2 or 3 months.
- As no specific treatment is available, the only option is to take general measures similar to those recommended for a cold: drinking plenty of fluids, analgesics, and rest. If there is a sharp pain in the upper left part of the abdomen (the site of the spleen), a doctor must be consulted urgently.

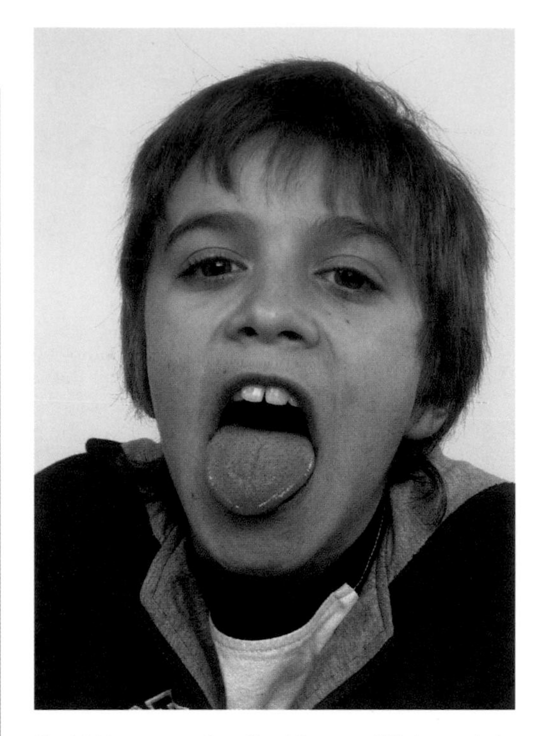

If a child has repeatedly suffered from tonsillitis in a period of 2 years (3–5 outbreaks), a specialist may consider the possibility of removing the tonsils, especially if there is a persistent presence of beta hemolytic streptococcus in cultures, despite taking appropriate antibiotic treatment.

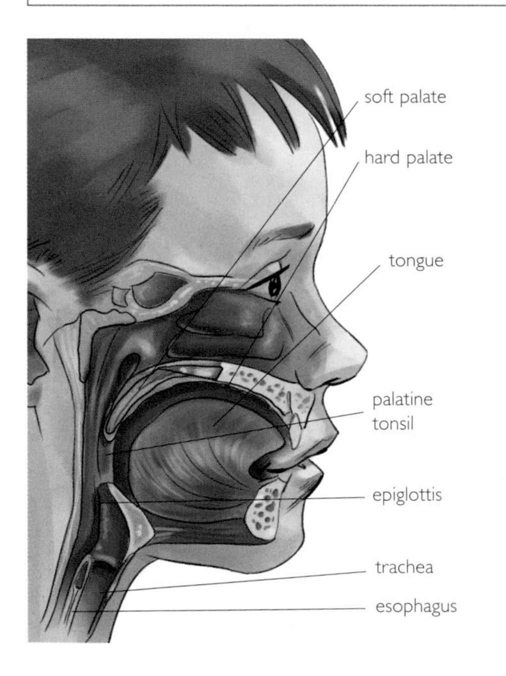

Tonsillectomy (surgical removal of the tonsils)

• The tonsils are 2 glandular structures situated on either side of the soft palate. They are made up of tissue that manufactures antibodies against infection (lymphoid tissue) and can be seen with the naked eye at the back of a child's mouth, by the neck, if his tongue is held down.

• When tonsillitis is recurrent and does not respond to medicines, the tonsils can be removed. This operation is normally performed in conjunction with removal of the adenoids.

• Although each case will be evaluated by a doctor on its individual merits, tonsillectomy is generally recommended:

– When hypertrophy of the tonsils (excessively large tonsils) is observed. In these cases, the tonsils are so big that they impede breathing, cause sleep apnea, and even make it impossible to swallow food.

– When a child has repeated throat infections.

OUTER, MIDDLE, AND INNER EAR

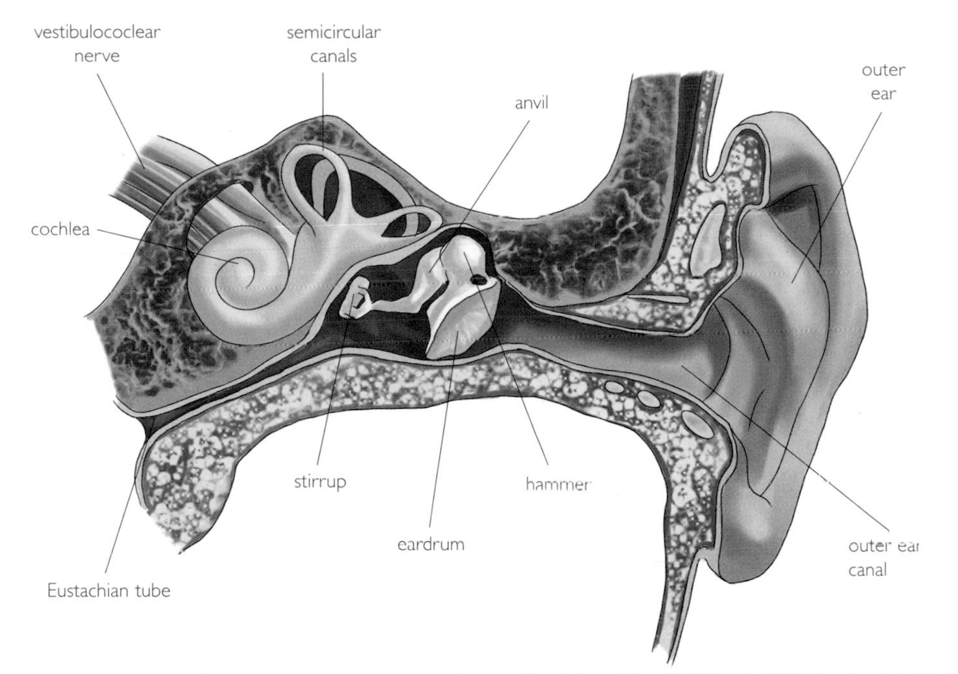

– When abscesses have appeared on the tonsils, as these tend to recur and are potentially serious.

– When tonsillitis causes feverish convulsions.

– When the size of the tonsils encourages the appearance of rhinitis and ear infections.

Inflammation of the middle ear

• The middle ear is connected to the pharynx via the Eustachian tube; this means that infections in the upper airways often give rise to complications in the middle ear. In some cases, however, these can become infected of their own accord.

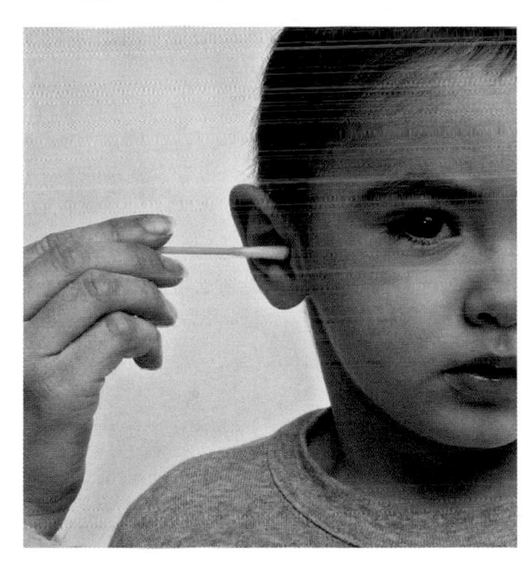

Lower airways

The lower airways start in the trachea and divide into the right and left bronchial tubes. These divide up in their turn to create a kind of tree which ends in the bronchioles, which open on to the alveolar sacs, the last part of the respiratory system. Here gases (oxygen and carbon anhydride) are exchanged with blood. The clinical picture varies according to how high up in the chest the infection occurs; the most frequent problems in childhood are acute bronchitis, typical and atypical pneumonia, and bronchiolitis.

• The middle ear becomes inflamed when the mucosa covering it produces a lot of mucus, which is trapped inside the Eustachian tube, causing intense pain and hearing difficulties (deafness in the most serious cases, if the treatment is inadequate). This inflammation can also be accompanied by fever, headache, and listlessness.

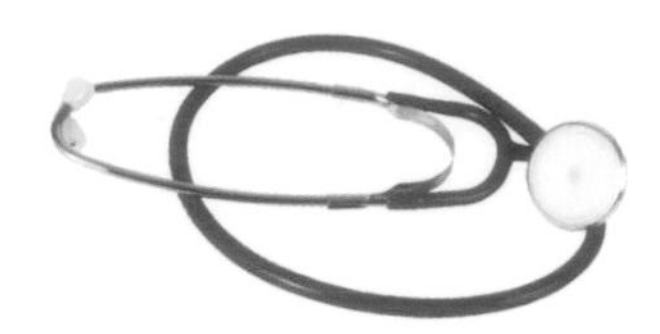

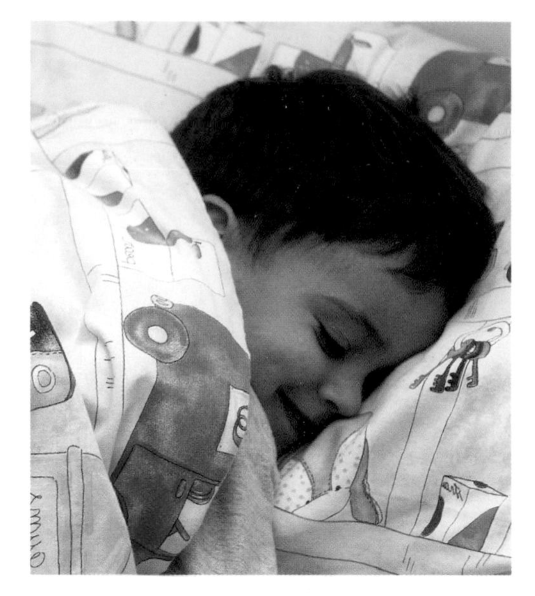

• The treatment focuses on eradicating the cause:

– If the infection persists, it should be treated with antibiotics, according to your doctor's advice.

– If the cause is an allergy, vaccinations and treatment with anti-histamines may be required, as well as environmental controls.

– If the adenoids are creating an obstruction by compressing the Eustachian tube, they need to be removed.

– If the inflammation has a number of causes and treatment proves difficult, the eardrum might need to be drained, using an implanted plastic tube, to ensure that the pressure of the liquid does not impair hearing.

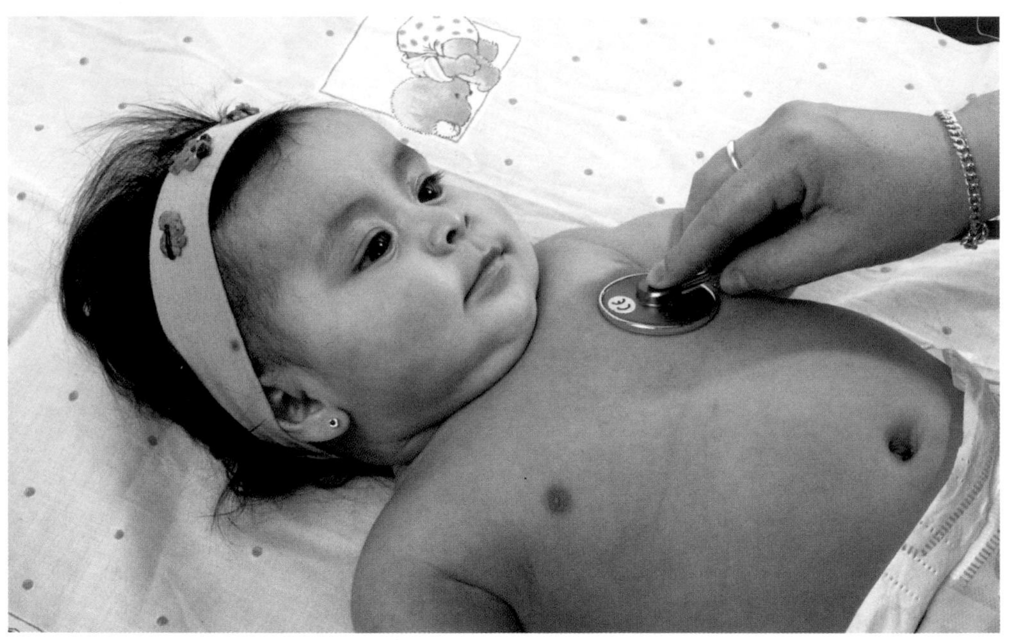

The clinical picture of acute bronchitis comprises a cough, with or without expectoration (mucous secretion eliminated by coughing), and fever. A physical examination does not normally reveal any abnormalities, and the same is true of a chest X-ray.

Infection of the lower airways

Acute bronchitis

• Inflammatory process of the tracheo-bronchial tree, generally complemented by an infection of the upper airways, or a complication of the latter.

• This is basically viral in origin, but can also be bacterial in a few cases (from Mycoplasma pneumoniae or Bordetella pertussis, which is responsible for whooping cough).

• The treatment is symptomatic, i.e. it focuses on the cough and fever. In some cases, particularly in allergic children, there can be a degree of bronchial obstruction, calling for the use of bronchodilators. Antibiotics should only be added if there is suspicion of bacterial infection, you should follow the advice of your doctor in this respect.

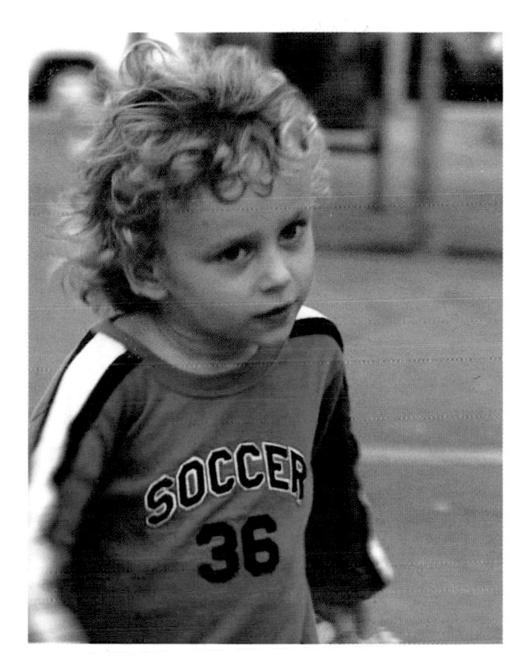

> Infections of the lower airways are of viral origin in 95% of cases in children aged between 4 months and 5 years. The most frequent culprits are the Respiratory syncytial virus, the Adenovirus, and the flu (Influenza) virus.
>
> Although viruses are still the most common cause of infection in children aged from 6–16, 30% of cases of pneumonia in this group are caused by the bacteria *Streptococcus pneumoniae* and *Mycoplasma pneumoniae*.

Whooping cough is caused by the Bordatella pertussis bacterium and is one of the most contagious of all childhood diseases. It is usually passed on as a result of direct contact with an infected person, or the inhalation of infectious particles ejected by coughing.

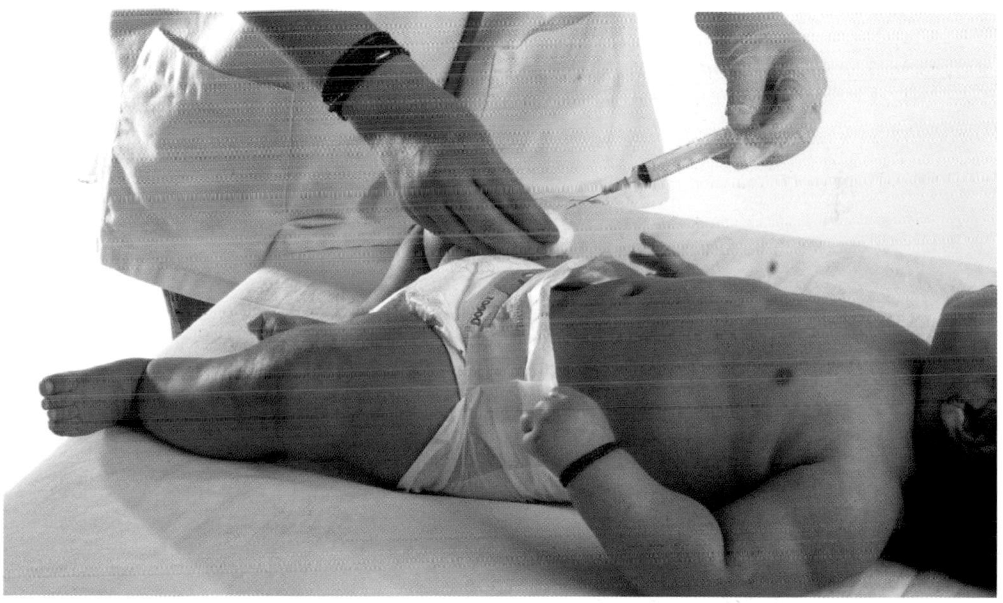

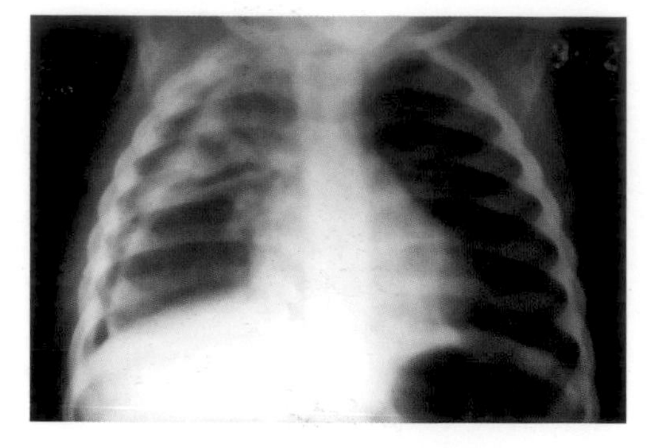

Pneumonia is an infection caused by the growth of micro-organisms inside the alveoli; these cause inflammation and lung damage. The inflammatory reaction creates secretions in the alveoli, which are clearly visible in an X-ray of the thorax.

Whooping cough

This is an infectious and contagious disease caused by the bacterium Bordetella pertussis.

• After an incubation period of 8–10 days, the child begins to show signs of bronchitis, such as coughing, particularly at night.

• About one week later, the catarrh goes through a convulsive period, characterized by a series of coughing fits, accompanied by a choking sensation. If one of these fits occurs while a child is eating, it may make him vomit and even cause a lung hemorrhage in serious cases. The cough gradually gives way to deep, noisy breathing.

The clinical picture of pneumonia can vary according to the type of germ involved.

• The complications depend almost entirely on the intensity of the attacks, which can cause pulmonary emphysema. In some cases, when the coughing fits are accompanied by vomiting, a child can become undernourished, making the situation worse and delaying his recovery.

• Infection is produced by direct contact with an infected patient, through the secretions expelled by coughing or sneezing. Although whooping cough can affect people of any age, it is most common in small children.

• Whooping cough can be prevented by means of a vaccination, which is administered in conjunction with vaccinations against tetanus and diphtheria (DTaP vaccine) at the ages of 2, 4, and 6 months, with boosters at the age of 18 months and 6 years.

Infant pneumonia

• Pneumonia occurs when a pathogenic micro-organism invades the tissue of the lung, through aspiration, via the nose or pharynx, inhalation, or the bloodstream.

• Under normal conditions, the airways are colonized by bacteria (bacterial flora). These bacteria do not reach the lung, as a result of immunological cells and the coughing reflex, activated by ciliate cells responsible for expelling any foreign bodies. If these

CHARACTERISTICS	TYPICAL PNEUMONIA	ATYPICAL PNEUMONIA (viral, mycoplasmic, chlamydophylics)
Onset	Often sudden	Usually gradual
Muscle pain–headache–discomfort from light	Mild	Severe
Shivering	Frequent	Rare
Toxic picture	Significant	Slight to moderate
Cough	Purulent expectoration or hemorrhagic sputum	Coughing fits, with merely a little mucous sputum or no expectoration
Sharp pain in the back	Frequent	Rare
Fever	Over 38.9%	Under 38.9%

Types of pneumonia

- **Aspiration pneumonia.** This is caused by the aspiration of stomach contents into the lung. This can occur in situations involving loss of consciousness, coma, etc.
- **Non-pneumococcic bacterial pneumonia.** Most pneumonia contracted outside a hospital is caused by pneumococcus, but many other bacteria can have the same effect, sometimes with a great potential for complications: Mycoplasma pneumoniae, Coxiella burnetti (Q fever), Chlamydia psittachi (psytacosis), Klebsiella pneumoniae, Legionella pneumoniae, etc.
- **Viral pneumonia (pneumonitis).** Many viruses can cause pneumonia (although in these cases the disease is normally referred to as pneumonitis): influenza, chicken pox, cytomegalovirus (CMV), Respiratory syncytial virus, etc.
- **Pneumonia caused by protozoa.** The most serious of these is triggered by Pneumocystitis carinii, which particularly affects patients with AIDS and other immunodepressive diseases.
- **Eosinophyllic pneumonia.** Strictly speaking, this is not really pneumonia, as there is no infection or infestation. Its variants include acute pulmonary eosinophyllia (Löffler's syndrome) and chronic eosinophyllic pneumonia.

defense mechanisms are weakened, the germs penetrate the lungs and cause infections.

• The symptoms of pneumonia are variable. In some cases, they conform to what is known as typical pneumonia, distinguished by the appearance, several hours or 2–3 days beforehand, of coughing with purulent expectoration (sometimes containing blood), chest pain, and fever with shivering. Pneumonia caused by pneumococcus usually follows these lines. Other types of pneumonia, classified as atypical, are marked by a more gradual onset of symptoms, such as slight fever, joint and muscle pains, tiredness and headache, a dry cough without any expectoration, and less severe chest pain. Some patients may present mild digestive symptoms, such as nausea, vomiting, and diarrhea. These symptoms are particularly characteristic of pneumonia caused by Mycoplasma, Coxiella, and Chlamydia.

• Any suspicion of pneumonia will lead a doctor to request a chest X-ray, to establish a diagnosis. If

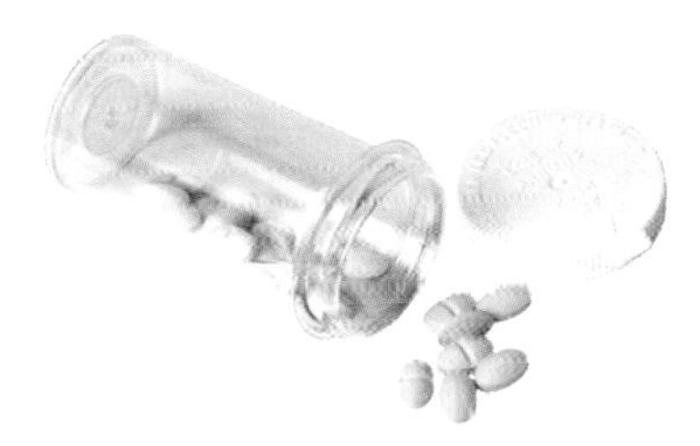

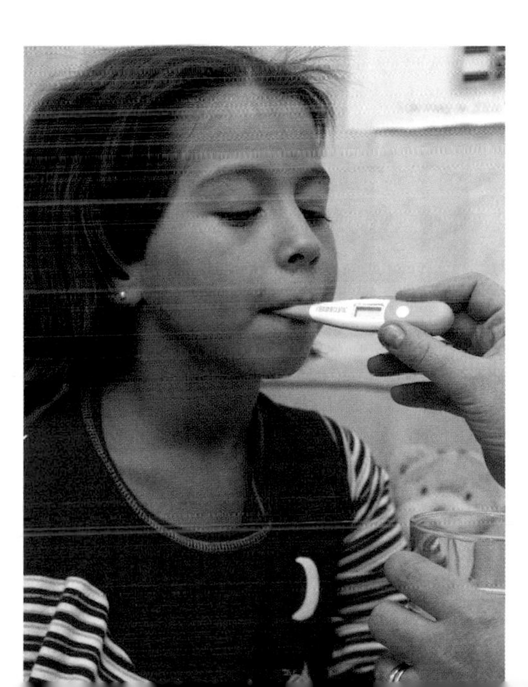

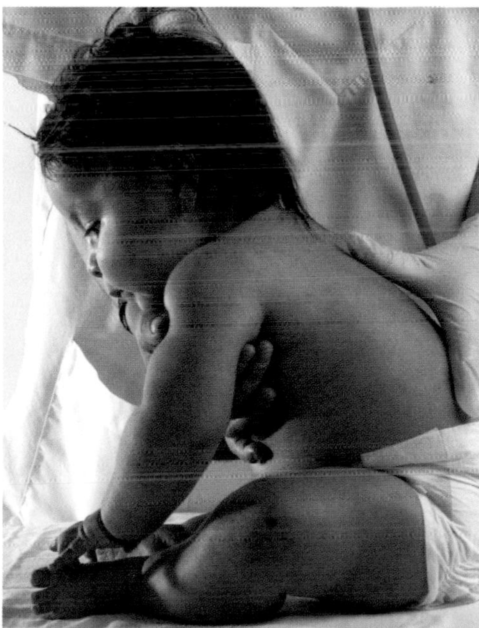

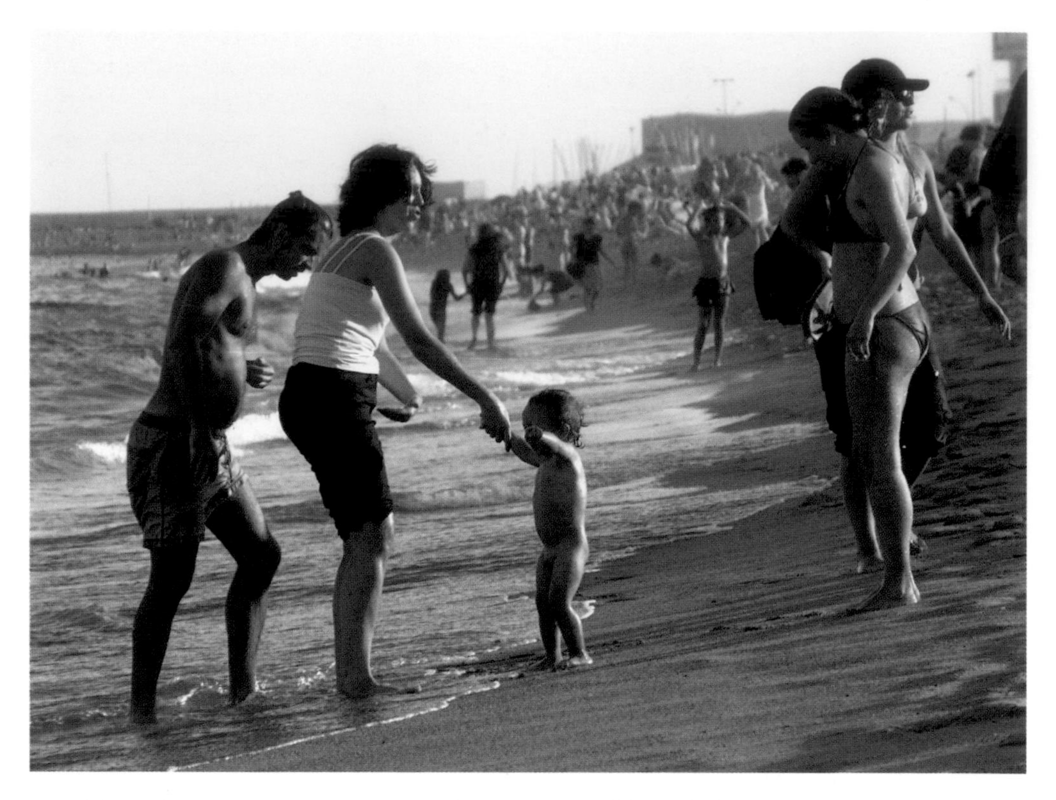

Acute inflammation of the outer ear is very frequent in summer, when children and adolescents flock to swimming pools and beaches.

pneumonia is confirmed, treatment must begin as soon as possible. Bacterial pneumonia requires the use of antibiotics.

• A large range of antibiotics are on offer, and the decision on which one to use will depend on the bacterium in question, the seriousness of the pneumonia, and the characteristics of the sick child. There is usually no need to identify the particular micro-organism responsible for the pneumonia, unless it is serious or fails to respond to treatment. In these cases, more tests may be needed, and the child is often admitted to hospital to ensure adequate monitoring and treatment.

Bronchiolitis

• This is an acute viral infection of the lower respiratory tract that can affect small children. After a bout of catarrh and a slight fever, the child starts to have difficulty in breathing, audibly wheezing and making crackling noises, and his cough becomes stronger and more persistent. There may also be retraction of the ribs and in extreme case the skin may turn blue because of obstruction of the airways.

• Bronchiolitis tends to appear in epidemics, especially in children aged under 18 months, with the maximum incidence being found in babies aged under 6 months.

No effective treatment is available for bronchiolitis. The use of corticosteroids are a subject of much debate and antibiotics are only prescribed in cases of additional bacterial infection. Drugs can be used to lower the temperature and improve the ventilation of the lungs, while serious cases that require hospitalization call for ribavirin, an antiviral medicine sometimes used in the form of an aerosol.

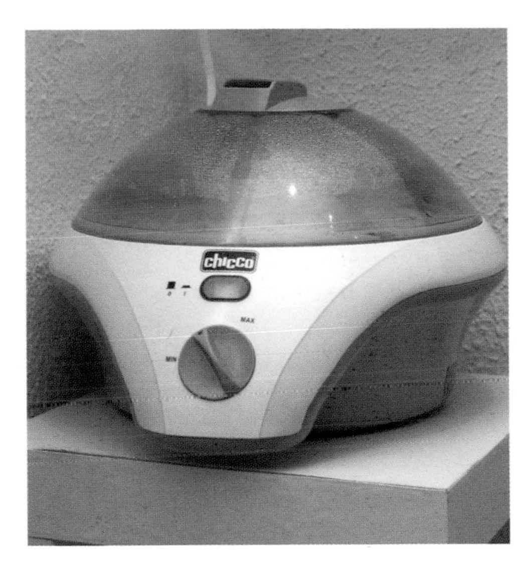

• The annual incidence during the first year of life is calculated as being 11 cases/100 children.

• The most frequent causes are the respiratory syncytial virus and the para-influenza 3 virus.

• Bronchiolitis spreads as a result of direct contact. The virus lurks in tiny drops in the breath and is easily passed on by sneezing and coughing. An affected child can disseminate the virus for 3–8 days, while the incubation period ranges from 2–8 days.

• The children most vulnerable to bronchiolitis (and the most serious cases) are babies born prematurely or with a congenital heart disease or immune deficiency

Other respiratory infections

Acute inflammation of the outer ear

• This affects the outer ear canal and is characterized by pain and itching.

• Excessive production of wax, an earful of water, or damage to the outer ear canal (through using cotton buds or earplugs) increase the likelihood of an infection.

• This is characterized by earache (which increases if the outer ear is touched or food is being chewed), itching, and secretion from the ear.

• Treatment involves a series of general measures, such as alleviation of pain with analgesics like paracetamol, aspirin, ibuprofen, or codeine, and the use of an antibiotic (ciproflaxicin, gentamicin, etc.) combined with an anti-inflammatory drug.

• If the eardrum is affected or the outer ear or glands are swollen, a backup with an oral antibiotic is necessary (amoxycillin/clavulanic acid, cefuroxim, etc.).

• It is not unusual for these problems to reoccur, particularly in summer. To avoid them, it is advisable to take the following precautions:

• Dissuade your child from putting his head underwater when swimming.

• Do not give him a shower or wash his hair without protecting his ears.

• Do not insert earplugs or cotton wool in his ears, as they retain moisture.

• Do not use cotton swabs, as these can damage the outer ear canal.

Laryngitis, epiglottitis, and croup

• This consists of an inflammation caused by infection of structures in the larynx.

• Laryngitis is particularly prevalent among children and is usually caused by viruses.

• A variant known as epiglottitis involves a swiftly expanding inflammation that can totally block the airway and prove fatal in the most serious cases. The main causal agent is the Haemophilus influenzae type B.

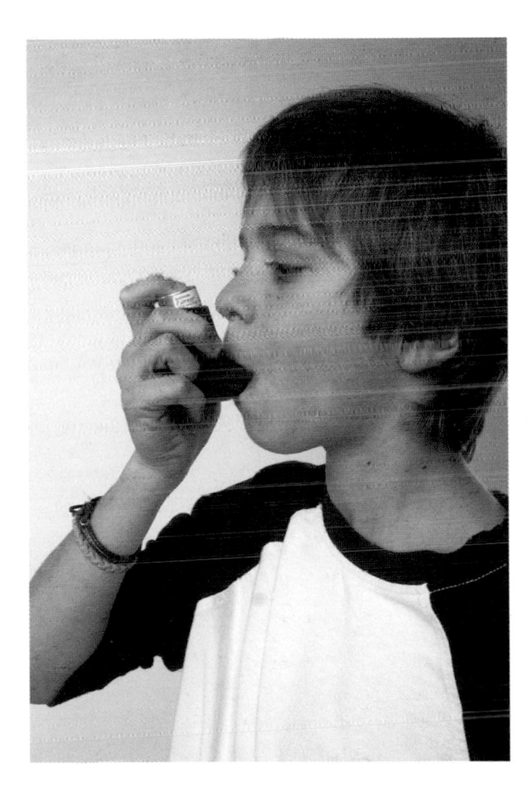

• Whistling in the larynx is one of the characteristic signs of this ailment; this is caused by difficulty in breathing resulting from the inflammation of the larynx and trachea, which prevents air from passing through the vocal cords. This symptom can also be triggered by various viral and bacterial diseases, chemical agents (caustics, irritating gases), physical stimuli (gases or hot liquids), or allergies (angiodema or angioneurotic edema).

• Croup is the most common cause of laryngeal whistling in children aged between 1 and 5. It consists of an inflammation that is generally of viral origin and leads to noisy and laborious breathing. Spasmodic croup often appears suddenly in the early morning: the child wakes up with difficulty in breathing and a very distinctive cough, similar in sound to a barking dog. This situation frequently occurs after the appearance of symptoms of catarrh or a cold; it is most common in autumn and winter, although this does not mean that it cannot arise at other times in the year.

If a child's difficulty in breathing is not too severe, you can try putting him in a bathroom full of steam for 20 minutes. More serious cases, however, require an immediate visit to an emergency room to establish a diagnosis and take the necessary steps as urgently as possible.

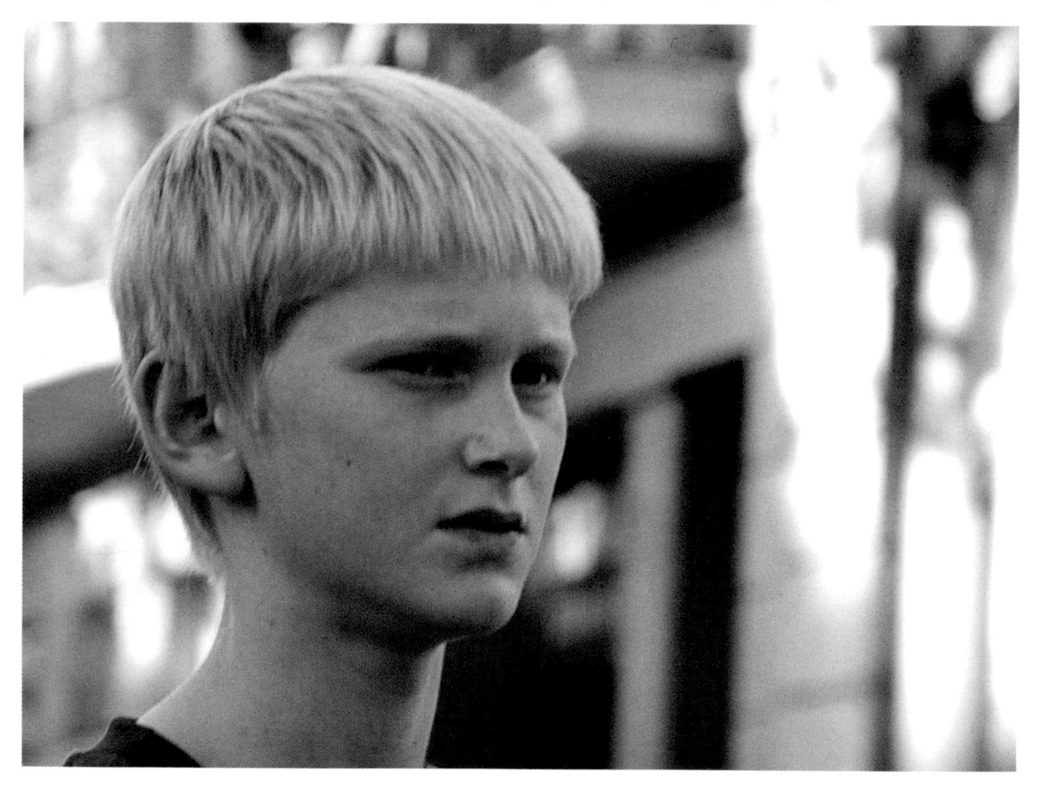

intestinal and urological disorders

A number of disorders, of varying origin and severity, manifest themselves through gastro-intestinal symptoms; for example, a urinary infection and tonsillitis can both be camouflaged by a complaint in the digestive system. As the symptoms involved are so similar, it is extremely difficult for parents to differentiate between colic from mild food poisoning and hepatitis, or between a urinary infection and appendicitis. The possibility of this confusion can lead to a disorder being over-dramatized or, at the other extreme, underestimated; both cases can result in an inappropriate reaction and, maybe, an untimely delay in treatment.

Intestinal and urological disorders

Food poisoning

• Food poisoning and summertime complaints customarily caused by salmonella are the types of gastroenteritis that most often result in visits to hospital emergency rooms.

• Gastroenteritis is a disease that affects the stomach and the intestines; it is caused by a bacterial or viral infection.

• This infection can be contracted after contact with an infected person – it can even take on epidemic proportions – or through the consumption of polluted water or food that has gone off.

• In both gastroenteritis and salmonellosis the symptoms generally appear 1 or 3 days after infection; they include diarrhea and vomiting, fever and stomach cramps.

Salmonellosis is a disease caused by bacteria from the Salmonella group, which live naturally in the intestines of both animals and human beings. The foods most frequently involved in this infection are raw or lightly cooked eggs (mayonnaise, whisked whites, soups or milk with egg yolk), undercooked poultry, and badly refrigerated or stored produce.

• The high-risk groups are children, elderly people, and sick people, who are all vulnerable on account of their propensity for dehydration, which can intensify gastroenteritis.

• It is important to take into account these preventive measures, especially during the summer months:

– Take care with eggs and dishes containing them: mayonnaise, salads, sauces, flans, and desserts.

– Salads and raw fruit or vegetables should be washed.

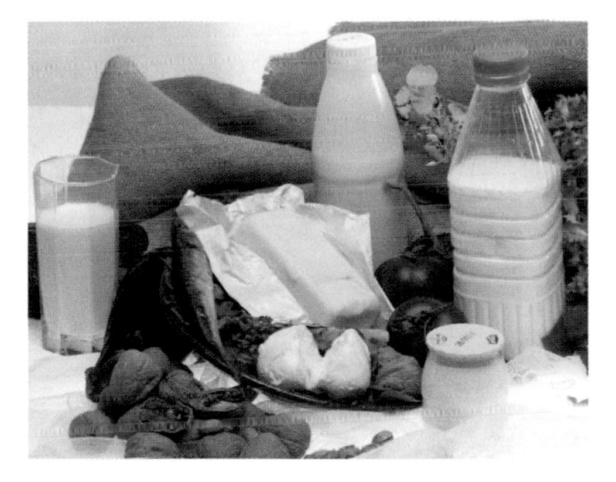

Botulism often occurs owing to poorly conserved produce, or homemade preserves made with equipment that has not been sterilized properly. It can also be caught from fresh fruit and vegetables grown in soil contaminated with Clostridium spores

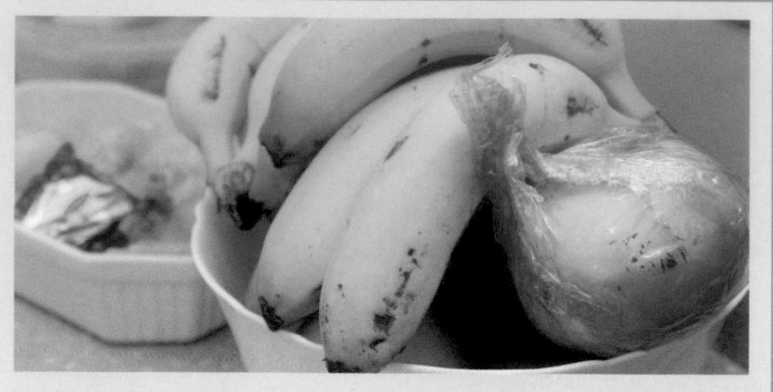

– If you are eating out, make sure that any poultry and fish have been properly cooked and refrigerated.

– Buy seafood from trustworthy sources.

– Take care with raw fish, sausages, and cold meats.

– A child's feeding bottle should be sterilized and kept meticulously clean.

– Drinking water should be bottled, or boiled beforehand.

Botulism

• This is an infectious disease caused by the toxin of the Clostridium botulinum bacillus, which results in paralysis of the nervous system. This can appear in 3 forms: food-borne botulism (consumption of food contaminated with the toxin); infant botulism (the micro-organisms colonize the intestine, where they release the toxin, which is absorbed and gives rise to symptoms); and wound botulism (colonization of a wound and subsequent germination of the Clostridium spores).

• The most frequent symptoms are a dry mouth, double vision and difficulty in seeing close up, and inability to swallow and speak.

• Abdominal symptoms such as nausea, vomiting, cramps, and diarrhea can also appear prior to, or at the same time as, the symptoms mentioned above.

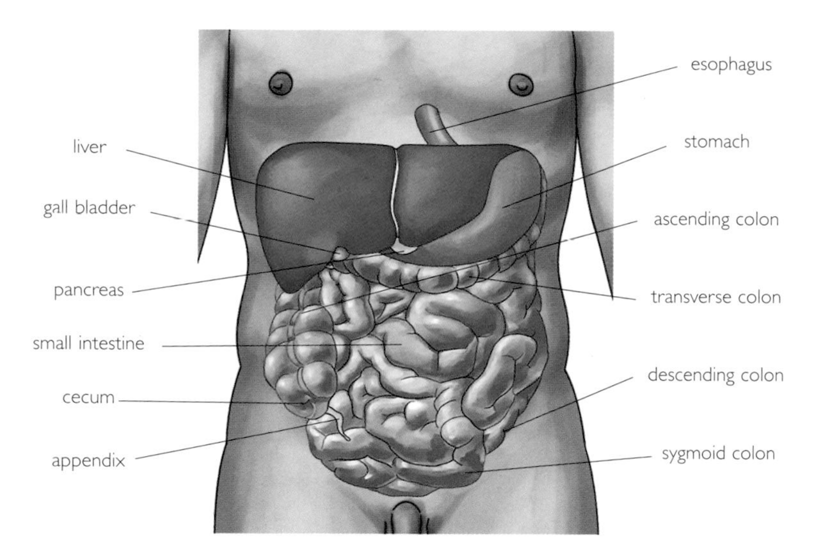

The abdomen can be divided into 9 regions that help a doctor determine the possible origin of a disorder, in accordance with the symptoms and physical examination.

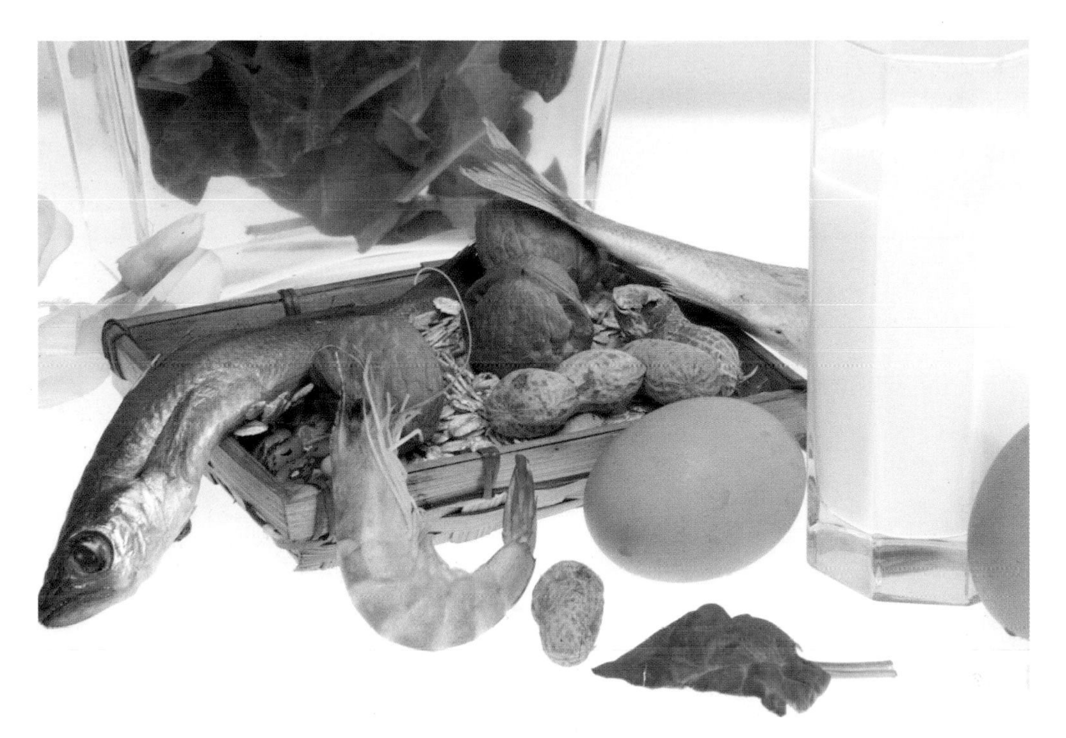

Acute and chronic abdominal pain, colic. Abdominal pain appears frequently in children, in a variety of forms and over varying lengths of time. It can have several causes:

– An acute pain (one that has recently appeared), may be caused by:

– Acute gastroenteritis.

– If abdominal pain strikes suddenly in babies, accompanied by crying, bent legs, pallor, listlessness, and vomiting or feces with blood, a doctor must be consulted immediately. It may only be the result of colic, but a medical opinion is needed to ascertain the exact cause.

– Accumulation of gases (meteorism).

– Appendicitis. A constant pain is complemented by fever, vomiting, and constipation; the pain gradually becomes concentrated in the lower right area of the abdomen.

– If it is accompanied by urinary symptoms and/or pain in the lumbar region, as well as fever, it can indicate a urinary infection (cystitis, pyelonephritis).

– Other causes: pancreatitis, peritonitis. In these cases, pain is accompanied by high fever, a very hard abdomen, and, overall, a very poor physical condition.

• When the abdominal pain becomes chronic (i.e. it recurs several times a month), once again there is a number of possible causes:

– It can be related to an irritated colon, especially in an excitable and temperamental child.

– It can also be a result of recurring pancreatitis, kidney or gall-bladder problems, colic, etc.

In cases of severe abdominal pain appearing for the first time, the doctor will decide, on the basis

Situations with abdominal pain that require urgent treatment

- Abdominal pain with fever and nausea (appendicitis, diverticulitis).
- Abdominal pain with nausea, fever, and diarrhea or constipation (intestinal obstruction).
- Abdominal pain with a hard or flat stomach (peritonitis).
- Abdominal pain with vomiting or diarrhea that contain blood.
- Persistent pain in the upper abdomen, with vomiting (pancreatitis).

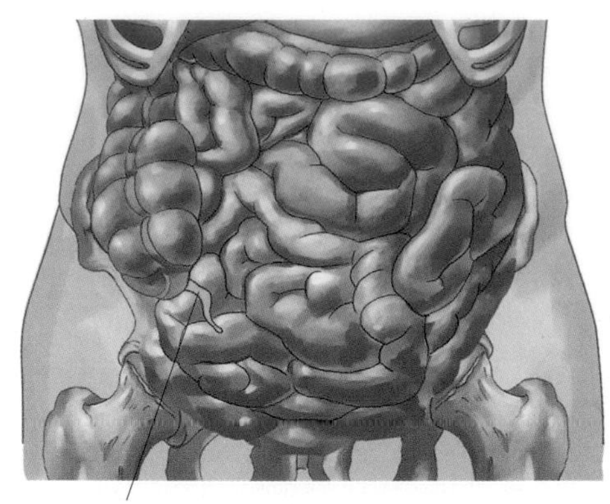

appendix

of a simple examination and the child's medical history, whether it is a question of an emergency requiring surgery, such as appendicitis, or simply a transitory disorder. Sometimes, however, it is necessary to monitor the situation for several hours before the correct diagnosis can be made.

Appendicitis

• Of all the common gastrointestinal disorders in the first 10 years of life, acute appendicitis is one of the most frequent.

• The appendix is situated very close to the abdominal entrails, particularly the intestine, which is covered by a coating called the peritoneum. Inflammation that starts in the appendix can spread quickly throughout the abdominal cavity to trigger peritonitis, which is serious and potentially life-threatening.

• The outstanding symptom of appendicitis is pain, which may not be very specific at first but eventually focuses on the lower right abdomen

Appendicitis is an inflammation of a structure linked to the initial portion of the large intestine (cecum): the appendix, situated in the region known as the right iliac fossa (the lower right area of the abdomen).

(iliac fossa). This pain can be either continuous or intermittent. The child may pull up his right leg to try to relieve it, but do not allow him to touch the painful area, which may be hard. He may also vomit or experience nausea (on occasions, prior to the pain). Other symptoms can include fever, headache, discomfort from light and noise, bad breath, and a smooth tongue.

Recommendations

• Do not give any medicines to ease the pain.

• Do not give your child any food or drink, as the vomiting could become more severe, heightening the intestinal tension still further.

• Allow the child to rest, without walking or moving.

• Ice can be applied to the painful area, but without exerting pressure.

• Consult a doctor as soon as possible.

Hepatitis

• This is an inflammation of the liver, usually associated with a viral infection. It can attain various degrees of severity, and even lead to the destruction of liver tissue.

• There is a wide range of viruses that can possibly cause hepatitis in children:

– Hepatitis viruses: 6 main types of hepatitis virus have been identified, including hepatitis A, B, C, D, E, and G.

– Cytomegalovirus (CMV), belonging to the herpes family; it can be passed from one person to another.

– Epstein-Barr virus (EBV), the virus most commonly associated with infectious mononucleosis.

– Herpes simplex virus (HSV), which mainly affects the face, the skin from the waist up, and the genitals.

– Varicella-zoster virus (VZV), also known as chicken pox, one complication that might arise from chicken pox is hepatitis.

– Enteroviruses: a group of viruses often found in children, such as the coxsackie virus, aphthous fever, and the echoviruses.

– Rubella (German measles), a rash caused by a virus from the rubivirus group.

– Parvovirus, often called the fifth disease, characterized by a facial rash that makes the cheeks turn red.

• Hepatitis A is the most common type of hepatitis found in children; it is caused by the virus of the same name. This type of hepatitis is normally propagated via oral-fecal contact or through food or water contaminated by feces containing the virus. Hepatitis A can also be passed on by sharing utensils used by an infected person.

Good hygiene is the key to the prevention of the spread of many diseases, including hepatitis.

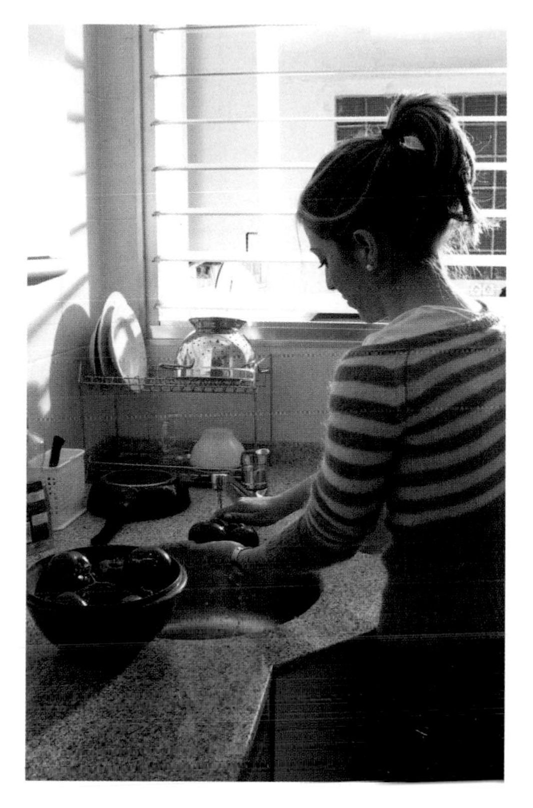

• Its symptoms include those similar to flu:
– Fever, nausea, vomiting, diarrhea.
– Loss of appetite, listlessness, pain or discomfort in the abdomen, joints, and muscles.
– Itchy, red spots on the skin.
– Dark urine and jaundice (yellow skin and eyes).
– The doctor will arrive at a diagnosis on the basis of the child's past history and laboratory tests. Ultrasound or hepatic biopsy are recommended in certain cases that do not correspond with the most usual forms of hepatitis.

Intestinal parasites

• Intestinal parasites are organisms that take advantage of nutrients in the human body to live in the gastrointestinal tract. Many such parasites can cause symptoms in the body, but, for the purposes of simplicity, they can be divided into 2 main groups:
– Protozoans, which are microscopic (Amoeba, Giardia, and Criptosporidium), or metazoans, which are worms, such as roundworms (oxyurides, ascaris, triocephalus, Ancylostoma, Necator, strongiloids, and Toxocara).
–The symptoms caused by parasites depend on the organism responsible – on many occasions they cause no discomfort at all. Protozoan parasites cause predominantly intestinal symptoms (diarrhea, distension, and abdominal pain); in contrast, the metazoans produce not only these symptoms, but they can also give rise to general discomfort or problems in other organs (weakness, pallor, weight loss, progressive nutritional deficiencies, anemia, chronic cough, anal itching, etc.).

Tips for avoiding parasites

- If there is any doubt about the purity of water, it should be boiled, filtered, and ozonized before drinking.
- Fresh food, especially fruit and vegetables, should be washed meticulously with drinking water before being eaten.
- It is important that your child washes his hands before eating, after going to the bathroom, and, above all, after playing with sand.
- He should not walk barefoot in dirty places that could be sources of infection.
- All the relatives of children affected by parasites should undergo a series of stools tests, even if they are free of any symptoms, as they may be healthy carriers of a parasite.
- The efficacy of home remedies has not been proven, so the use of purgatives, coconut or pineapple ice cream, enemas, or other such measures is not recommended

Urinary infection

• This refers to infection of the urinary system. It is usually of bacterial origin, and the most frequent disorders are infection of the urethra (urethritis), the bladder (cystitis), and the kidneys (pyelonephritis).

• Urinary infection is more common in childhood (especially the first 2 years) than in any other period of life. Furthermore, it is in childhood that this disease can be most serious: in babies, generalized infection, sepsis, and meningitis can appear; in older children, urinary infection, particularly if it is recurring, can affect the functioning of the kidneys and lead to chronic renal problems.

• In small children (age 1–2), the only symptom may be fever. Other symptoms can be cloudy, foul-smelling urine, limited weight increase, vomiting, excessive crying, etc. As the symptoms of urinary infection are not clearly distinguishable in small children, doctors often need to analyse the child's urine to confirm a diagnosis.

• In older children, the symptoms are linked to the action of urinating: burning and a continual, urgent desire to urinate, sometimes with the presence of blood and/or cloudy, foul-smelling urine. When the infection affects the kidneys (pyelonephritis), there can also be fever, vomiting, and pain in the right-hand and/or left-hand side of the lumbar region (the lower part of the back, on either side of the spinal column)

• The doctor will decide which laboratory tests are needed to identify the infection and the type of antibiotic to be prescribed. In all cases, it is advisable for the child to drink plenty of fluid. If he has a fever, use the customary antipyretic drugs (paracetamol, ibuprofen, etc.).

The bacterium Escherichia coli is responsible for 90% of urinary infections. A urine culture will determine its presence and enable the selection of the appropriate antibiotic to fight against it.

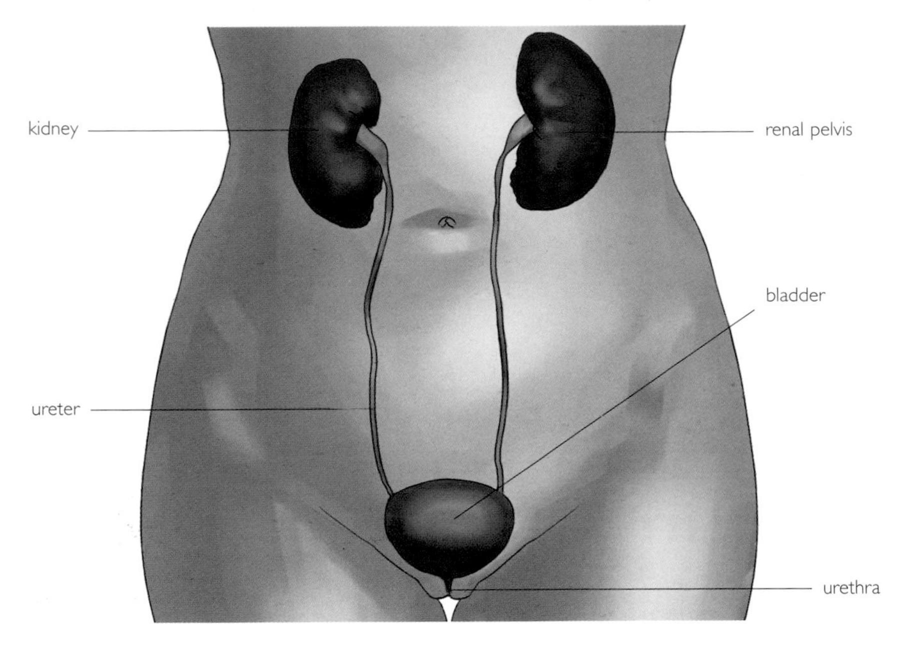

diseases with skin rashes

Infections typical of childhood (although not exclusive to it), which are characterized by rashes or spots on the skin are becoming less and less common nowadays, owing to the emergence of vaccines for several of them. This does not mean, however, that they are no longer of any concern to parents; they are not always easy to differentiate and it may be difficult to decide on the appropriate treatment for them and the need or otherwise for quarantine.

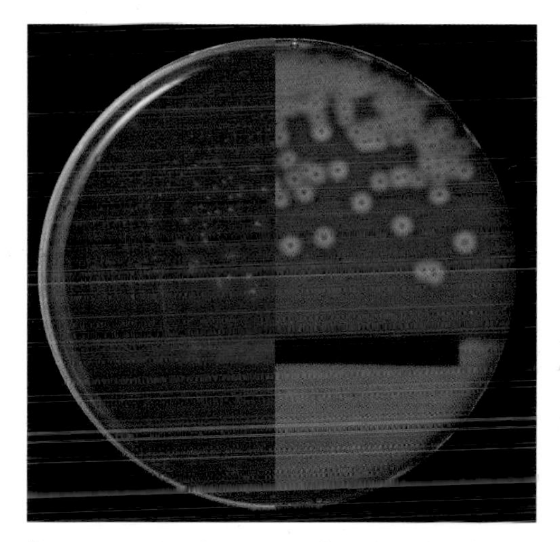

The beta hemolytic Streptococcus is the bacterium that causes scarlet fever, along with some types of tonsillitis and, more seriously, rheumatic fever and kidney complaints (glomerulonephritis).

Diseases with skin rashes

Scarlet fever

• Scarlet fever is an infectious disease caused by the streptococcus bacterium. Its symptoms are fever, tonsillitis, swollen neck glands, and marks on the skin, which also flakes off in thin layers. It is most common in children between the ages of 2 and 10, generally in winter or spring. There is a 20:1 chance that a child with a sore throat and fever is suffering from scarlet fever.

• The incubation period is short (generally 1–2 days). The marks appear 1 or 2 days after the onset of the disease, generally on the neck and chest, and then spread over the rest of the body. The eruption can last for a week and, as the marks

Diseases distinguished by skin eruptions vary in their degree of severity, depending on the individual case, but they are generally benign and free of serious complications.

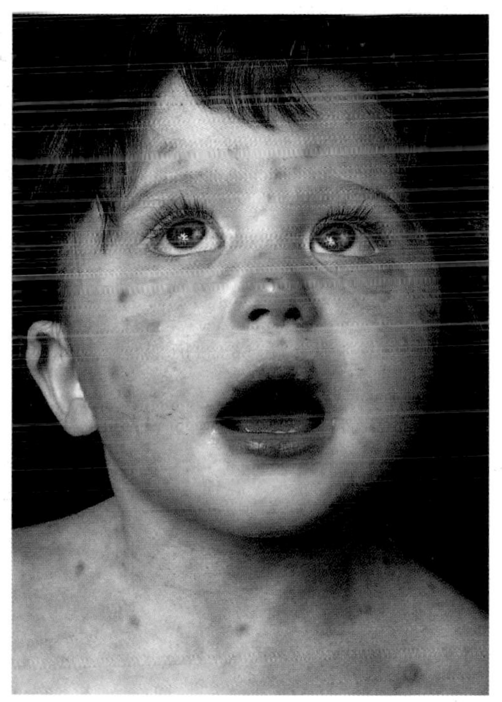

disappear the skin in the groin and around the tips of the fingers and toes might peel.

• It is treated in the same way as a throat infection: therapy with antibiotics to destroy the bacteria responsible for the infection, rest, plenty of liquids, analgesics, and antipyretic drugs.

• If no antibiotics are taken, scarlet fever (just like tonsillitis) can unleash ear infections, sinusitis, swollen neck glands, and pus on the tonsils. The most serious possible complications are rheumatic fever and lesions in the kidneys (glomerulonephritis) or heart (rheumatic cardiopathy). The most effective preventive measure is vaccination.

Rubella (German measles)

• Rubella is an acute, contagious viral infection characterized by spots or marks on the skin and swollen glands. It can appear during childhood and is usually benign. It can be significant in a pregnant woman, however, as it can lead to damage to the unborn baby.

• The incubation period varies from 10–23 days, while infection takes place 1–2 days prior to the appearance of the rash until 6 or 7 days after its disappearance. Rubella can be practically free of symptoms, or accompanied by a very slight, intermittent fever. A mild pinkish rash appears (although this can take various forms), starting on the face and chest, and then spreading over the whole body in about 24 hours. The rash generally disappears after 1–5 days. It is often complemented by swollen glands, which sometimes prove painful.

• There is no treatment available for Rubella. When it is accompanied by fever and discomfort, it is advisable to use drugs to treat these symptoms. Vaccination with the MMR vaccine guarantees life-long protection against Rubella. It is important to realize that this vaccination protects against both suffering from and transmitting the disease, and therefore prevents congenital Rubella in newborn babies.

Measles

• Measles is an infectious disease caused by a member of the paramyxovirus family. It is extremely contagious and is passed on by direct contact with an affected person, or via the air (through sneezing, for example).

• Measles is generally contracted in childhood (between the ages of one and four), although vaccination campaigns have now made it uncommon.

• The incubation period is about 10 days, and the maximum infection level is reached during the fourth and fifth days prior to the appearance of any signs of sickness. Measles usually lasts about 10 days, from the onset of the first symptoms. Once a child catches measles, he is immune for life.

The most serious problems associated with Rubella arise in women who contract the disease during pregnancy, or in the months prior to it. It is very important that women of child-bearing age are vaccinated against it.

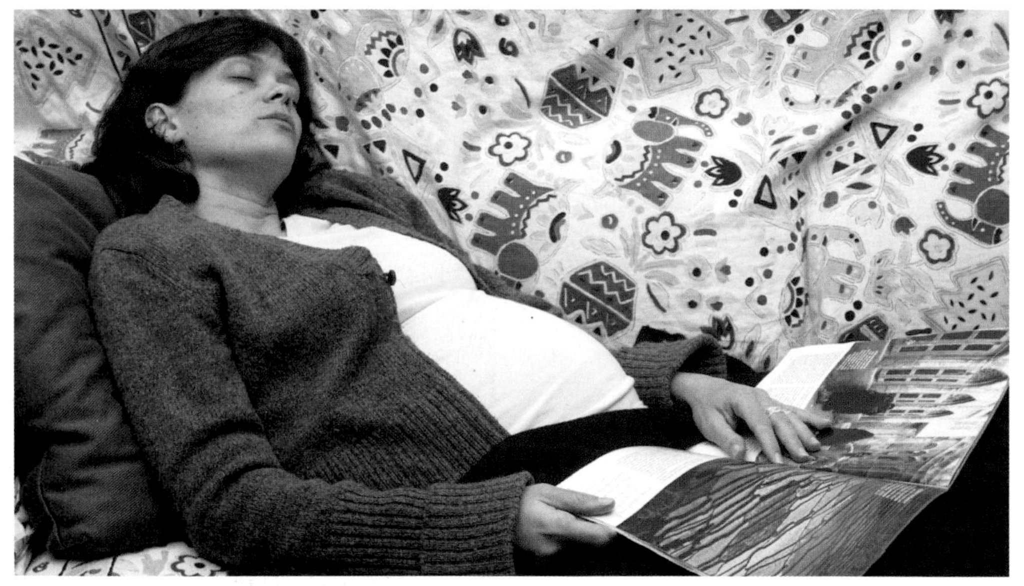

Rubella (German measles) and pregnancy

The most serious risk associated with Rubella is to pregnant women who might contract the disease during pregnancy, or in the months prior to it. In these cases, there is a high risk of the fetus developing the syndrome of congenital Rubella, which can cause sight problems or even blindness, hearing loss, cardiac pathologies, mental retardation, cerebral palsy, or walking difficulties.

Babies with this syndrome have a low body weight at birth, along with diarrhea, pneumonia, and meningitis. The fetus is most vulnerable in the first 8 weeks of pregnancy, as this is the most important phase of fetal development, and as such involves the greatest risk of abnormality.

Specialists recommend that women of a fertile age are vaccinated against the disease to avoid the syndrome of congenital Rubella, or, if they are anxious, to undergo tests before becoming pregnant to detect the presence of antibodies against the disease. The vaccine should not be given during pregnancy, or during the months immediately before conception. It is important for pregnant women to stay away from people with Rubella, to avoid any possible infection.

Comprehensive vaccination programs to protect children against measles have saved around one million lives a year worldwide. Although developing countries like India have not achieved such a wide reach, the WHO reckons that measles will have been eradicated in 2007. CLOSE BOX

• The spots appear 4 or 5 days after the onset of the disease. First, there is fever, listlessness, catarrh, sensitivity to light, conjunctivitis, and a dry cough.The fever can reach levels of 104 °F (40 °C), but it gradually goes down.Two or three days after the appearance of spots on the cheeks, a rash breaks out on other parts of the body, starting with red spots behind the ears and on the neck, before spreading to the rest of the body in less than 2 days. During this phase, it is probable that the child has a high fever and, in some cases, abdominal pain, diarrhea, and even vomiting.

• The most frequent complications of measles, especially in babies, are infections of the middle ear and respiratory diseases like pneumonia. It rarely causes neurological problems.

• Today's vaccination programs make it difficult to catch measles, but if it does break out, the recommended treatment is rest and drugs to bring down the temperature and alleviate the cough.

Chicken pox

• This is a contagious disease caused by the varicella-zoster virus (VZV), which is responsible for shingles in adults aged over 65. Of all the diseases accompanied by a skin rash, it is currently the most common.

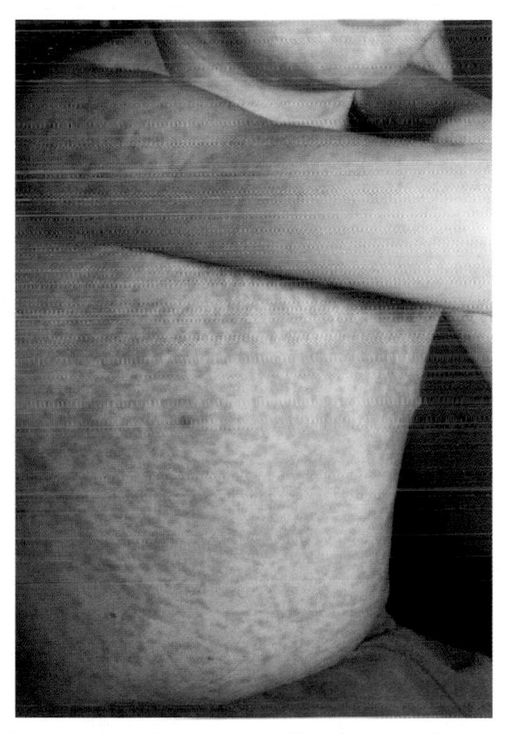

The most characteristic symptom of measles is the presence of white spots surrounded by a red circle (Koplik spots).

The MMR (mumps, measles and Rubella) vaccine

This combined vaccine against measles, Rubella, and mumps is one of the immunizations typical of early childhood. In most countries, this vaccination is a prerequisite for admission to a school. The first dose is recommended at the age of 15 months, but it can be prescribed before that in case of an outbreak (at 12 months). The first dose cannot provide total immunity and so a second one is recommended before starting primary school (age 4–6) or in early adolescence (age 11–13). Vaccination is also advisable for adults unsure of whether they received it in their youth. One dose of the MMR vaccine protects 90–98 percent of people who receive it from contracting measles, mumps, or Rubella throughout their life; a second dose guarantees 100 percent protection. Side effects are very rare, apart from minor problems like feeling off-color or reddening of the injection site. The benefits far outweigh any adverse effects, on account of the complications associated with these 3 diseases.

A child affected by chicken pox will be immune for life, although the virus can remain hidden in the body and manifest itself years later as shingles, a painful, blistery rash. Shingles is more common in adults than in children.

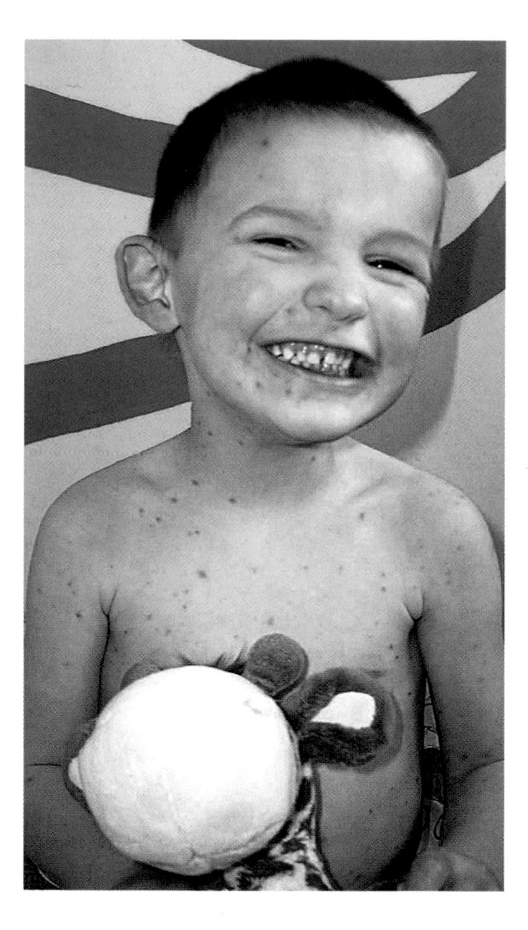

- The chicken pox virus is particularly prevalent among children aged between 2 and 8, in cycles running from January to May. Adults can only be infected if they have not previously had the disease.
- The incubation process is asymptomatic and lasts about 2 weeks. It is followed by sudden fever and listlessness, then blisters on the body and face, which continue to emerge over the course of 3 or 4 days, before spreading over the whole body. As the disease develops, the blisters dry up until they form a crust and eventually disappear.
- Chicken pox is mainly transmitted via direct contact with the rash, in the stage prior to the formation of the crusts, as the liquid inside them contains high concentrations of the virus. The disease can also be spread through the air, via respiratory secretions from an infected person. The most contagious period starts one or 2 days before the appearance of the rash and continues for 5 days after this event.
- The most frequent complications of chicken pox are opportunist bacterial infections on the blisters, most commonly caused by Staphylococcus aureus and Staphylococcus pyogenes. Lesions can also appear in the liver, caused by the chicken pox virus itself; although these rarely give rise to symptoms, they can have neurological repercussions. Chicken pox can also lead to pneumonia in adults.

Pregnant women who have not had chicken pox need to take extra precautions. If the disease is contracted in the first months of pregnancy or just before giving birth, the fetus can suffer from various disorders and even abnormalities.

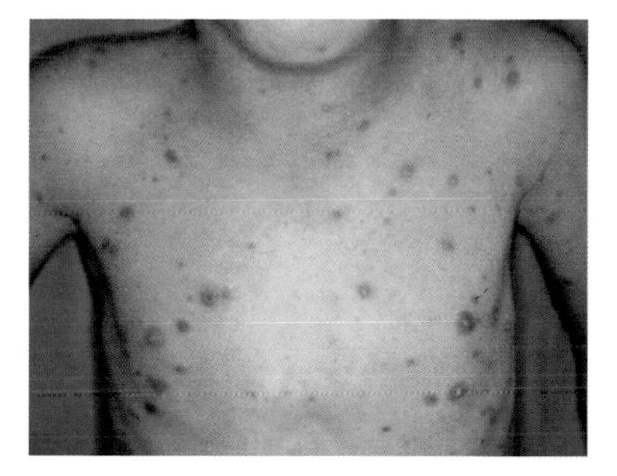

People affected by immunodepression or under treatment that suppresses their immune system (chemotherapy, corticosteroids) are at greater risk of developing severe forms of chicken pox, along with pneumonia and other complications. Children rarely have any serious complications.

• Treatment is usually based on alleviating the itching caused by the rash and, if necessary, treatment with Aciclovir, a specific medicine for the varicella-zoster virus.

Infectious erythema or fifth disease

• Infectious erythema or megaloerythema is characterized by a distinctive rash, with very red cheeks and spots on the chest and arms. The striking rash on the face has led this sickness to be known as "slapped cheek disease".

• The virus that causes the fifth disease is a Parvovirus. Before the rash breaks out, catarrh or pharyngitis can appear, along with a slight fever. The rash can persist intermittently for weeks or even months, sometimes as a result of stimuli like sunshine or heat.

• When it occurs in adults, it causes a burning sensation in the face, joint pains, and even signs of arthritis. If the fifth disease is contracted by a pregnant woman, there is no danger of deformations in the fetus, although there is a risk of a miscarriage.

Roseola or sixth disease

• Roseola, also known as exanthem subitum or sixth disease, is caused by the herpes virus type 6 and is characterized by high fever and a skin rash.

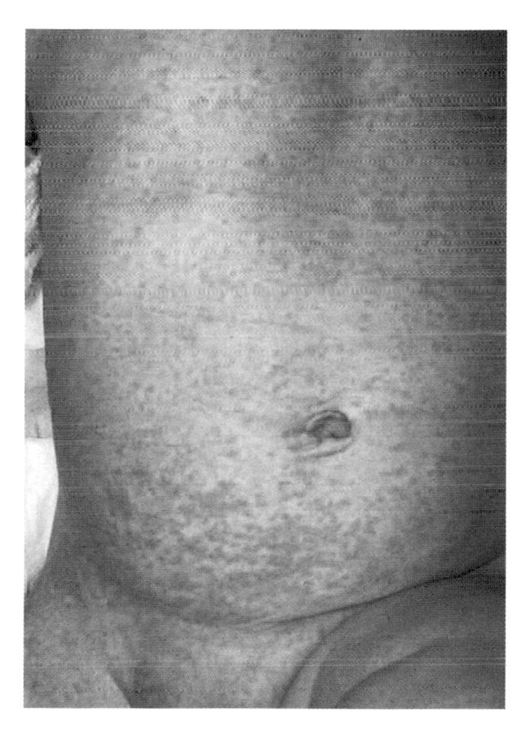

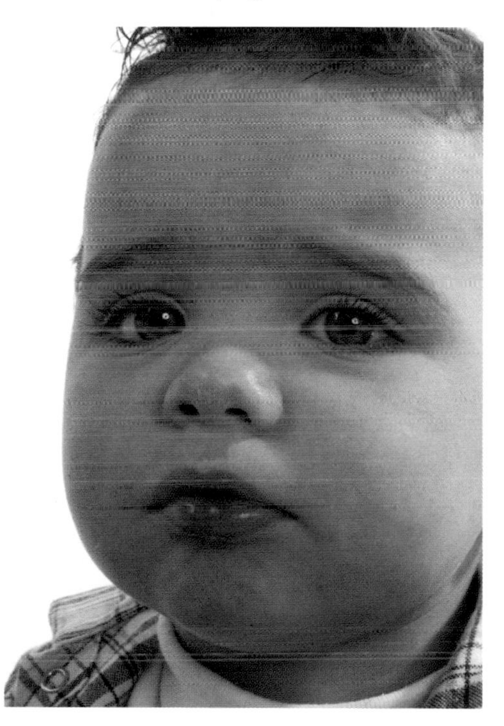

It is a common disease that affects about 30% of babies aged between 4 and 24 months, although it can also be found, albeit rarely, in older children.

• The incubation period ranges from 5–15 days. The disease itself is easy to diagnose once the rash appears along with a high temperature. The fever lasts 3 or 4 days, and once it fades it gives way to pinkish spots, which start to appear on the chest before spreading to the face, abdomen, and, to a lesser extent, the limbs.

• Roseola is a benign complaint that can be diagnosed retrospectively, once the rash has appeared. This means that it can be confused with pharyngitis or an ear infection when the fever starts to appear, complemented by a sore throat or earache.

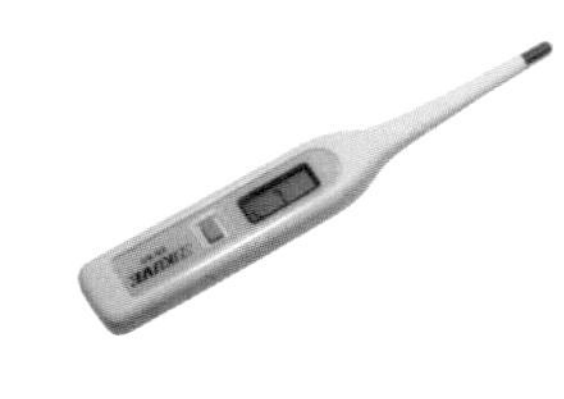

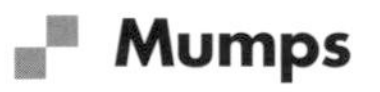

Mumps

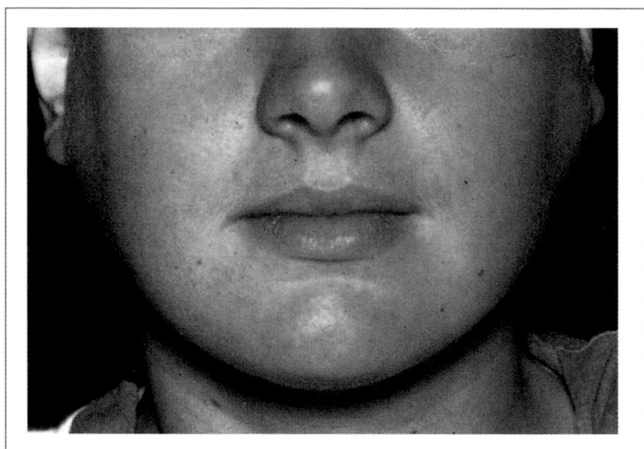

Although mumps is not a disease associated with a skin rash, it is a contagious, viral disease that can be prevented by means of the MMR vaccine, which also covers measles and Rubella, as outlined above.

The virus affects the salivary glands, especially the parotid glands (situated below and in front of the ears), although, when complications ensue, it can also encroach on the pancreas and testicles (20–30 percent of cases) or lead to meningitis or encephalitis. Mumps is spread by direct contact with saliva and discharges from the nose and throat of infected subjects. Its incubation period ranges from 12–25 days.

The most effective measure against this disease is ensuring that the immunizations levels remain as high as possible. Children with mumps should not go to school and adults should not go out while they are contagious.

herpes and athlete's foot

There are a number of skin lesions of infectious origin whose cause, characteristics, form of presentation, and location are very different, but are grouped together, because they are transient, benign ailments, as well as being very frequent in childhood (although they are also found in adults). These lesions are the work of the herpes simplex viruses and are mainly situated on the lips and feet (a superficial mycosis known as athlete's foot).

Herpes

• The herpes viruses form a family that includes the herpes simplex virus (HSV), which cause a series of manifestations on the skin and mucous membranes; in isolated cases, they can spread and lead to serious problems.

• Herpes mouth sores. These affect the mucous membranes of the mouth, gums, and lips. It is caused by the Herpes simplex virus type 1. It is a frequent complaint among children aged bet-

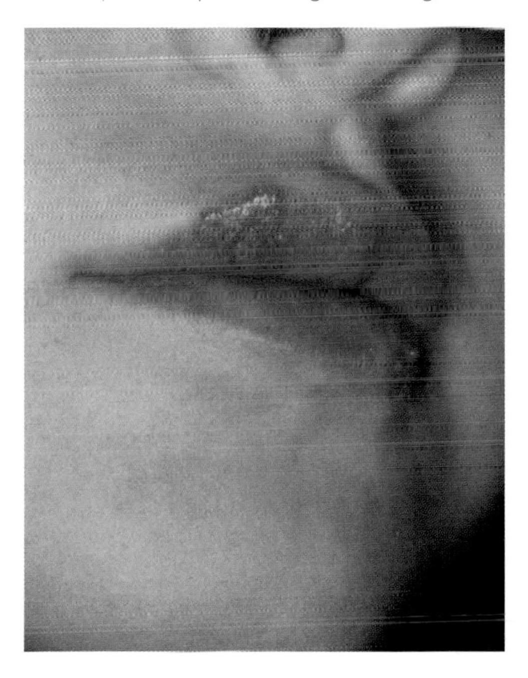

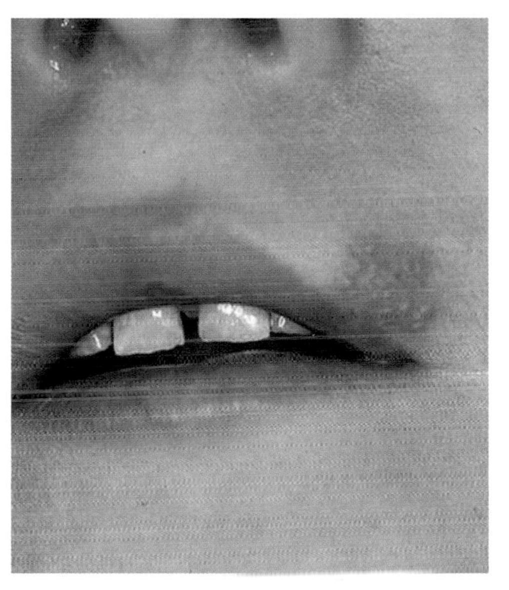

The most frequent manifestation of infection by a Herpes simplex virus in childhood is a mouth sore; this is most commonly observed in children aged between 6 months and 5 years.

Various other childhood diseases, such as Coxsackie viral infection and recurrent aphthous ulcers, are distinguished by mouth ulcers, without being triggered by herpes viruses. In these cases, a doctor is needed to make an exact diagnosis and prescribe the appropriate treatment.

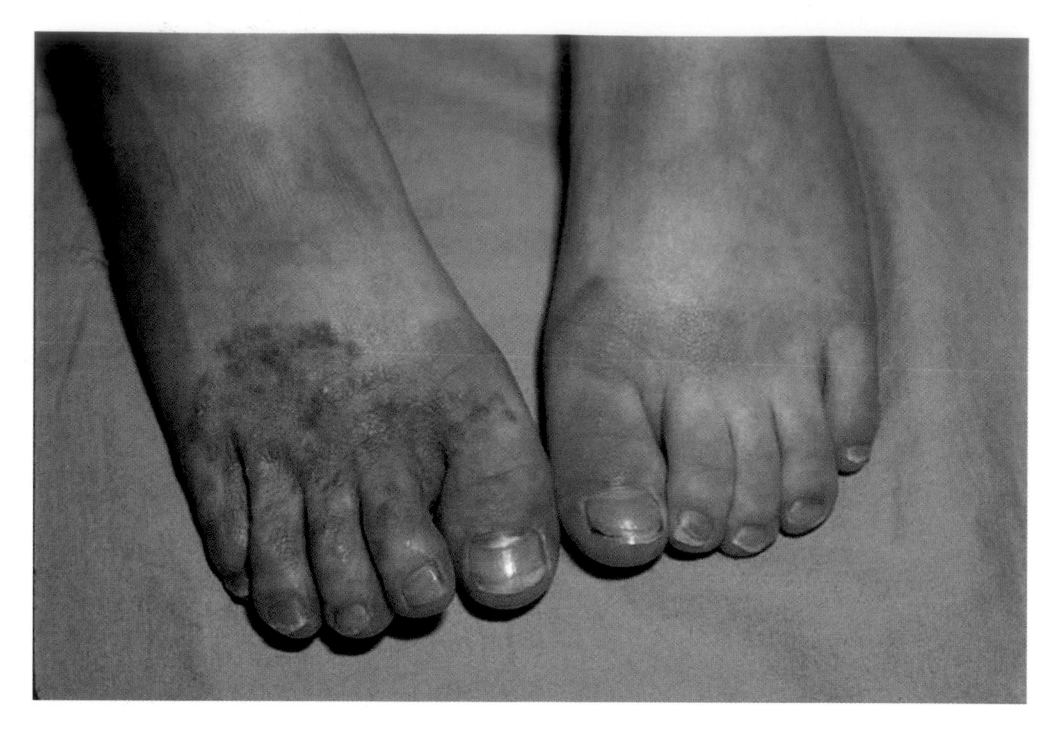

ween 6 months and 5 years. They start off being irritable and tearful, with no desire to eat or drink. This is followed by the appearance of small blisters, which join up to form a larger, painful ulcer. This is a grayish color, on a red base, and usually measures between 1 and 3 mm. In severe cases, ulcers can spread to the pharynx, palate, gums, tongue, and lips. They develop a crust, which later

Athlete's foot is almost always caused by anthropophylic fungi (i.e. ones that affect human beings), such as Trichophyton rubrum, Trichophyton mentagrophytes, and Epidermofitos floccosum, which can act in combination, either simultaneously or consecutively. The fungi are almost invariably passed on indirectly, particularly from the floors of public showers and swimming pools, towels, carpets in hotels, etc., or through the use of the same socks and shoes by various people. These factors explain why the infection can reappear so readily, and why it is more common in young people.

falls off and allows the healing process to take its course (1–2 weeks). The gums can redden and become very inflamed, with a propensity to bleeding, and the child also has bad breath. The glands in the neck and under the chin swell up and can be painful. Excessive salivation, localized pain, and difficulty in swallowing may be other symptoms. Your child may have fever for 3–5 days, while the other symptoms can last for up to 2 weeks. Treatment,

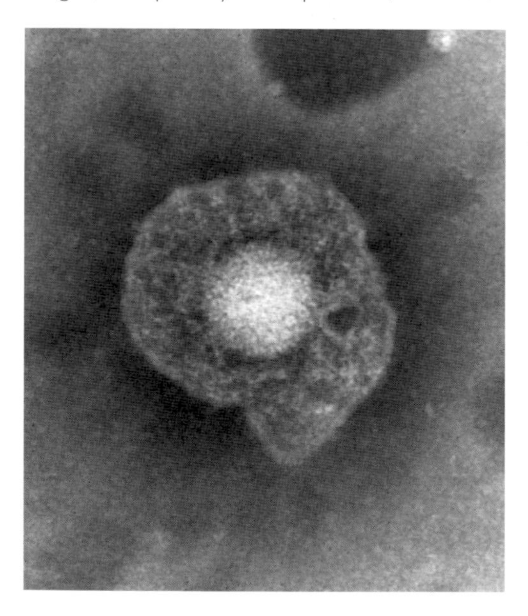

Microscopic image of one of the herpes viruses.

focused entirely on the symptoms, is based on analgesics, antipyretics, and gels applied topically to the lesions. Your child should follow a diet with no citric fruit or condiments, and plenty of cold fluids; if necessary, specific anti-viral drugs, such as Aciclovir, can be given.

• Although most infections caused by the herpes viruses are asymptomatic infections that go unnoticed, in other cases the virus can remain latent throughout a child's life and occasionally be activated, after exposure to the ultraviolet radiations of the sun, emotional and physical stress, menstruation, a respiratory disease, or an injury.

Athlete's foot

This is the fungal infection most commonly found in young people. It is extremely infectious and comes in irregular outbursts that can be extremely itchy. It affects the foot, between the toes and on the sole or, occasionally, on the upper part.

• There is a greater risk of this disease if the foot is damp as a result of the use of socks or shoes that do not allow it to breathe (sneakers or boots).

• Athlete's foot is rare in young children but it is more common in primary school pupils and adolescents.

– Children affected by athlete's foot sometimes also have fungal infections on their hands, as well as an additional bacterial infection that can complicate the situation still further.

• Treatment

Avoid wearing closed leather footwear in summer.

– A doctor has to decide whether a child needs specific treatment with anti-fungal medicines like micomazol, econazol, clotrimazol, ketoconazol, etc. which are usually applied in the form of creams and powders. In serious or recurrent cases that resist the action of topical preparations, the administration of oral anti-fungal drugs may be necessary.

–The doctor will also evaluate the need for antibiotics for lesions that have become infected by bacteria.

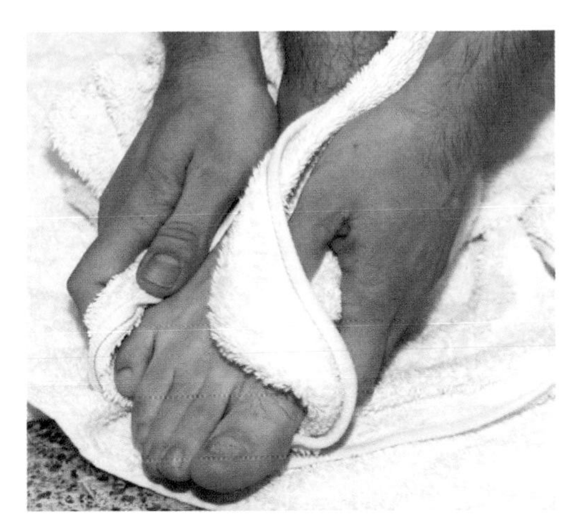

Treatment should be based on good hygiene, thorough drying of the feet, and the use of footwear in public showers and swimming pools (campsites, clubs, hotels, etc.). Anti-fungal talcum powders may be required as a preventive measure by people particularly susceptible to this complaint or constantly exposed to areas where the presence of fungi may be suspected (such as public pools).

Athlete's foot. A doctor should be consulted immediately if

- The foot is swollen and hot, particularly if red lines are also visible, as these are signs of a possible bacterial infection. Fever and pus or other types of secretion are also warning signs.
- A diabetic gets athlete's foot.
- If the symptoms do not disappear within a month after taking personal hygiene measures.

AIDS

Acquired immune deficiency syndrome (AIDS) is a chronic, progressive disease that affects both adults and children infected by the human immune deficiency virus (HIV). The process starts with an initial latent period without symptoms (which may last for years), during which a subject is called a healthy carrier. The first children's AIDS cases were described in the United States in 1982; since then, their incidence has never ceased to increase and now constitutes a veritable worldwide epidemic. No vaccine against HIV is available as yet, so prevention is the key factor.

AIDS

Transmission routes

• Horizontal route. Two mechanisms are responsible:

– Via blood or objects that have been in contact with blood, i.e. shared razor blades, syringes, or toothbrushes; blood transfusions with no medical controls; tattooing and piercing instruments used without sufficient hygiene, etc.

– Via sexual relationships, which for our purposes cover sexually active adolescents and victims of sexual abuse.

• Vertical route. This refers to mother-child transmission, which is responsible for 80% of the cases of AIDS in children and can take place in 3 different ways:

– Prenatal transmission: HIV can cross the placenta and infect the fetus. This can occur from the 8th week of pregnancy onward.

– Perinatal transmission: a baby can be infected just before being born, or during the delivery. This transmission seems to take place via an infected mother's vaginal secretions or blood resulting from her uterine contractions during childbirth. For this reason, HIV-positive mothers are now given a cesarean section.

– Postnatal transmission: like other viruses, HIV can be excreted in a mother's milk and thereby infect her baby. Breast-feeding is therefore contraindicated in HIV-positive mothers.

The HIV action mechanism

The white corpuscles and antibodies normally act and destroy a foreign body that enters the body. This response is coordinated by cells known as CD4 lymphocytes. HIV, however, uses these cells to replicate, i.e. to copy itself and thus multiply and propagate itself. When the new copies of the virus pass from the lymphocyte into the blood stream, they

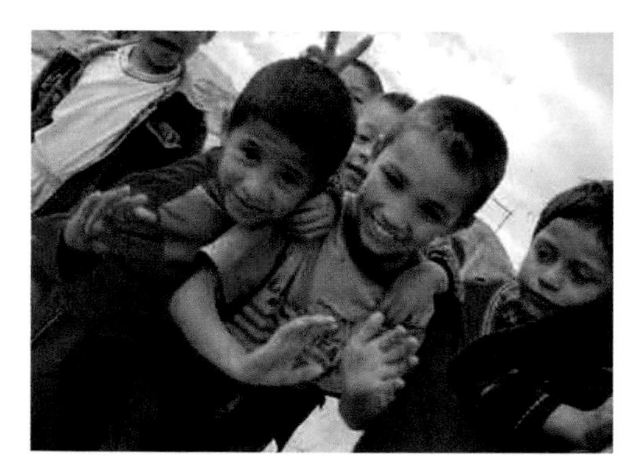

If no significant changes occur in the near future, in 2010 a quarter of all the orphans in the world will have lost their parents because of AIDS. In sub-Saharan Africa, this figure will be 50%. Although no exact figures are available, it is estimated that, in 2005, one in 5 children aged under 15 in sub-Saharan Africa will have lost their father or mother, or both – mostly on account of AIDS.

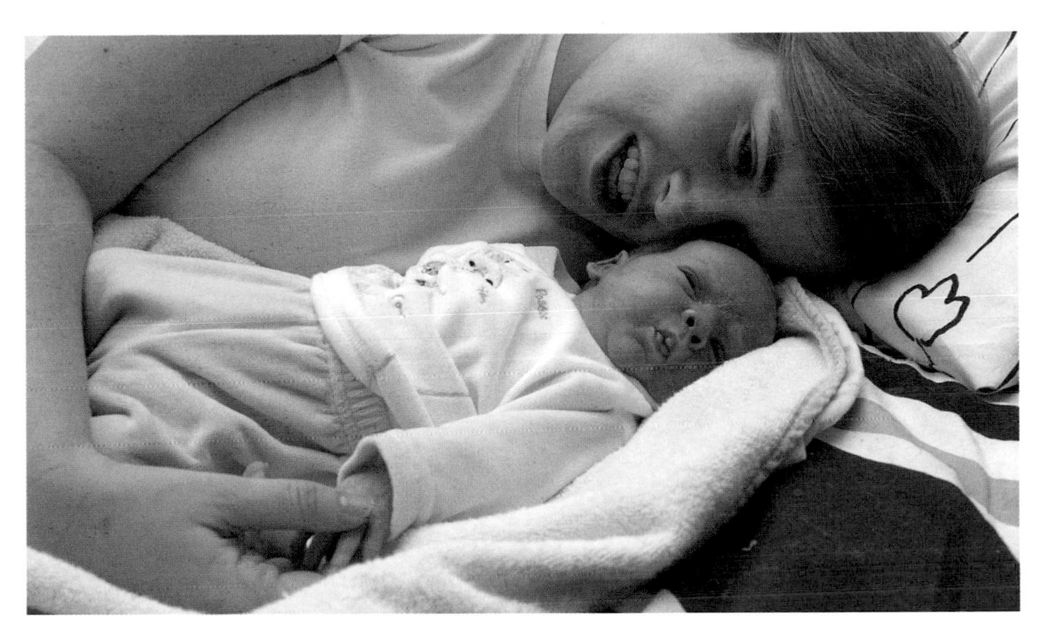

The possibility of transmitting the virus via mother's milk rules out breast-feeding in mothers who are carriers of HIV.

look for other lymphocytes in order to continue propagating themselves. Meanwhile, the CD4 lymphocytes used in the virus' reproductive cycle die.

This cycle is repeated constantly, resulting in further new copies of the virus and thus a spreading of the infection. Although the body reacts by producing more CD4 lymphocytes, the virus increases its presence in every cycle and so destroys more and more lymphocytes and gradually reduces their numbers (leading to immune deficiency). This drastic undermining of the body's immune system means that an infected person cannot react to other infections, leaving them vulnerable against viruses, bacteria, and diseases such as cancer. This is why HIV-positive patients are so susceptible to infections, which severely debilitate them and can be fatal.

Clinical manifestations

Pediatric AIDS can take 2 forms:

• Precocious: in 20% of infected children, the clinical manifestations of the syndrome appear in the first months of their life and the diagnosis can usually be confirmed at about the age of 12 months. The most common manifestations are:

- encephalopathies
- pneumonia caused by Pneumonocistis Carinii
- serious bacterial infections
- very low weight and small stature.

These children generally die before their third birthday.

• Slowly progressive: the remaining 80% of infected children present symptoms later on, in a less aggressive manifestation. The most common symptoms are:

- interstitial pneumonia
- infiltration of the parotids (salivary glands)
- thinner and smaller than uninfected children
- dermatitis
- less serious bacterial infections.

The average age for the diagnosis of AIDS is 3, and the prognosis depends on the emergence of opportunist infections. The retroviral treatment (triple therapy) available today has significantly altered the course of the disease in these children.

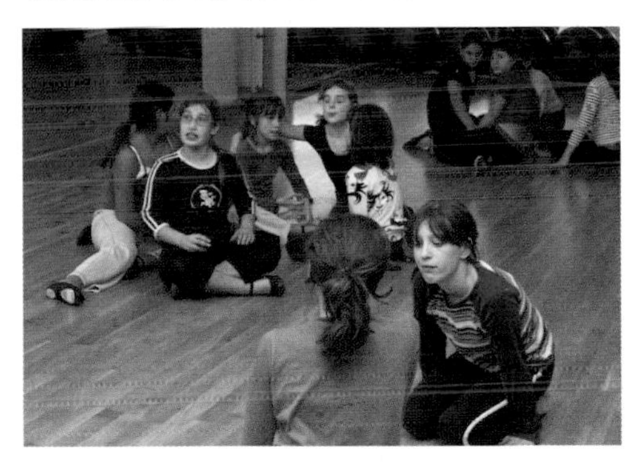

At the moment, children have not been considered priority targets for access to antiretroviral treatment, even though over 3 million children have died all over the world as a result of AIDS-related diseases. It is estimated that 1,800 totally avoidable infections of children occur every day. The vast majority of children with HIV acquired the virus through perinatal transmission. An antiretroviral treatment "suitable for children" does exist, but it is very expensive, difficult to store, and complicated to administer, especially in poor countries (which, coincidentally, have the highest levels of infection).

Difficulties in treating AIDS

AIDS develops more quickly in children than in adults, with more serious consequences. These problems aside, there are several specific reasons why AIDS is more difficult to treat in children:

- Drugs prepared in a form suitable for pediatric use are not always available. Many children cannot swallow pills, so their medicine has to be administered in syrups or liquids. Some of the drugs used to treat AIDS are not soluble in water however, or they have a very unpleasant taste.
- Moreover, the treatment demands strict compliance in the taking of 3 or more drugs, taken in combination 2 or 3 times a day, year in, year out, if resistance to these drugs is to be averted. This discipline is not easy to achieve in children. In addition, tests on new therapies are invariably carried out on adults and so pediatricians receive no clear guidelines about their use or dosage in children.
- At first, babies with AIDS were not treated until a few weeks after birth. It has now become clear that it must start immediately, to impede the multiplication of the virus. The diagnosis cannot always be confirmed straightaway, however, as it is only possible to detect the virus when it has acquired a significant concentration in the blood (although increasingly sensitive tests are being developed). Some specialists recommend starting treatment in the babies of mothers with AIDS as soon as they are born, even though a good many of these children may not be infected; in contrast, other experts prefer to wait for the results of tests.

Antiretroviral treatment for children comprises the same medicines as those used by adults, even though they often have not been approved for small children and dosage recommendations are not always available.

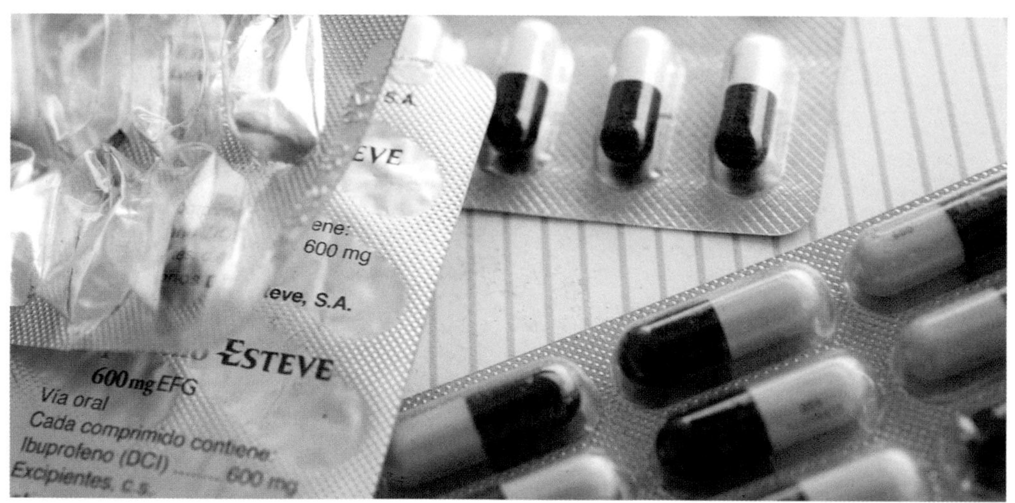

acquired neurological disorders

This term groups together a series of neurological problems that are common in childhood and generally of readily identifiable origin, such as headaches, whose causes can range from simple myopia to a brain tumor. These are complemented by diseases of infectious origin, such as meningitis, polio, tetanus, and even adverse reactions to medicines, such as Reye's syndrome. Knowledge of the general characteristics of these disorders is always useful for parents, for reference purposes, in medical consultations, or to take preventive measures.

Acquired neurological disorders

Childhood headaches

• Headaches are the second most common chronic complaint in children after obesity. A headache should not be merely considered a symptom, however, as it can have many causes, ranging from an eye problem, such as undetected shortsightedness, to a serious brain tumor. Migraines are particularly worthy of note, on account of their high incidence in children and adolescents.

Types of headache

1. Primary headache: these are normally caused by tense muscles, dilated blood vessels, or inflammation of the cerebral structures. This type of headache includes:

– Migraines: these can appear in children between the ages of 5 and 8, normally in families with a history of migraines. Some adolescent girls can have migraines related to the menstrual cycle. Although every child can experience symptoms in a different form, the most common ones are:

– Pain on one or both sides of the head or, in smaller children, in the whole head. The pain can

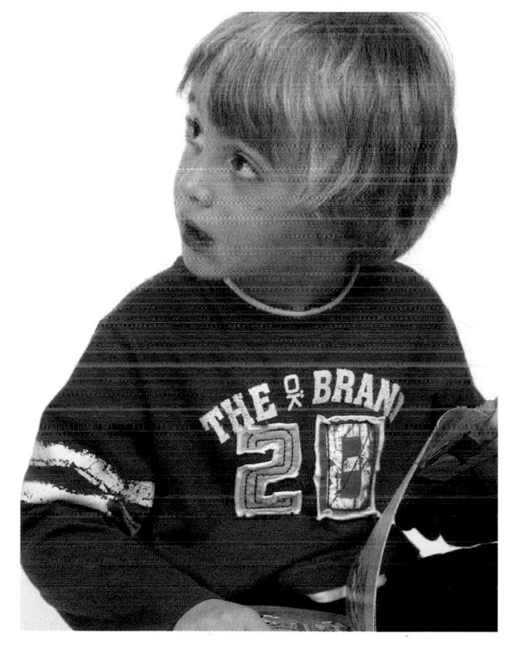

Headache is a common symptom in some visual disorders, so an annual visit to an ophthalmologist is well worth the effort.

Tension headaches often affect children aged between 9 and 12. They are frequently caused by stress, nervousness, and depression.

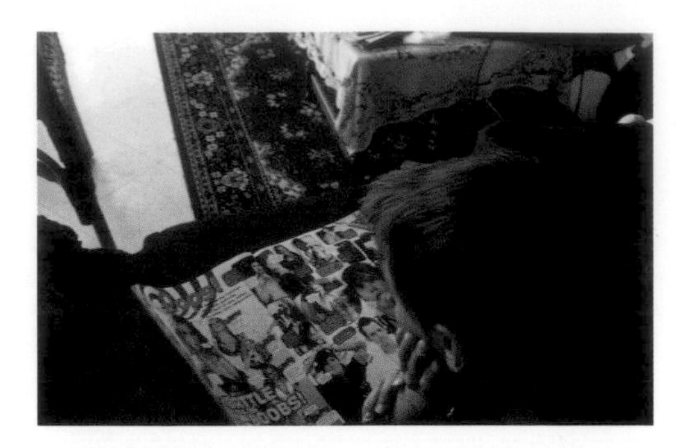

be throbbing or continuous (although younger children may not be able to describe it accurately).

- Sensitivity to light or sound.
- Nausea, vomiting, or both.
- Abdominal pains.
- Sweating.
- Before a migraine, some children experience perceptual changes, such as the sensation of seeing flashing lights or changes in their field of vision, or of noticing strange smells.

– Tension headache: this is the most frequent type of headache. The symptoms can vary from one child to another, but the most common ones are:

- Slow but progressive onset.
- The pain is normally located on both sides of the head.
- There is a dull pain, like a band around the head, or in the back of the head or neck.
- The pain is slight to moderate, but not strong.
- Disruption of sleep patterns.
- There is normally no nausea, vomiting, or sensitivity to light.

– Headaches in series: these are generally found in children over 10, particularly adolescent boys. Headaches can recur over a period of weeks or even months, and these series may reappear every year or two. The most common systems are:

- Strong pain on one side of the head, normally around the eye. The eyelid may drop and even become red and inflamed, and the pupils may dilate.
- Blocked or runny nose.
- Swollen forehead.

2. Secondary headaches:

This type of headache is the least common; it has an organic cerebral cause, related to structural and functional problems which need to be diagnosed. Recognizing headaches related to a condition is critical not only because treatment can eliminate headache but also because the condition causing the headache could be life–threatening.

Meningitis

- The nervous system, brain, and spinal cord are covered by membranes known as the meninges. These membranes not only play a part in the nervous system but also act as a barrier against toxins and micro-organisms. If this barrier is crossed, the result can be meningitis, a term that embraces all inflammatory diseases affecting the meninges, regardless of its cause, although it usually refers to the serious, infectious or bacterial meningitis.
- The most frequent cause is usually infection by Haemophilus influenzae type b (Hib) or Neisseria meningitidis (groups A, B, C, Y, W-135).
- Meningitis of viral origin (aseptic meningitis) is often seen in children and is less serious than the bacterial form. The most common viruses enter through a child's mouth, multiply inside his body, and are eliminated in his stools. Dirty hands can pass it on to somebody else (a process known as fecal–oral transmission). They can continue to be transmitted for weeks after the infection has been overcome.
- The most frequent symptoms of meningitis are:

– Fever.
– Headache.
– Stiff neck.
– Blocked nose.
– Vomiting.
– Sensitivity to light.

- Symptoms that imply a greater degree of seriousness or danger include:

– Sleepiness and exhaustion.
– Skin rash.
– Convulsions.
– General muscle pains.
– Occasional diarrhea.
– Accelerated breathing.

- Preventive measures.

– Avoid infection by using handkerchiefs and avoid the coughing and sneezing of anybody who may have meningitis.

– Anybody in close contact with a meningitis patient should ask a doctor about preventive treatment with specific antibiotics.

If meningitis is suspected in a child a lumbar puncture may be taken to analyze the cerebrospinal liquid to determine the cause of the infection. Other tests, such as a brain scan, may sometimes be recommended to ensure that he does not have any other significant illness.

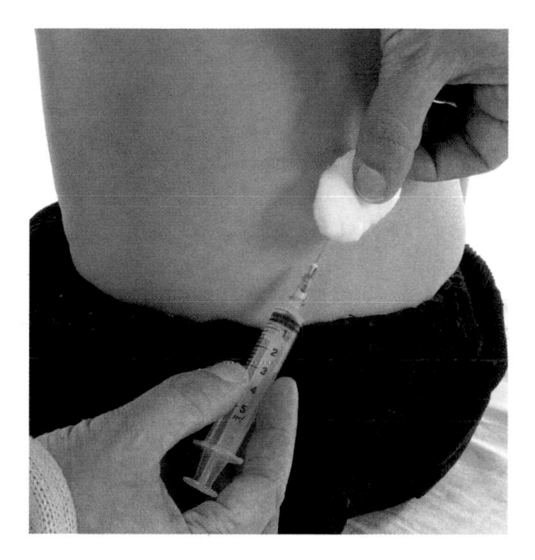

– Vaccination. Children with immunodepresssion or in an epidemic situation (10 cases per 100,000 inhabitants) can be given the vaccine against Neisseria meningitidis (groups A, C, Y, W-135). Vaccines against Haemophilus influenzae and other bacteria responsible for meningitis are also available.

– Treatment depends on what micro-organism is involved, but it always requires hospital admission. There is no specific treatment for viral meningitis, but this is usually benign. In other cases, the doctor will take account of the disease's origin to prescribe the most appropriate antibiotics, as well as various measures for the child's general healthcare.

Reye's syndrome

• Reye's syndrome is an inflammation of the brain (encephalopathy) and liver, accompanied by fever and caused by viral infections or chicken pox in children treated with acetylsalicylic acid (aspirin). Although Reye's syndrome does not appear in all children treated in this way, they are 30 times more likely to succumb to it than others in a similar situation. The exact reason for this phenomenon is still unknown, but it could be linked to genetic factors.

Meningitis can occur at any age, but over half of those affected by the disease are aged under 15. Babies under 8 months are particularly vulnerable.

THE MENINGES

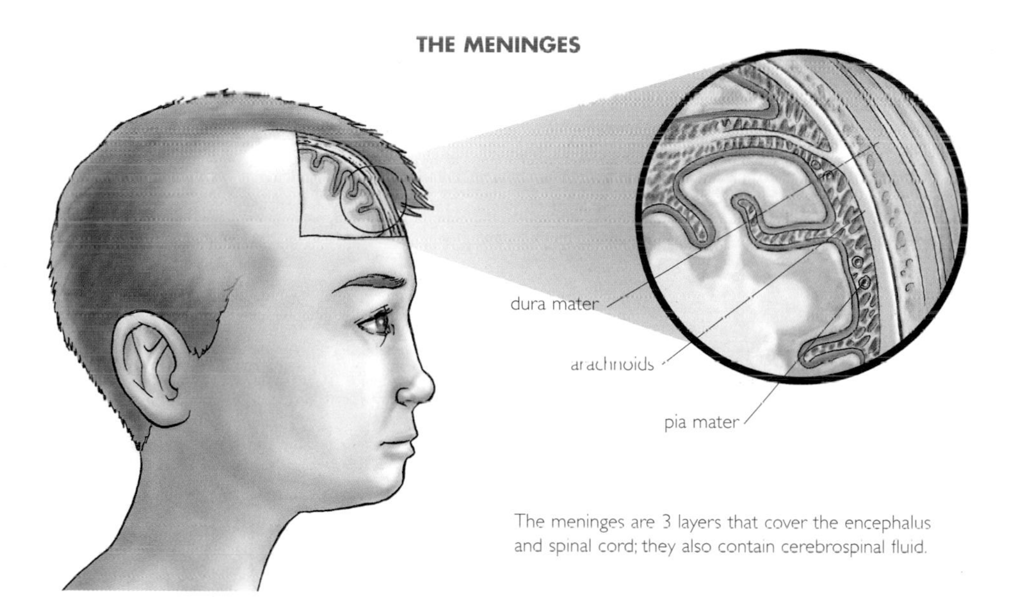

The meninges are 3 layers that cover the encephalus and spinal cord; they also contain cerebrospinal fluid.

POLIOMYELITIS

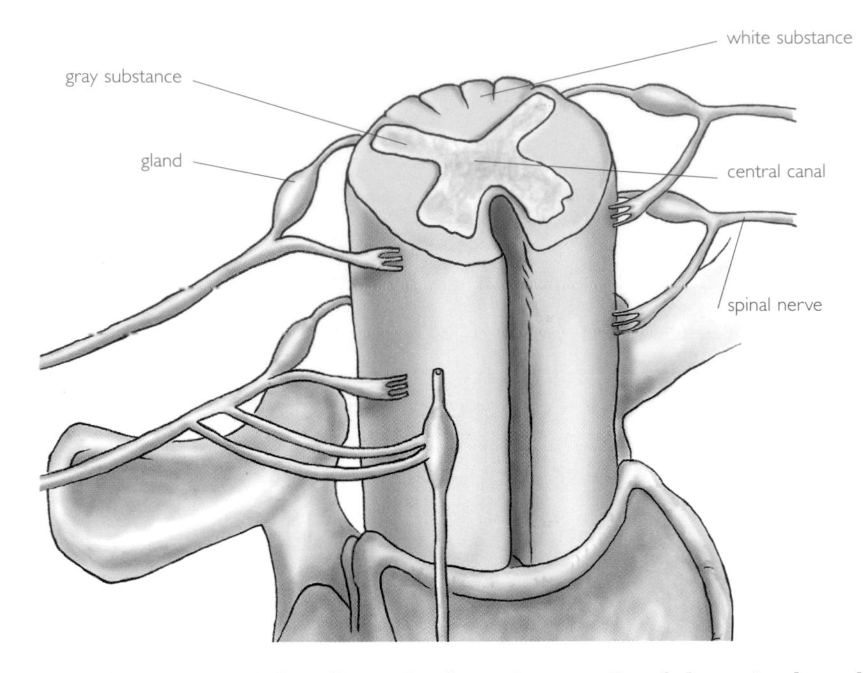

The polio virus mainly affects the front horn cells of the spinal cord, at the root of the motor nerves that trigger muscular action.

• In children of all ages, Reye's syndrome usually appears about one week after flu, chicken pox, or an infection of the upper airways. It can be complemented by vomiting, changes in behavior, great excitability, delirium, sleepiness, loss of muscular strength, and loss of consciousness, rapidly leading to convulsions and coma, and can even be fatal.

• Treatment is very intensive and so hospital admission is essential. It involves the administration of serum with salts and glucose, as well as cortisone to reduce cerebral inflammation. Despite this, it is usually necessary to monitor breathing and in some cases a child may need a respirator. Eighty percent of patients recover without any problems, but for the remainder the outlook is very grim, or even fatal. If there are sequels to the disease, their characteristics will depend on the intensity of the initial outbreak and the progress of the treatment.

Poliomyelitis

• This is a disease caused by a virus (poliovirus type I, II, and III), which attacks the front horn cells of the spinal corn, the starting point of the motor nerves responsible for conveying the cerebral response to the muscles, thereby triggering their reaction. If these motor impulses are blocked, the skeletal motor is not stimulated and therefore does not work, becoming atrophied and degenerating.

• Polio mainly affects children under 3, but it can strike adolescents and even adults.

• The poliovirus is transmitted from person to person via secretions from the nose or throat and via the fecal/oral route. Polio can also be contracted indirectly by eating food or drinking water contaminated by the virus. Once a person has been infected, he can become a carrier and continue spreading the virus via his stools for several weeks.

• The incubation period gives way to the first symptoms: gastrointestinal disorders, fever, joint pains, heavy limbs, etc. Then, a total or partial paralysis sets in; this recedes, but it can leave some muscles damaged, while others recover their capacity for movement. The affected muscles start to atrophy, arresting growth (especially in children) and leaving physical deformities.

The use of aspirin should be avoided in the treatment of the fever and discomfort associated with viral infections, flu, and chicken pox in children and adolescents (under 18). Paracetamol and ibuprofen are recommended alternatives.

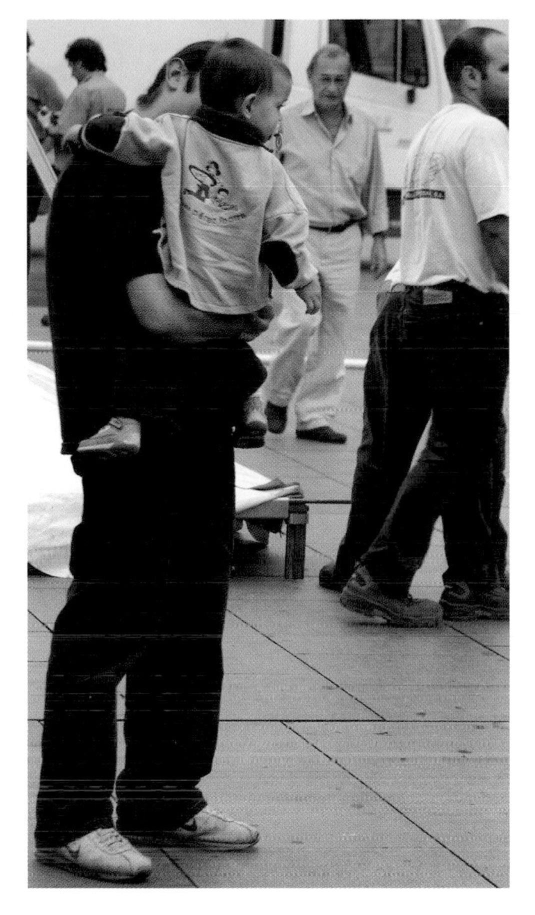

Tetanus

• Tetanus is an acute disease, characterized by the presence of intense but intermittent muscular spasms and paralysis, resulting from the action of a powerful toxin produced by the bacterium Clostridium Tetani. This disease is often deadly, especially in children and elderly people, but it can be forestalled by appropriate medication and vaccination.

• Tetanus is a complication that can appear after a cut, laceration, bite, or other type of wound, however minor.

• The disease can develop days or even weeks after the wound, give rise to stiff muscles, particularly in the jaw, and even convulsions and severe difficulty in breathing.

• A tetanus infection can be avoided:

– By consulting a doctor immediately after any cut or wound.

– By monitoring your child's vaccination program along with your doctor, to ensure that he is fully protected.

– By carefully cleaning any wound, removing any remains of tissue and leaving it open, without any sticking plaster or stitches, to allow the air to reach inside (the tetanus bacterium dies on contact with oxygen).

– Some antibiotics can help to eliminate the tetanus bacteria, but they may be useless if the

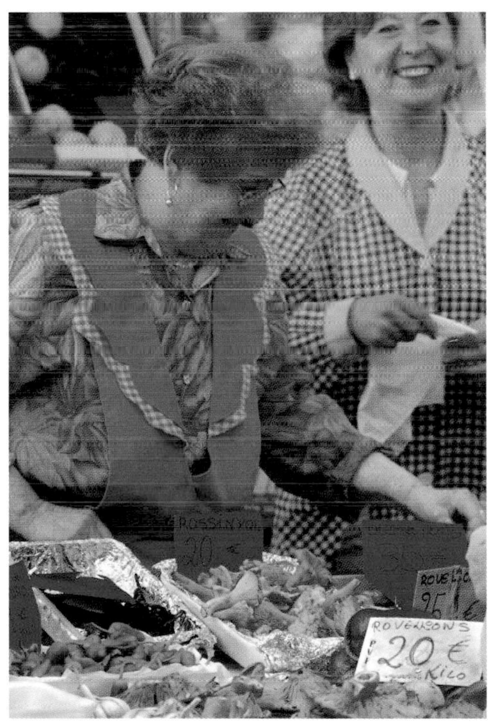

Polio is a terrible disease but it can easily be prevented with meticulous hygiene, the avoidance of fecal contamination of water and food, and vaccination. At the slightest suspicion of polio, go to a hospital immediately.

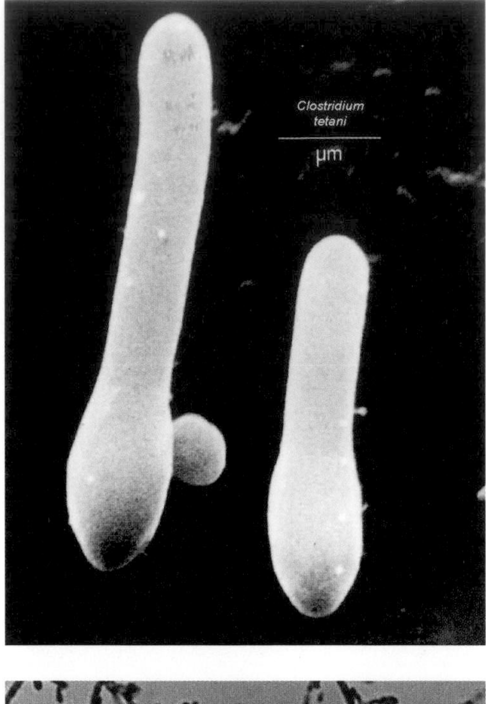

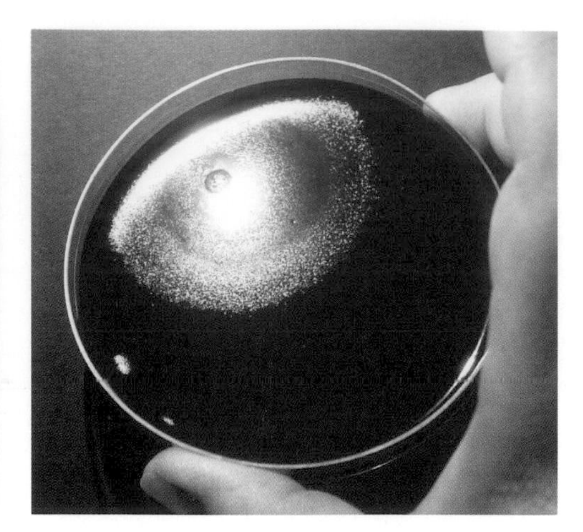

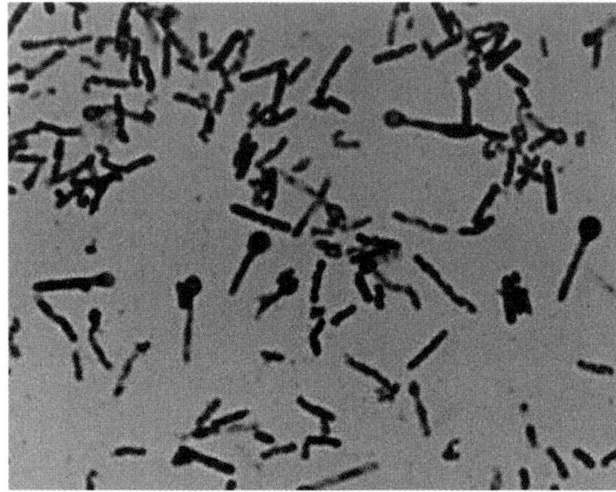

wound has not been treated properly and if the child has not received the appropriate immunization.

– The vaccine against tetanus for children is included in the DTaP vaccination (against diphtheria, pertussis, and tetanus). Older children are usually given a booster in the double vaccine (DT: diphtheria, tetanus).

The tetanus bacterium generally lives in the ground, but it can be found almost anywhere. If its spores enter a wound, beyond the reach of oxygen, they germinate and produce a toxin that interferes with neuromuscular control. A tetanus infection is extremely serious and can be life-threatening, if the wounded person has not been previously vaccinated.

cancer in childhood

Children represent between 1 and 3 percent of all cancer cases. For some time now, new therapies have made it possible to significantly improve the survival rates, and the quality of life, in these children. Nevertheless, it is the second highest cause of death in childhood. On the positive side however, statistics indicate that 76 percent of cases can be cured, and this figure rises to 90 percent in some types of cancer.

General aspects and most frequent types

• The initial stages of cancer can manifest themselves in children with supreme subtlety, making it very difficult to diagnose. This is one of the reasons why it is so important for a child to have regular medical check-ups, and for his parents to remain on the alert for any warning sign that their child may be sick. These warning signs include: lack of energy, frequent headaches, loss of appetite, persistent fever, aching bones, unusual spots, lumps, or inflammations, etc.

MOST FREQUENT TYPES OF CANCER IN CHILDREN

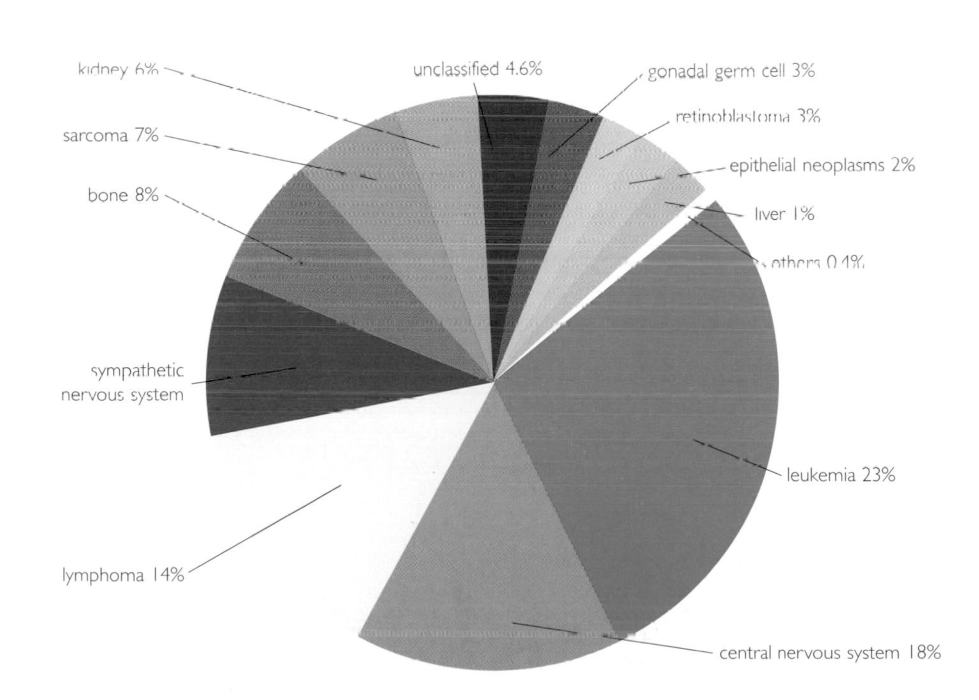

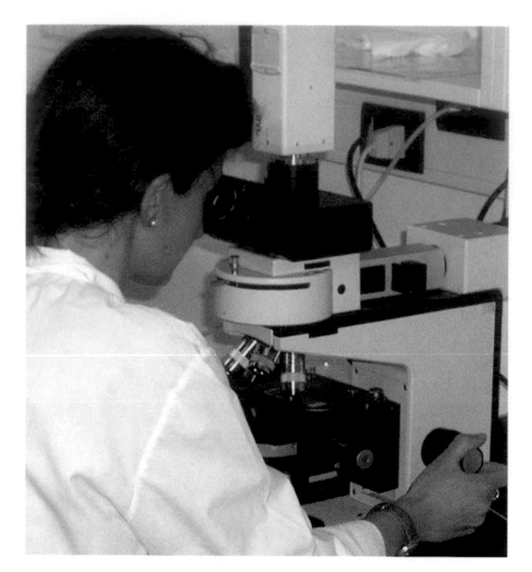

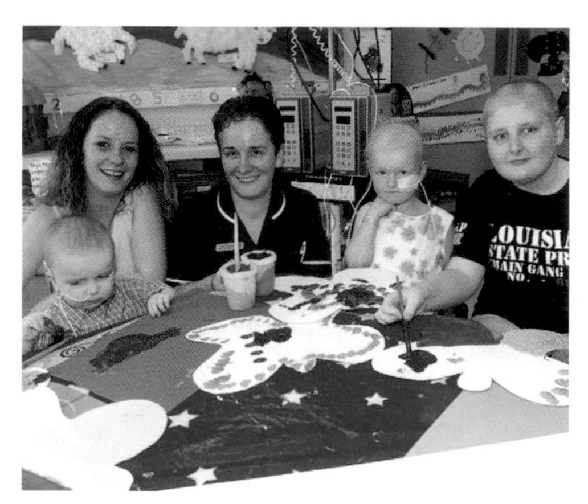

A child's physical appearance can provide a constant reminder of how different he is from others and this can undermine his confidence, leading to regressive behavior or withdrawal and reluctance to go to school. A medical team's psychological support for both the child and his family are of primary importance in this respect.

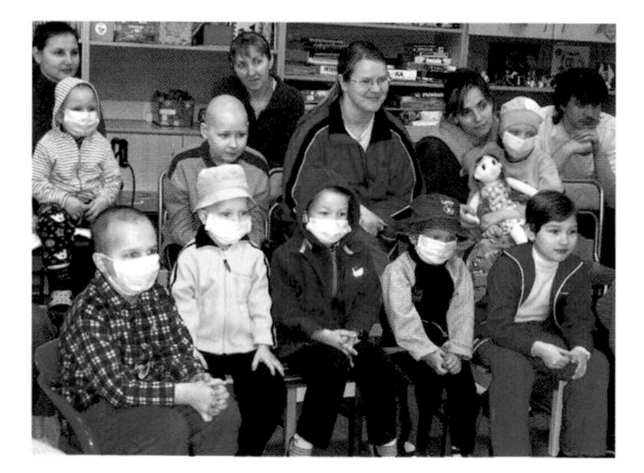

Most childhood tumors appear between the first and fourth years of life; they are more common in boys than in girls.

The definitive diagnosis of cancer is provided by microscopic examination of the damaged tissue from a biopsy – of the bone marrow, for example. Once the pathological anatomy results are available, it will be possible to confirm the diagnosis and choose the treatment most suited to the particular patient.

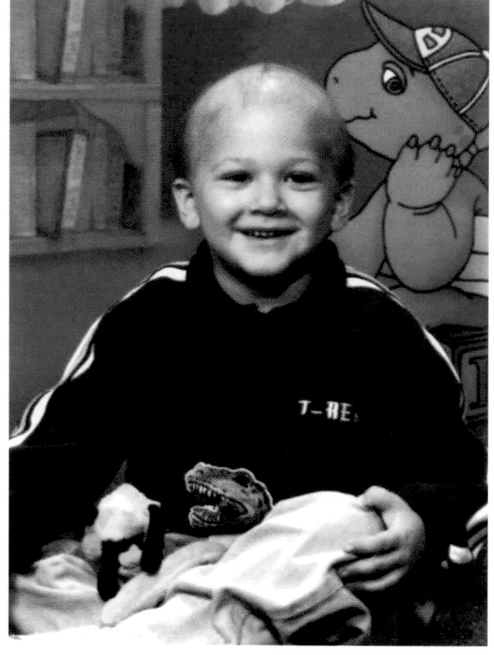

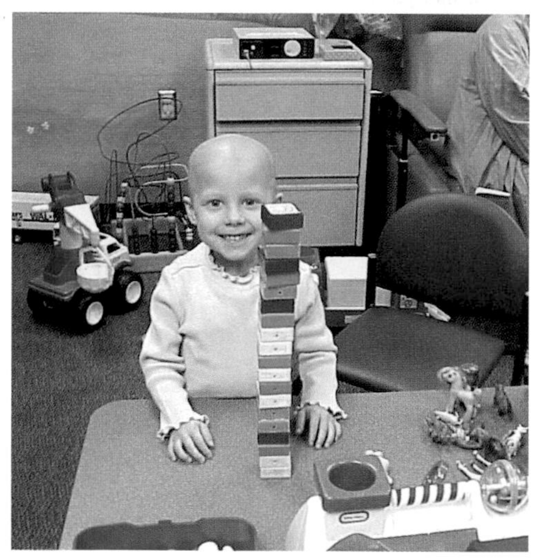

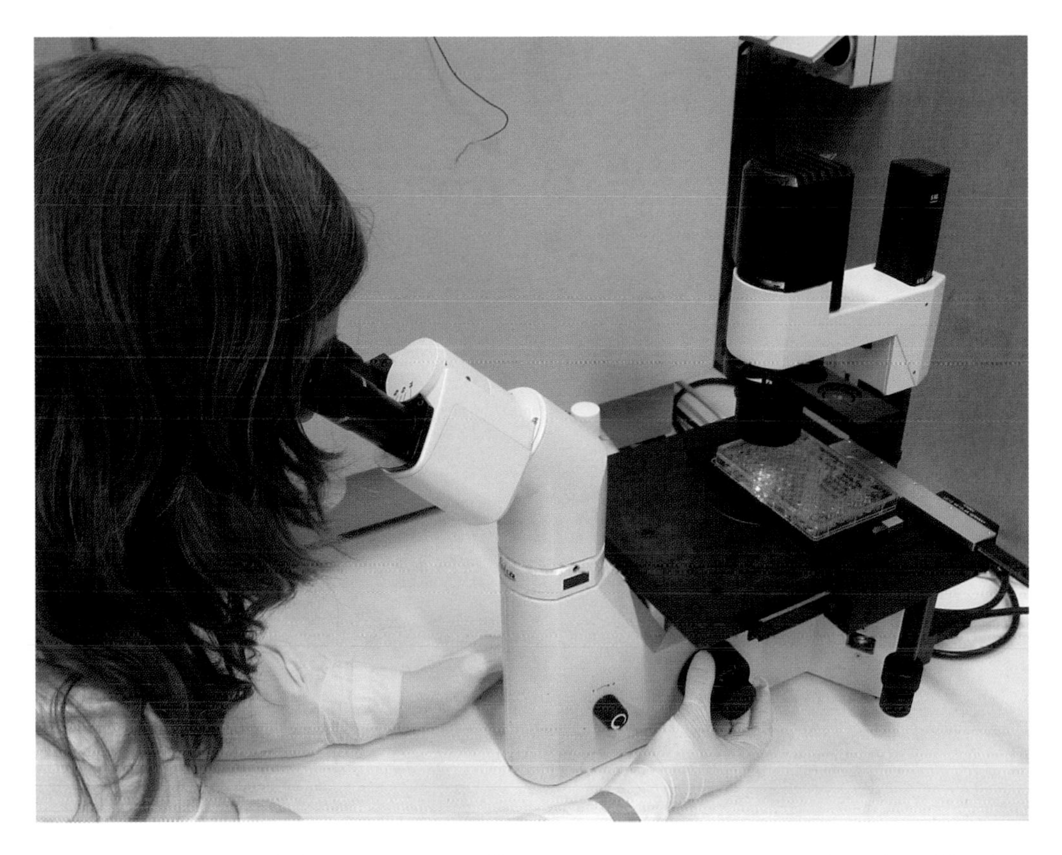

It is important for a child to return to his normal life as soon as possible. Going back to school is particularly important, as it plays a key role in a child's everyday life. His teachers need emotional support, as well as information about their pupil's disease, as their attitude is crucial to the child's full integration with his classmates.

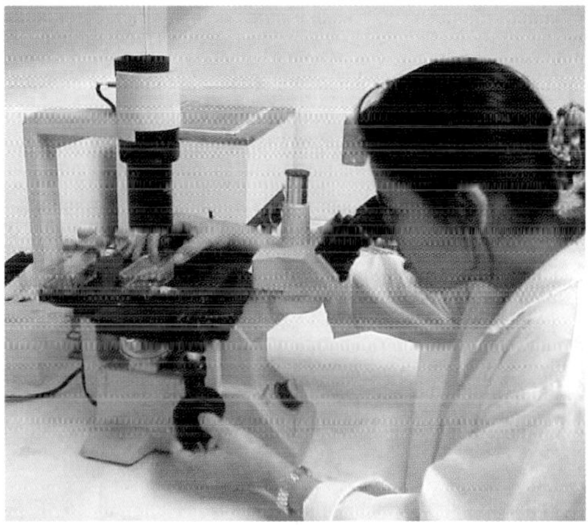

• If the presence of a tumor is suspected, the doctor will request a blood analysis, X-rays, and other more specific tests, to identify the type of tumor and find out how far it has spread.

Types of cancer

• **Leukemia.** This is the most common type of cancer in children, accounting for about 23% of the total cases. Of these, 80% correspond to acute lymphoblastic leukemia (ALL), which originates in a lymph cell in the bone marrow, which loses its characteristics and its function to become a tumoral cell (lymphoblast). There are various classifications of ALL, depending on the type of lymph cell in which the tumor originates.

• **Lymphomas.** These tumors have the third highest incidence rates in children; they are divided into two types: Hodgkin's lymphoma and non Hodgkin's lymphoma.

How much should a child know about his sickness?

- Although this is a subject of great controversy, many experts recommend telling a child what is going on, to avoid any misunderstandings, assuage fears, and obtain a greater degree of collaboration. It is up to his parents, however, to decide on the best moment to talk to him, what to explain to him (and how), whether they need psychological assistance or support, etc.
- Children aged under 6. It is difficult for a child of this age to fully comprehend a disease or diagnosis, so his parents need to try to reassure him by making him understand that it is not a punishment and that he has not done anything wrong. What most preoccupies these children is being separated from their parents, as well as any pain or discomfort to which they may be subjected. It is important for a child to feel secure and happy, with a positive frame of mind: distract him with toys and colorful objects, try to create a cozy environment in the hospital room (possibly with some items from his bedroom at home), play with him constantly, and praise his good behavior when he undergoes tests or receives treatment.
- Children aged between 7 and 12. They begin to understand that getting well depends on taking medicine, hospital monitoring, and following the doctor's instructions. They are increasingly aware of their sickness and understand indignities like losing their hair. A child's parents and relatives should answer all his questions sincerely, keep up their sense of humor, make an effort to keep him entertained, ask the medical team what exercise he can do, make sure that he sees his classmates, friends, siblings, etc.

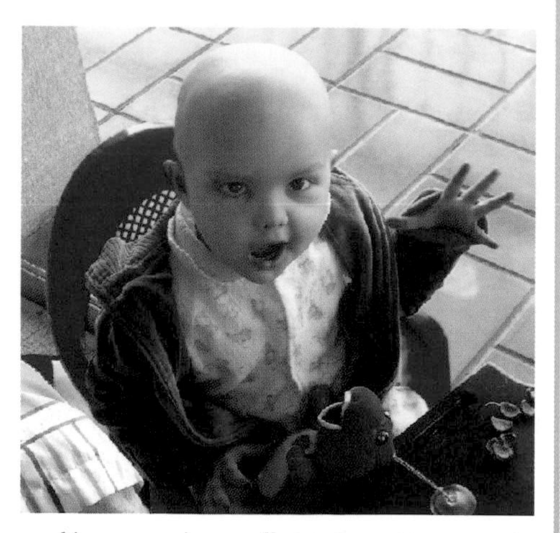

- Children aged over 13. Adolescents are particularly concerned about social relationships and realize that some aspects of their sickness prevent them from leading a normal life like their friends. Feeling different can be very painful in this phase, and going back to school can involve stress and anxiety. A young adolescent needs to be allowed to participate in the decisions and discussions about his disease, so encourage him to ask about anything on his mind, while respecting his privacy and even allowing him to talk to the doctor by himself. A sense of humor can be a useful tool for relieving his frustration.

Children can have a wide range of reactions to disease, depending largely on their age and degree of emotional and intellectual development. Ultimately, however, they all share the same concerns: the possibility of pain, the duration of their sickness, and the separation from their parents and siblings.

A non-Hodgkin's lymphoma is caused by an immature lymphocyte, although in this case it attacks not only the bone marrow but also the lymph glands, which play a role in the immune system. For all practical purposes, non-Hodgkin's lymphoma can be considered leukemia with lumps.

Hodgkin's disease is particularly prevalent in adolescents, and it has been related to the Epstein-

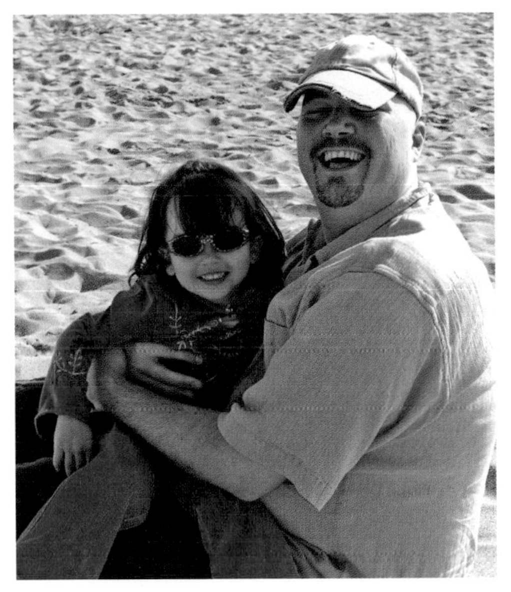

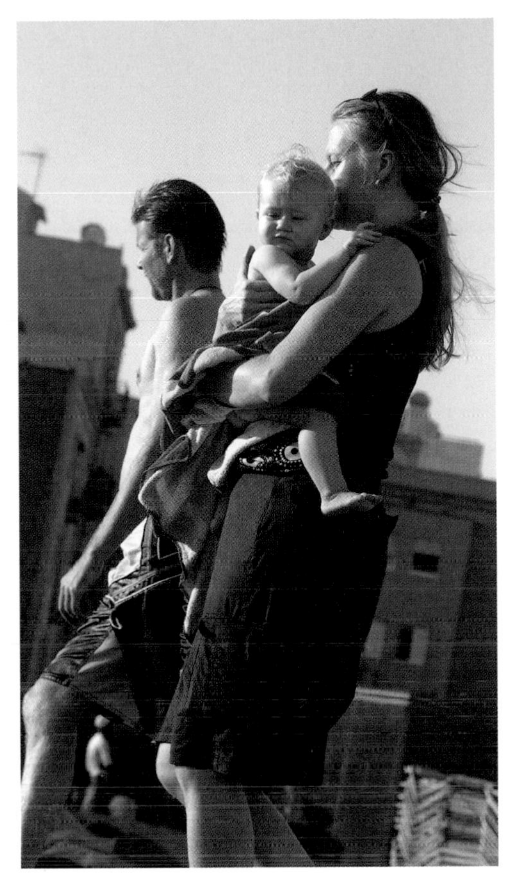

Barr virus. Of all types of cancer, this has one of the best prognoses for recovery.

• **Brain tumors.** This is the most common type of cancer after leukemia. Brain tumors can be benign or malignant; their prognosis and treatment depend on the type of cell in which they originate, as well as a wide range of other factors, such as the location of the tumor, the extent to which it has spread, the child's age, and his general state of health.

Treatment

The main treatments for cancer in children are surgery, chemotherapy, radiotherapy, and immunotherapy. A single treatment is often insufficient, so a combination may be required.

Chemotherapy is a systemic chemical treatment that affects the whole body, which means that it can also encroach on healthy cells and tissues. It is this organic effect that gives rise to some of chemotherapy's most distinctive side effects: hair loss, ulcers, diarrhea, vomiting, etc. The most alarming – and the most closely monitored – side effect, however, is myelosuppression. This denotes a reduction in the number of cells in the immune system, along with a similar scarcity of red blood cells and platelets. So, a child receiving chemotherapy is particularly vulnerable to infections that may require a stay in hospital. He may also need blood transfusions if he has anemia, or transfusions of platelets, if there is a risk of hemorrhages.

Radiotherapy is usually used in conjunction with one of the other two therapies; it destroys cancerous cells with high-energy radiations.

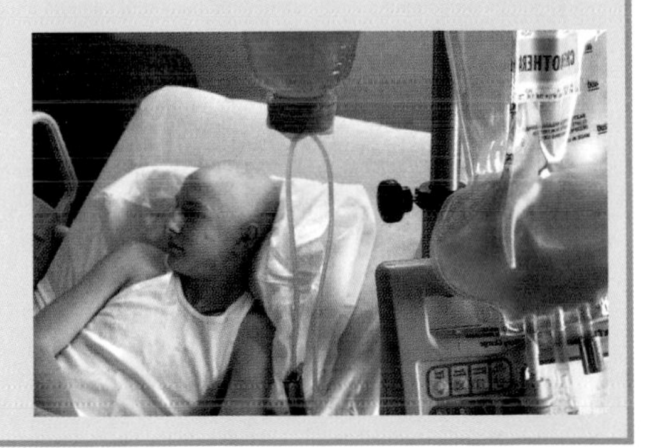

• **Neuroblastoma.** This tumor, often diagnosed in the first year of a child's life, originates in the sympathetic nervous system, situated along the spine and in the suprarenal glands, just above the kidney. The tumor itself is often found in the thorax or abdomen; in some cases, it compresses the spinal cord and weakens the limbs or alters the function of the sphincters.

• **Retinoblastoma.** This cancer of the eyes is not very common, but it is considered responsible for about 5% of cases of childhood blindness. It can be diagnosed before the age of 5. It is one of the tumors with the greatest possibility of being cured, but its prognosis and treatment, as well as the child's chances of recovering his eyesight, depend on how far the cancer has spread.

• **Wilms tumor.** This can appear in one or both kidneys and generally affects children aged between 2 and 3. It accounts for about 10% of pediatric cancers, and it is curable in most cases.

• **Osteosarcoma.** This is the most common type of bone cancer in children and adolescents. It usually appears on the tip of long bones (femur, tibia) and in the knee area.

• **Ewing's tumor.** This is the second most common malignant bone cancer, after osteosarcoma. It originates in the parasympathetic nervous tissue and can also be found away from bones.

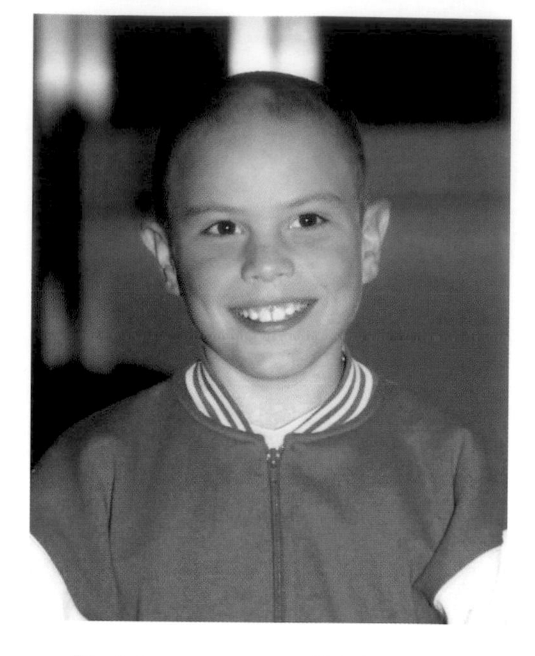

• **Rhabdomyosarcoma.** This is the sarcoma most often found outside the bones. It always affects muscles, and it is responsible for between 4 and 8% of cancers in children.

Despite the high recovery rate, cancer is still the second greatest cause of infant mortality in developed countries, after accidents.

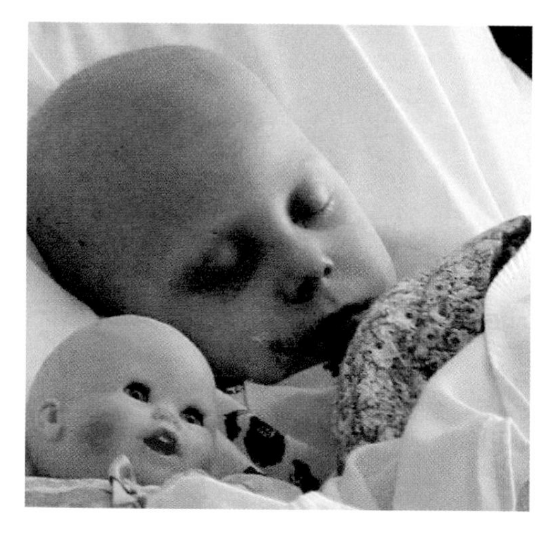

A sick child will ask why he goes into hospital so often, why he feels so tired or so much pain, why he has so many tests, etc. The better informed such children are, the less stress they feel and the more cooperative they will be during treatment. Every case is unique, however, and a child's parents are the best judges of how and when to speak to him.

bonding and education

The education of a child is as wide-ranging as life itself. Parents are responsible for laying the foundations and marking the boundaries that determine the course of this never-ending process. There are no magic formulas or secret recipes: every child poses a new and formidable challenge.

The great adventure

• Educating a child is an adventure. In most cases, this task is undertaken with the desire to achieve a precious goal: the happiness of your child. There is no infallible guide to success, however, and even less to instant triumph. Education involves constant uncertainty; this has its advantages, as it prevents parents from resting on their laurels and becoming bogged down in routine, or from turning into slaves to their own selfish needs and desires. Parents are

Educating children is as simple and as complex as knowing oneself and reaching maturity. There are no instruction manuals or guarantees; the adventure of being a parent begins and ends with every step, at every moment.

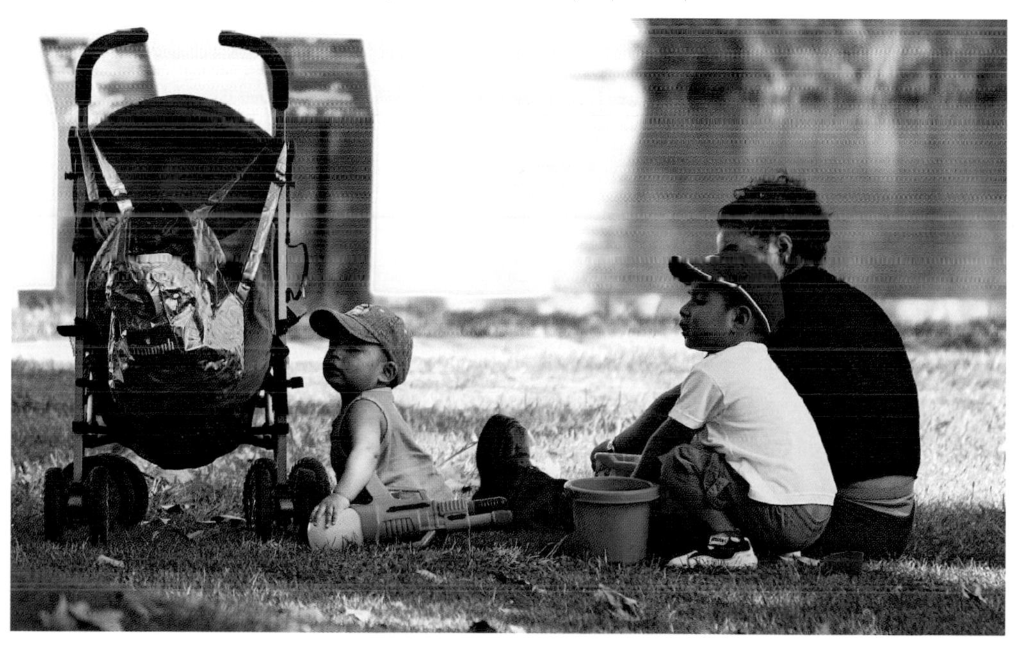

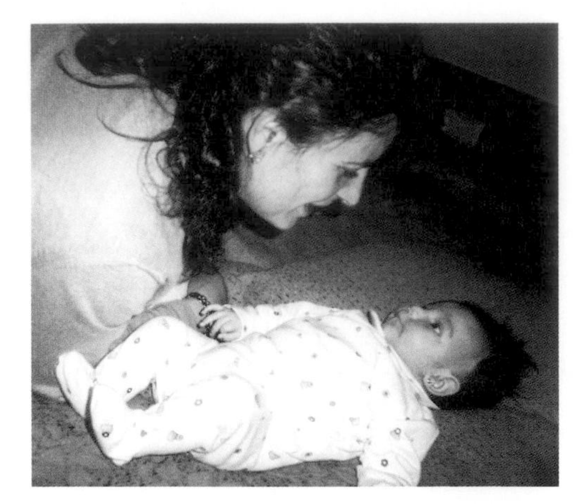

Like all relationships, the parent–child bond is a two-way affair: both parties give and take. The same is true of education: children learn from their parents, and parents from their children, on a daily basis.

under permanent pressure to give the best of themselves, from the first to last minute of every day.

• As with every bond, success and failure does not always flow in one direction. Children learn from their parents, but parents also learn constantly from their children. Among other things, they learn that not everything can be controlled, that personal traits and reactions cannot always be fathomed, that it is possible to subordinate personal interests. Every child is a distinctive person who will forge a bond with her parents that is unique and unrepeatable, but there are no perfect parents nor perfect children. For this very reason, there is always room for improvement in their relationship.

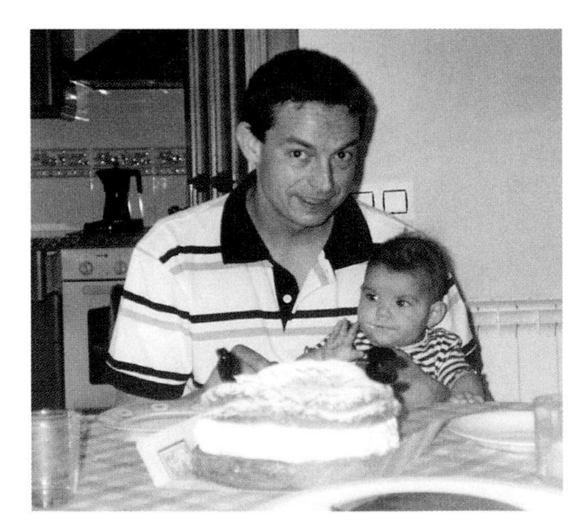

Parents, children, and society

• Education is transmitted not only when it is being consciously imparted, but also in day-to-day living. Children often learn more from what they observe than from formal instruction. The unconscious attitudes of their parents provide models for their children to follow and imitate, especially during the first years of life. In this way, their personality is gradually formed and molded, allowing them to acquire self-awareness and self-esteem. It can therefore be said that the evolution of children begins with the evolution of their own parents – their personal histories, prior to their children's birth, and even before they met each other. This process means that both strong points and shortcomings are passed on and perpetuated from generation to generation.

• Similarly, although perhaps to a lesser extent, the specific social and cultural circumstances of a time and place also shape children and provide them with role models. Seemingly unremarkable occurrences can become the points of reference against which children measure their own experience and development.

• The guarantee of a good education lies in a loving relationship between parents and children; this serves as a basis that can be extended to relationships with the rest of the family and people in other social settings. This experience will mark all the relationships that a child establishes, as well as her own view of herself.

Distinguishing between care and overprotection

• Parents instinctively protect their children. They see them as dependent and defenseless; they hug them when they cry, they keep them out of danger, they show them what they can and cannot do, they console them when they are feeling sad, etc. Similarly, parents constantly worry about what could happen to their children: even when they are asleep, particularly when they are small babies, parents check on them to make sure they are breathing properly; they tend to their cuts and grazes when they fall over, and consult a doctor whenever they fall sick. This is of course all perfectly normal and responsible behavior.

• Sometimes, however, normal vigilance can turn into an excessive concern that leads parents to overprotect their child. They hang on to her every need

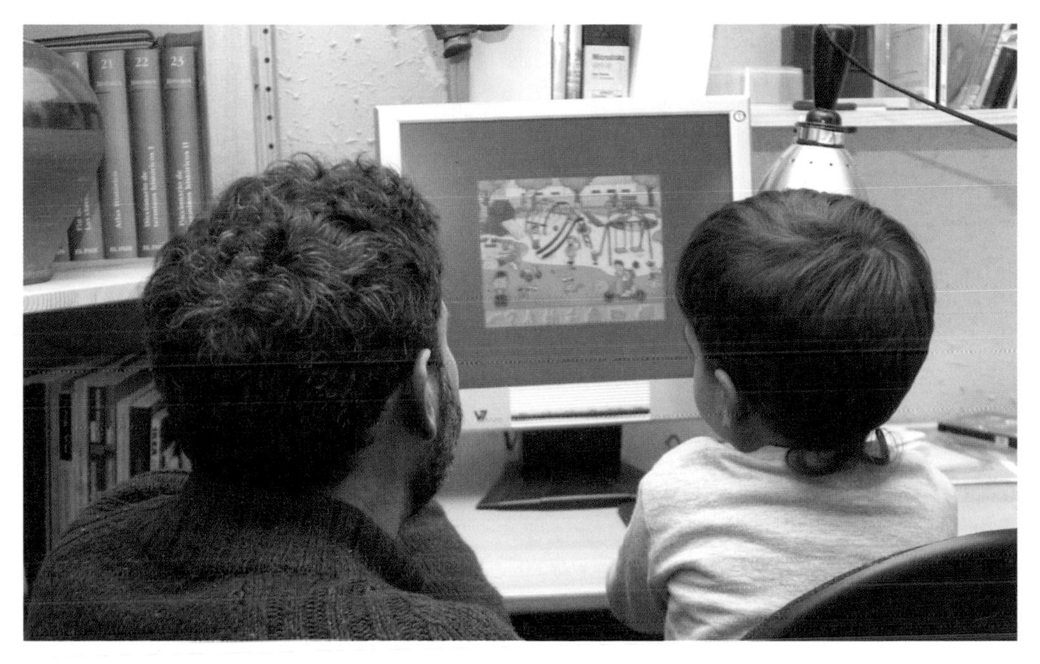

Parents should not be discouraged by the number of outside factors that can impinge on the education and development of their children. Such influences should serve instead to make them aware that, given the impossibility of monitoring every situation, a child's primary experience, and the basis of her education, lies in the family unit.

around the clock: whether she is hungry, whether she is cold, whether it is time to get dressed, whether she could fall over, whether she should have a bath, etc. Such parents can go without sleep if their child is sick or sad, and fail to understand that she might sometimes prefer to be left alone in her room. The end result is a spoilt brat, accustomed to having everything done for her. She does not know what it means to become frustrated and overcome setbacks. Even if she is given some responsibilities, she will tend to shirk them.

The reasons for such overprotective behavior in parents might include.

• An experience of overprotective parenting in their own childhood, so they follow this pattern because they know no other way.

• A desire to shield their children from the experience of a lack of affection that marked their own strict upbringing and so they go to the other extreme of consenting to everything and demanding nothing in return.

• An experience of early trauma that makes them adopt an overprotective attitude, to avoid a repetition of this situation.

• Being adoptive parents who seek to compensate for the lack of biological parenthood by doting on their child.

• being older parents who play the role of permissive grandparents rather than being parents responsible for their children's education.

• Having an only child on whom they lavish attention and devote all their available time to.

• Feeling guilty about spending most of their time away from their children on account of overwork or divorce, and trying to make up for absences by spoiling their child.

Being overprotective can have the following consequences for the child:

• The child is not expected to act her age.

• She is prevented from taking on responsibilities.

• She has not been taught how to be independent.

early stimulation

Early stimulation aims to take advantage of the adaptability of a young child's brain and her capacity to learn. Exercises and games are used to provide stimuli that enhance cerebral functions that will be essential in later life. This is not merely a question of honing intellectual abilities like reading and adding up, but also of furthering a child's physical, sensory, and social development.

Early stimulation

Cognitive development

- From the third month of life, a baby displays a great desire to explore and investigate. Her increased mobility allows her to take in her surroundings more fully and classify her perceptions.
- By the end of the first year, her mobility has been greatly enhanced, opening up new fields of exploration. She is capable of carefully observing

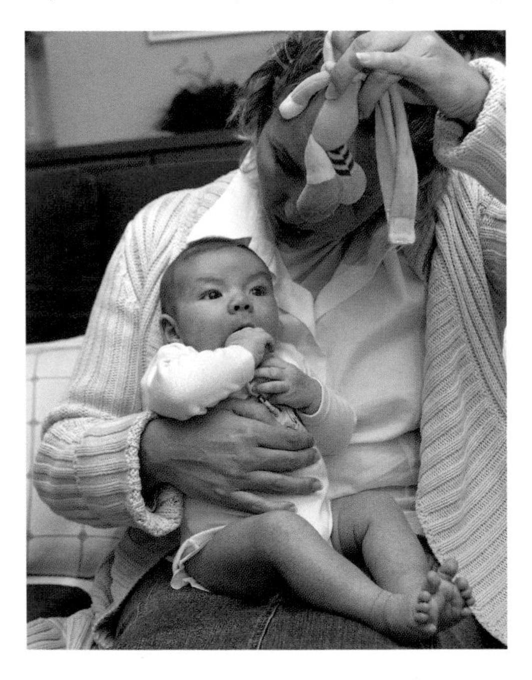

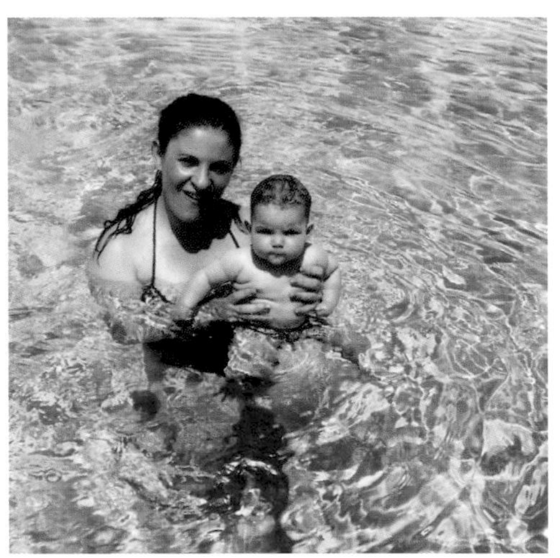

A stimulation program can of course be tedious and repetitive for parents, as it demands dedication on a daily basis. Some experts question its effectiveness but in any case, the time spent with your children will certainly be rewarding.

Early stimulation consists of the stimulation of various physical skills to encourage a child's self-control by developing confident and uninhibited movements, as well as broadening her mental capacities by improving dexterity. This process will encourage a child to exercise her curiosity and use her imagination by playing.

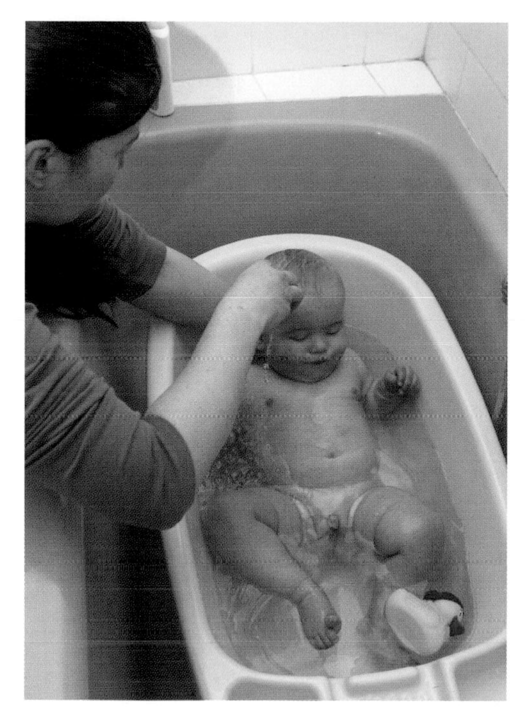

A baby ceaslessly investigates the world around her from the moment she is born. Any arousal of her senses that allows her to perceive stimuli and relate them to each other encourages her intellectual capacities.
Caresses, massages, breast-feeding, continuous explanations, and bathing all help to stimulate a baby.

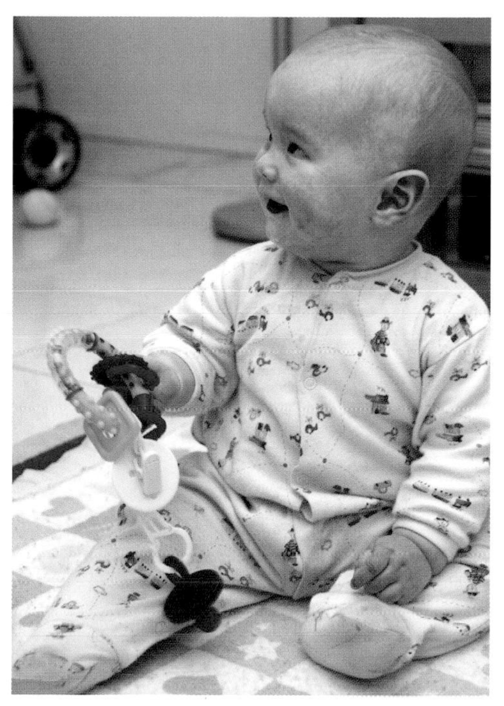

Motor control develops in a downward direction, i.e. a baby first learns to control her head, then her trunk, and finally her limbs. It is very important to seek information about the sequence of your child's development in each area, so that you can learn how to stimulate her latent capacities.

something that interests her for a considerable time. This is a good time to teach her new concepts, as she is very predisposed to learn.

• Language is very important. Talk to her as you go about your everyday activities, explaining what you are doing; sing and read to her as well. A child's learning progress is sequential (i.e. one skill helps the acquisition of another new skill) and progressive (i.e. functions of increasing complexity are accumulated). All the various parts of the nervous system act in a coordinated manner to facilitate this process, with each area interacting with the rest to ensure the orderly evolution of the child's capacities.

Gross motor development

• The first skill a child has to master is that of lifting her head. The ideal posture for stimulating this ability is a face-down position; she will discover how to support her body with her arms and thrust forward her head and upper trunk.

• Once a child can keep her head up and support herself on her arms, she has to learn how to turn over. To develop this skill, put her on her back on a sturdy surface, attract her attention so that she turns her head to one side and help her to place her arms and legs in a position from which she can complete the rotation. Once she is face down, help her to continue turning over by showing her the easiest position for this movement. This sequence can be repeated 10 or 15 times in both directions. Once she acquires the knack, give her less help, so that she can complete the action on her own.

• When a child is able to turn over on her own, it is time for her to learn how to sit. To do this, sit her down on a sturdy surface, supporting her hips and helping her to lean forward on her hands. Once she is seated, play with her by gently pushing her forward and sideways, to improve her balance.

• When a baby first starts dragging herself around, all the effort comes from her hands. If you position yourself behind her, you can guide her legs so that they move in synchronism with her hands. This tactile stimulation will notably improve her ability to coordinate her movements and keep her balance. It is worth encouraging her to crawl and delay the transition to walking as much as possible.

• Once a child has mastered crawling, she will start walking in no time. To improve her sense of balance, put her near a small table and, holding on to her, play at seeing how long she can keep her balance. You should ensure that she adopts an erect position, with the feet in line and the back straight, so that she can walk comfortably, using a stable chair or large toy as a support, with her arms stretched out in front of her.

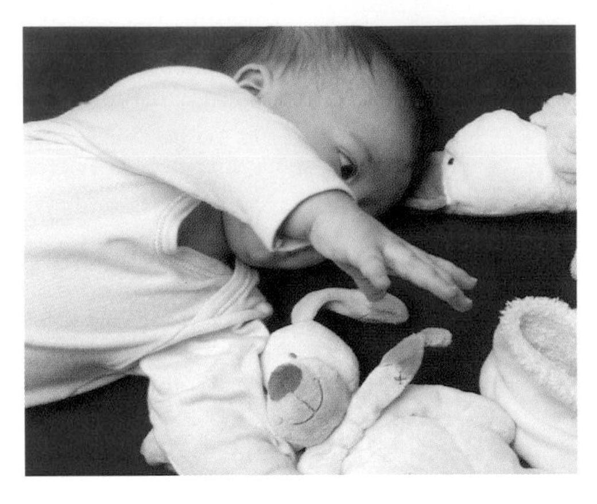

Fine motor control begins in the first months of a baby's life, when she discovers her hands and gradually learns how to use them through experimentation. Leave toys within reach, to encourage her to grasp them.

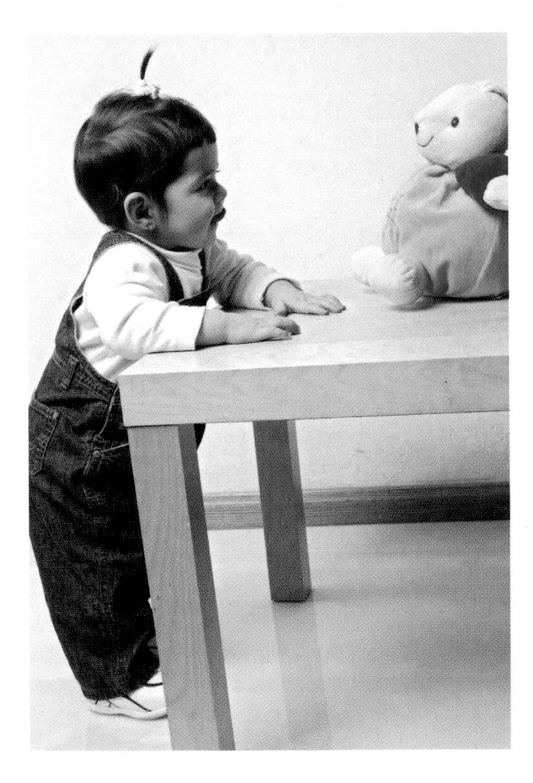

• Play games involving rocking, turning over, jumping, and swinging; these all provide stimulation for the mechanisms responsible for a child's sense of balance, and also help improve the coordination of her body movements.

• In all these situations, you must be sure to hold her securely. If these activities do not particularly appeal to your child, they should be undertaken only briefly and then gradually prolonged. Remember that the key to all these learning techniques is making them fun for the child.

Fine motor development

• Once a child has managed to coordinate her vision with her hands, she will start to pick up objects, at first with the entire palm of her hand.

• After the first year of life, a child can pick up objects with greater dexterity, using her fingers as a pincer; by now, she also knows how to throw objects! She will try to scribble and turn the pages of picture books.

• All these factors are proof that her level of perceptive-motor coordination is increasingly approaching that of an adult, as the movements she uses to grasp, push, release, and hurl objects are becoming increasingly sophisticated.

• She will gradually learn the skills of putting a spoon in her mouth, of brushing her hair, and of putting a telephone to her ear.

Learning to overcome the force of gravity depends on the organization of all the senses, and particularly the balance system, which helps a child to automatically recognize the correct position of her body and its relationship to her surroundings.

infant sleep disorders

A baby's sleep patterns change as she grows older and gradually learns that she should be awake during the day and asleep at night. Many children learn this automatically, but others need their parents to guide them.

Sleep disorders

The phases of sleep

• Sleep is a physiological state, maintained by both the brain and body, that does not imply any truncation of the functions proper to wakefulness, although these are modified: cardiac rhythm, blood pressure, respiratory frequency, body temperature, etc. are all reduced. The patterns of sleep and wakefulness undergo various changes as a child grows up until, on the verge of adolescence, they acquire characteristics similar to those of an adult.

• Generally speaking, there are 2 types of sleep: rapid-eye movement (REM) and non-rapid-eye movement (NREM). Each has its own characteristics:

• NREM. This occupies most of the time spent asleep. It is usually divided into 4 phases, related to the depth of the sleep. The starting point for their classification is 0, which corresponds to "wakefulness."

Night-time sleep is typically made up of the repetition of a cycle of 90–110 minutes of REM and NREM sleep. Almost 80 percent of this cycle consists of 4 phases of NREM, which become increasingly deep. Our metabolism and vital functions slow down during these phases. REM sleep, in contrast, is characterized by the intensification of cerebral activity. Around 90 percent of people who wake up during the REM phase state that they were dreaming. The REM periods become increasingly longer as the night goes on.

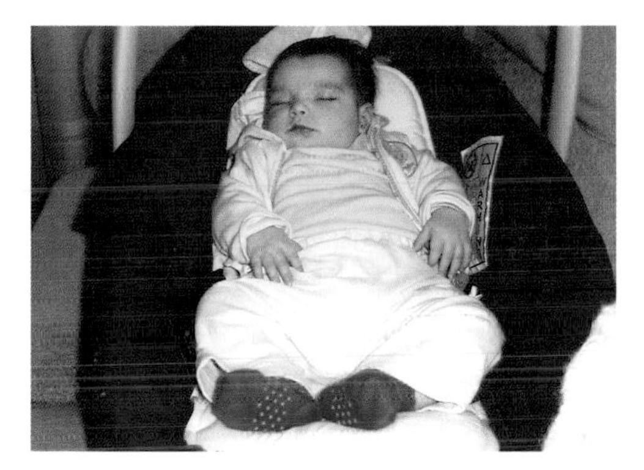

The first 3 months of a baby's life are governed by cycles of roughly3 hours each, as she needs to feed, sleep, and excrete frequently. In this period, a baby will sleep an average of 16 hours per day.

Phase 1: initial sleepiness when a person starts to doze off.

Phase 2: the next step into a deeper sleep is the longest of these phases.

Phase 3: this is deeper still – it is difficult to wake somebody up during this phase.

Phase 4: the deepest phase of all – it can take several minutes to wake a person up in this phase.

• REM. This consists of a single phase marked by fast sideways movements of the eyes, in combina-

During NREM, the brain lacks the capacity to store information in the memory, making it impossible to remember any dreams from this phase.

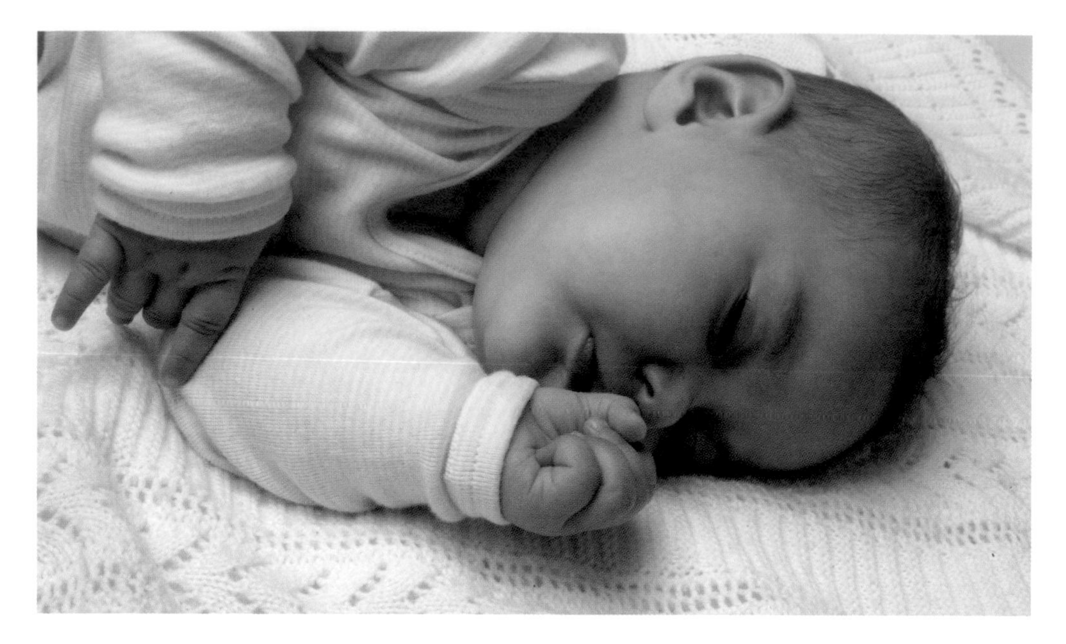

Sleep habits, like other forms of behavior, are learnt and can be taught. The available data suggests that 98% of children with sleep disorders were not taught this habit correctly.

tion, usually occurring between phases 1 and 2 of NREM sleep. It is impossible to move the voluntary muscles (arms, legs, face, and trunk), but respiratory, intestinal, cardiac, and muscular activities are maintained. The memory also remains in operation, which is why we can remember our dreams.

Changing sleep patterns in infancy

- In the first month of life, the daytime and night-time pattern of the cycles of sleep and wakefulness are very similar. In about the second month, sleep becomes deeper and longer-lasting at night.
- At the age of 1 year, a child usually sleeps 12–14 hours per day and takes 2 naps.
- Between the ages of 12 and 18 months, she starts to skip the morning nap, but she may continue taking a post-lunch siesta up to the age of 4.
- Between the ages of 4 and 12, a child's sleep patterns start to resemble those of an adult, with an average of 10 hours sleep a day, without any naps. Some researchers have noted a change in the sleep patterns of adolescents, which manifests itself in greater sleepiness during the day, precipitated by heightened daytime activity and late nights at the weekend. It is important to allow them to sleep in later, but remember that there is no "catching up" when it comes to sleeping, so a long daytime nap can make it more difficult to sleep at night.

Infant sleep problems

- Refusing to go to bed. Children can resort to excuses and/or manipulative behavior to delay the moment when they have to go to bed. Many ask their parents to stay with them until they fall asleep, or even to sleep in their parents' bed. They can also develop rituals, such as asking for water,

A baby's sleeping patterns are determined by a small group of cells in the brain that work like a clock. This internal clock has to be stimulated by routines and sleeping habits. These routines are established by parents so that a baby gradually adopts new sleeping patterns. In 70 percent of cases, her internal clock will adapt perfectly with little outside help; the remaining 30 percent can need more active encouragement.

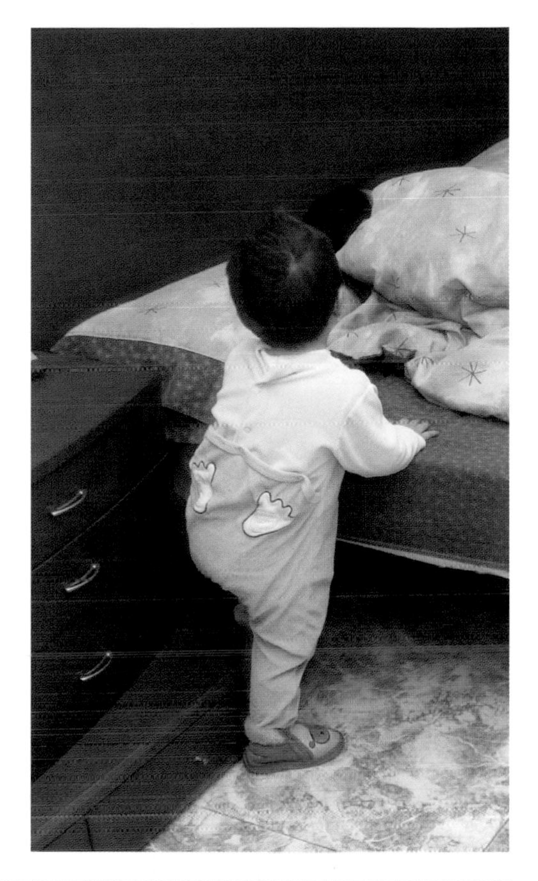

Children can pester people to achieve what they want. It is important to establish norms and not permit a child to deviate from her bedtime routine.

a goodnight kiss, etc. In all these cases, the child is trying to attract attention and take control of the situation by manipulating the people around her. This is a behavioral issue and should be treated as such.

- Getting up during the night. This can be a corollary to refusing to go to bed. The excuse is usually fear, but a child's ultimate aim is to sleep with her parents or persuade one of them to come to her own bed. In these cases, the child is also seeking attention and manipulating the situation to her own ends. Once again, this is a functional disorder.

It is normal for a child to have nightmares if she has seen an adult movie or TV program featuring monsters, witches, suspenseful situations, or harrowing scenes. The images are archived in her mind and later prevent her from sleeping or they reappear in the form of vivid dreams.

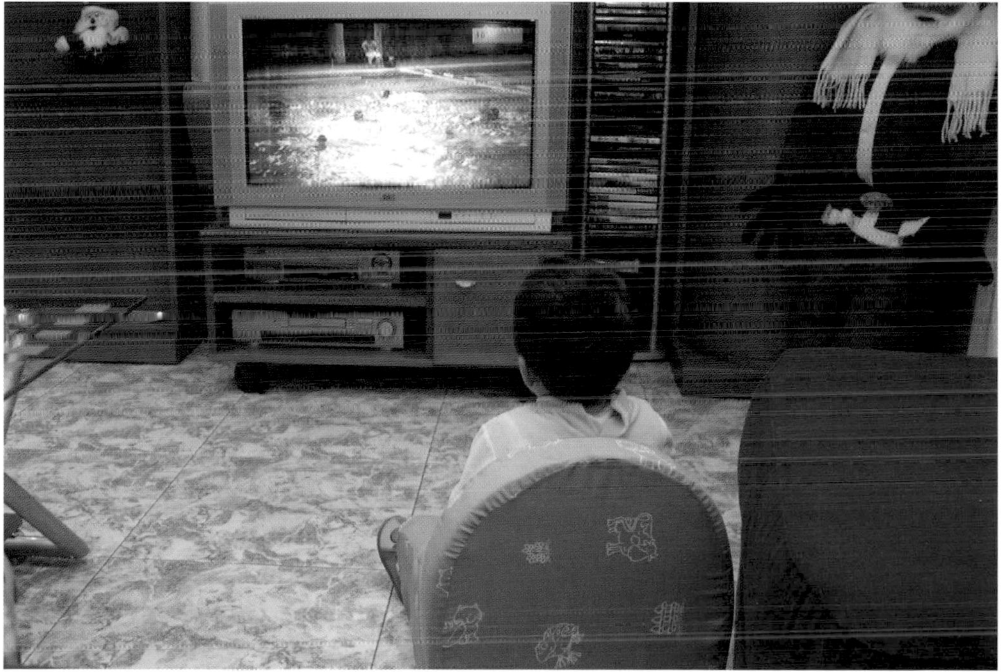

• Night-time terror. Night-time fear involves recurrent episodes of sudden awakening, during the first third of the main period of sleep (phases 3 and 4 of NREM), and starts off with a cry of panic. Every episode is accompanied by intense anxiety and physical manifestations like tachycardia, dypsnea, and sweating. The child generally answers questions incoherently, appearing confused and disorientated, as well as making stereotyped movements like clinging to the pillow. If she goes back to sleep before this distress has abated, it is highly likely that she will not even remember the incident the following day. In most cases, this is a harmless, transient disorder that does not require treatment. If there is no improvement, a neuro-physiological examination may be in order.

Nightmares. These are often a trigger for night-time panic. The child wakes up crying or shouting, but it is easy to communicate with her and provide reassurance.

Sleepwalking. Without waking up, the child gets out of bed and walks round her room or the rest of the house. This is considered a disruption to the sleep rhythm caused by immaturity in the mechanisms inducing relaxation and immobility. It can be studied by using a continuous electroencephalogram (EEG) during sleep. If a child does not walk in her sleep repeatedly and is in no physical danger, she will usually stop doing it without any need for treatment. If the problem is more serious, it may require treatment with a drug like carbamacepin (single night-time dose).

• Insomnia. Difficulty in falling sleep, or waking up in the middle of the night without being able to go back to sleep again, is associated with anxiety disorders and depressive conditions. It can also be linked to complaints such as adenoid infections, which have a suffocating effect when a child lies down, or with some anti-influenza drugs like teophyllin, ephedrine, and beta-adrenergics. Insomnia can also

Narcolepsy, a specific form of hypersomnia, is a sleep crisis that occurs in daytime, either occasionally or repeatedly. It is usually accompanied by a sudden loss of muscle tone (cataplexy), hallucinations, and paralysis (inability to wake up, except to breathe). Electroencephalographic analysis has revealed that these crises start with a REM phase.

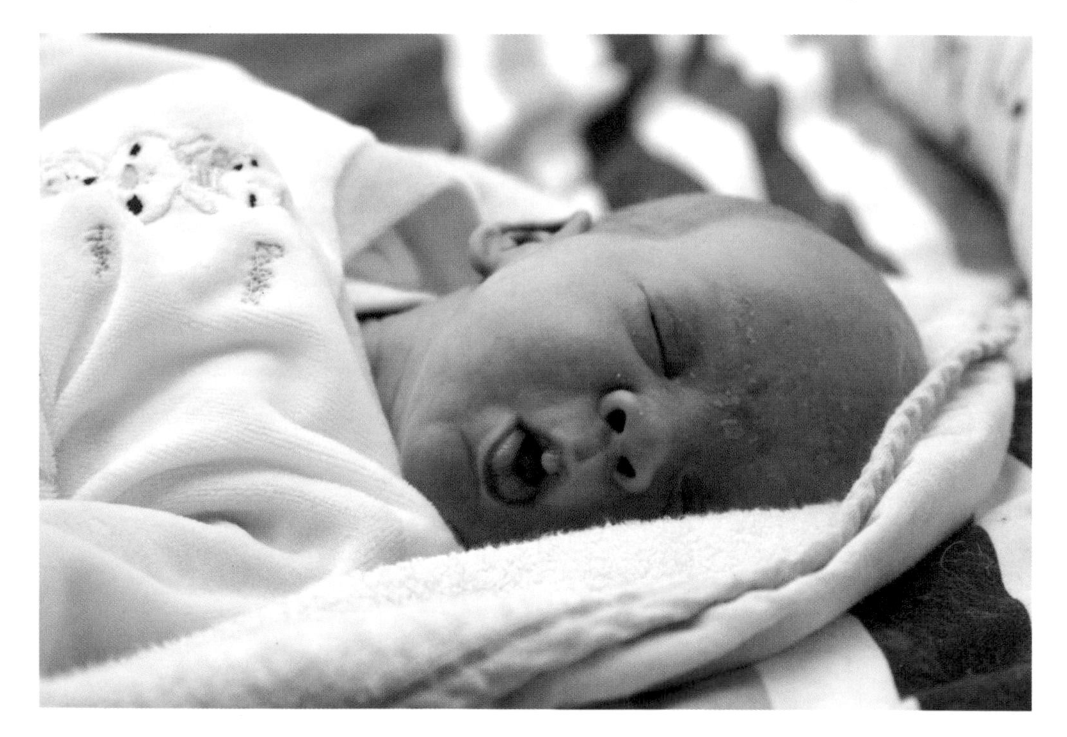

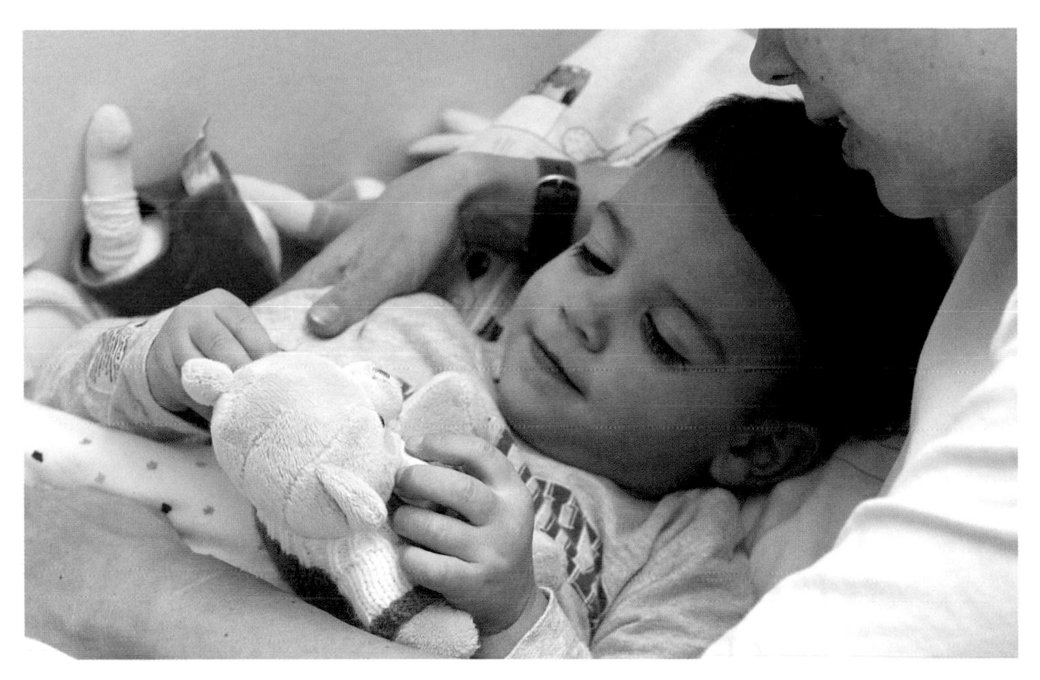

Parents need to be aware of how to educate their children with respect to sleeping, as it is a task that requires a clear head and plenty of patience. Both parents should agree on a strategy to avoid the intrusion of bad habits that could disrupt a routine. The aim is that a child learns to go to sleep alone, in his own bed, with the light out, since if he wakes up during the night, these are the conditions he will encounter and his parents will not be on hand to help him sleep again.

be triggered by analgesics containing caffeine, and nose drops with pseudo-ephedrine. A child may be unable to sleep after being very excited before going to bed, in tense situations, or after staying up to watch late TV shows or programs unsuitable for her age, etc. Stressful circumstances, such as sickness, hospitalization, or problems at school, can also lead to insomnia in a child. If insomnia persists or recurs, some professional psychological help may be needed.

• Hypersomnia. The child tends to sleep during the day. Sometimes connected to insomnia, this often proves to be nothing more than a reaction to changes in sleeping patterns or apnea. It can also appear during the course of depressions. A doctor will check whether the child is taking a drug that induces sleepiness: tranquilizers, antihistamines, antitusigen, certain cough medicines, ciproheptadine, etc. If hypersomnia proves to be persistent or recurring and has no apparent cause, it may be worth undertaking a neuro-physiological study (continuous EEG during sleep).

Learning the sleeping habit.

• Some research suggests that 35% of children aged under 5 suffer from sleep disorders, of which only about 2% have psychological causes that need treatment. The remaining 98% can generally be attributed to the acquisition of bad sleeping habits.

A few tips

- The learning process starts as soon as a baby is born, even though he will not start to regulate his sleep until the third month of life. It is very important to respond to night-time crying immediately and to accustom the child to sleeping in his crib, not in your arms, with the light out. If he falls asleep in somebody's arms, he will expect to still be there when he wakes up, so he may be confused and frightened.
- Babies should not associate food with sleeping. This is why it is advisable to make sure there is light, music, or another stimulus when you are nursing him, to prevent him from falling asleep.
- It may be useful to add objects to the crib so that they can remain there all night and become associated with sleeping: soft toys, drawings, bedclothes, etc.
- Like all learning processes, it is enhanced by a routine, which can start with a bath, followed by dinner, and concluding with bedtime.
- It is advisable to put a baby to bed at the same time every night – between 8 and 9 pm is a good time – as this will make him better prepared to go to sleep.
- Create a soothing ritual that he can associate with sleep, such as reading a story or saying a prayer.
- It is important to explain even to a very young child that his parents are teaching him how to sleep properly and so he cannot get into their bed or stay awake longer.
- Parents should always leave a child's bedroom before he falls asleep.
- If he cries, his parents should enter at short intervals (maximum wait of 5 minutes) to reassure him and talk to him quietly, not to make him be quiet or go to sleep, but to let him know that he has not been abandoned.

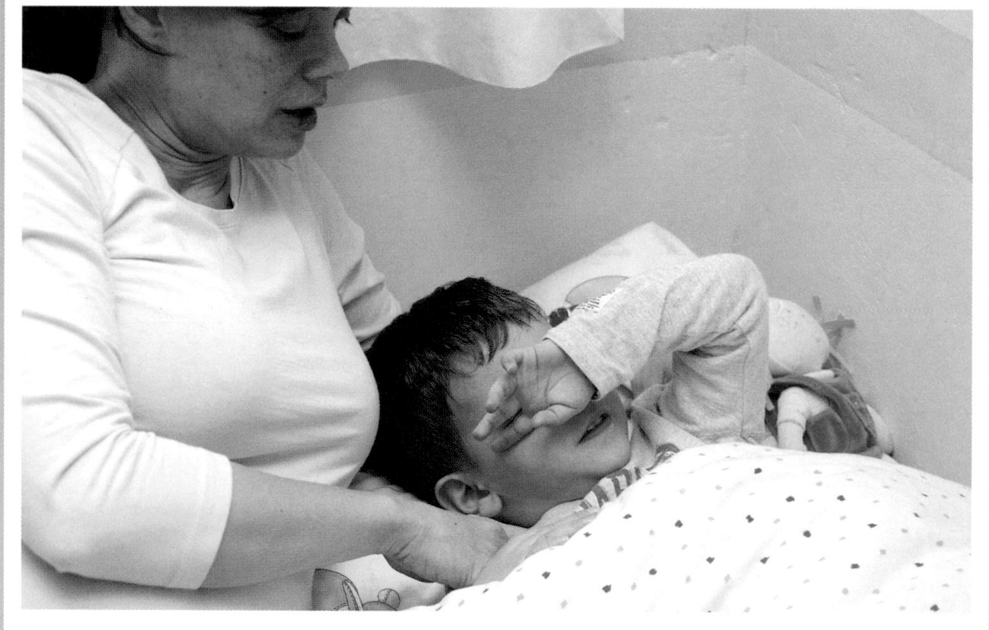

Educating a child how to sleep can take several weeks and sometimes demands great perseverance; he will reap the benefits, however, for the rest of her life.

problems at school (I)

When a child starts going to school, his entire family passes an important milestone. In the first years of his life, he has grown and acquired sufficient maturity to cope with the challenges of this new phase. He will be put to the test in various ways and it is therefore likely that he will encounter setbacks of varying degrees of importance. Both parents and teachers play an essential role in detecting any problems at an early stage.

Going to school

Children who do not want to go to school

• Going to school is usually fun for small children, but it can induce fear or even panic in some cases, often causing a child to feign sickness or exaggerate physical symptoms so as to stay at home and avoid school. A child aged between 5 and 10 who behaves in this manner is suffering from a paralyzing fear of leaving the security of his home and family.

• This irrational fear can appear for the first time in children attending a kindergarten or play school, but it is more common in primary school. The child will generally complain about a headache, sore throat, or stomach pain just before it is time to set out for school. The sickness improves when he is allowed to remain at home, but it reappears the next morning. In some cases, a child categorically refuses to leave the house.

• A child with an irrational fear of attending school may also display some of the following traits:

– insecurity when left alone in a room.

– inordinate concern about something bad happening to his parents.

– a tendency to following his mother or father around the house and be excessively clingy.

– difficulty in going to sleep.

– a propensity for nightmares.

– an exaggerated fear of animals, monsters, or thieves.

– fear of being alone in the dark.

– tantrums when he is obliged to go to school.

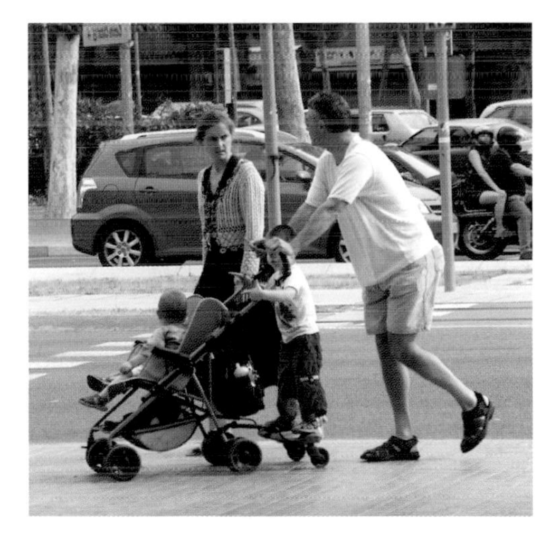

Starting school is difficult for many children, as the transition from their home or kindergarten to a primary school represents a big leap. It is possibly the first time that a child really has to cope without his parents, and he may see his encounter with so many unknown children as an ordeal rather than an opportunity.

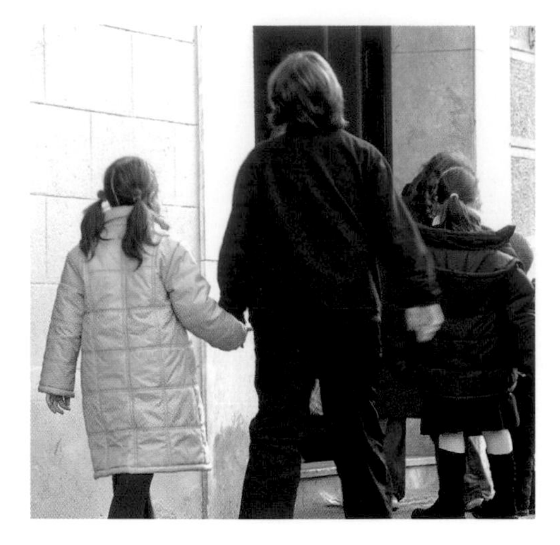

Primary-school children are usually very eager to learn and absorb knowledge easily. Their powers of observation become sharper and their ability to memorize is at its height. Their sense of identity grows and they become increasingly aware of their gender.

These fears are common in children suffering from an anxiety disorder. The potential long-term effects (i.e. in adulthood) can be very serious if such children do not receive professional attention. They can have serious academic and social problems if they stop going to school and go for long periods without seeing their friends. Before this situation arises, parents can help their child by taking him to a child psychologist, who will work on getting him back to school and into his daily routine as soon as possible.

Specific learning difficulties

- It is not easy to spot a child's learning difficulties in the pre-school phase, but these problems can be readily detected if they appear at school.
  – Inability to reach the reading level expected of children of his age, or problems in other academic

Boys' and girls' gender roles tend to be clearly defined. Boys normally enjoy playing rough games, while girls prefer less rowdy activities like skipping or playing with a ball or with dolls. At this age, children often tend to play with members of their own sex.

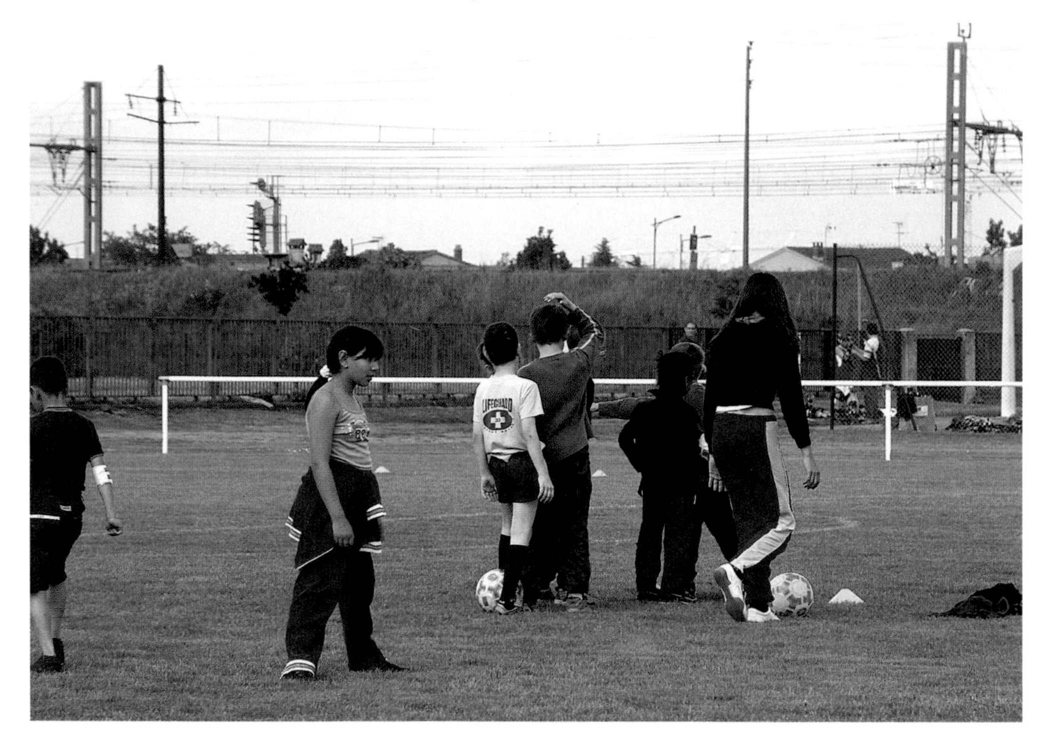

A child can have difficulties that make him fall behind his classmates academically. Reading is one of the most common problem areas. Roughly 1 in every 10 children has difficulties in keeping up the rhythm of the rest of his class in reading and writing. These children will not only have difficulties with their own language but will also be at a disadvantage when they study other subjects. They can lose interest in school and believe that they are not cut out for studying.

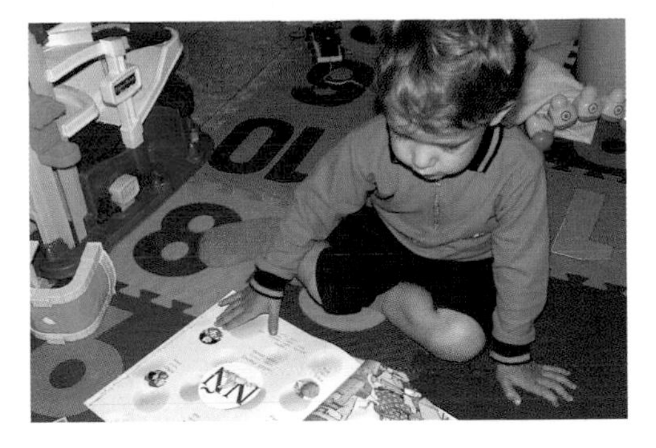

fields, despite having an adequate IQ and receiving a good education.

– Problems with language or speech that persist and change over time. For example, a child who starts talking late can go on to have problems with the pronunciation or usage of certain words, as well as having difficulties in expressing his ideas.

– Slow and unclear writing.

– Problems of memory and concentration.

– Low self-esteem and frustration with academic results.

School years form a period with many demands, and some children can develop signs of physical and nervous disorders that may cause them problems throughout life. Fortunately, however, most children see school as a place for exciting and enjoyable challenges.

If a child is set very demanding targets in the first years at school, she may not be mature enough to meet them. It may take a great deal of time, effort, and energy to achieve results that other children obtain with relative ease. This can lower her self-esteem and make her insecure. These problems can give rise to symptoms of nervousness, such as sucking her thumb or biting her nails, as well as irritation, lack of concentration, and difficulty in sleeping.

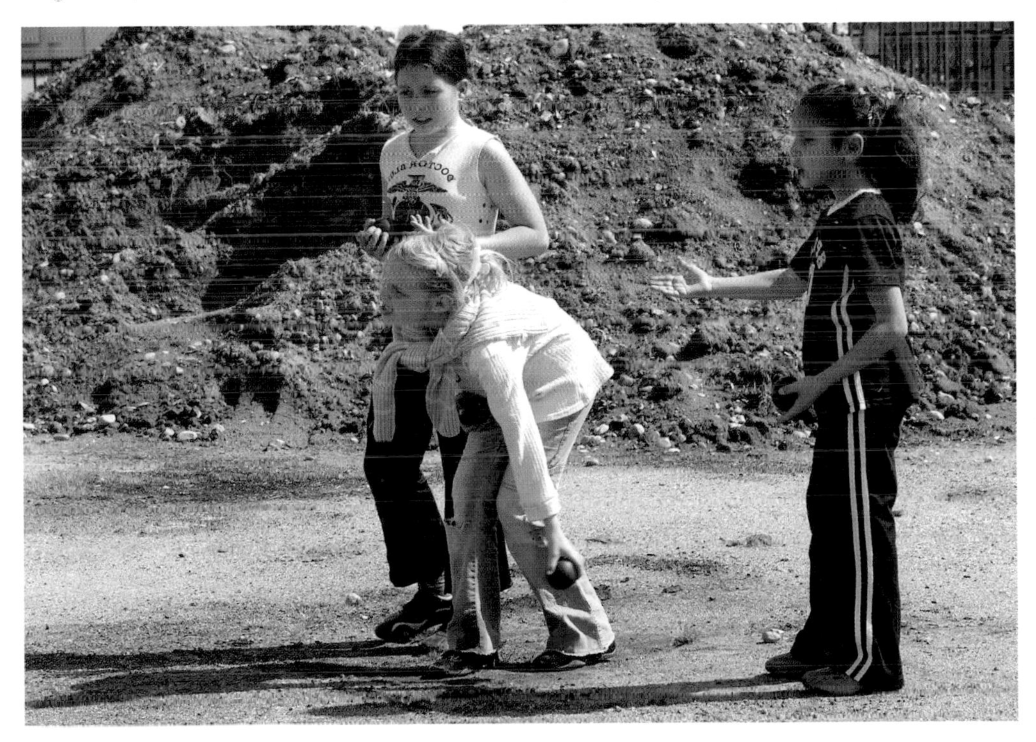

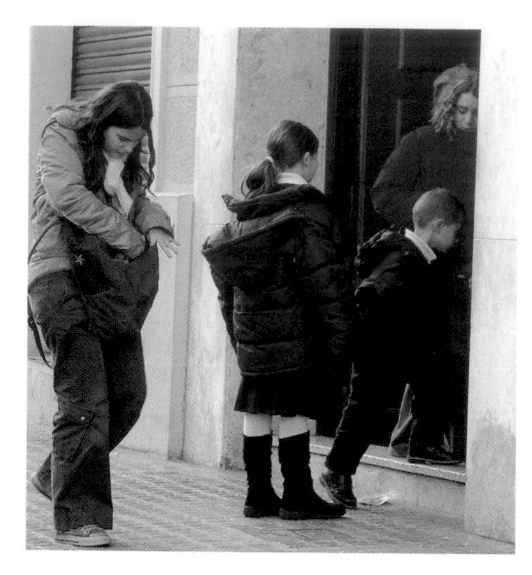

Refusal to go to school generally occurs after long periods at home, such as vacations, a long weekend, or a sickness. It can also occur after a distressing event, such as the death of a relative or pet, or a change of school or home.

– Family history of difficulties with learning and language.

• Although the exact causes of these learning difficulties are unknown, the latest research points toward a slight cerebral disorder or arrested development of certain parts of the brain.

• Children understand what they are reading through the interpretative skills of their brain. The interpretation of perception is different from the registration of information by the sense of sight. The brain relates visual images to past experiences. Specific learning problems might indicate defects in this process, and do not indicate problems with eyesight.

• Acquired dyslexia and other learning difficulties can result from brain damage caused by infections (encephalitis, meningitis), lesions (cerebral traumatism, contact with and/or abuse of a toxic substance), premature birth, chemotherapy, etc. Learning difficulties can also arise as a consequence of mental deficiency, abnormalities in sight and hearing, emotional disorders, or unfavorable environments (dysfunctional family, inadequate education, truancy, or economic problems), although these problems do not fall under specific learning difficulties.

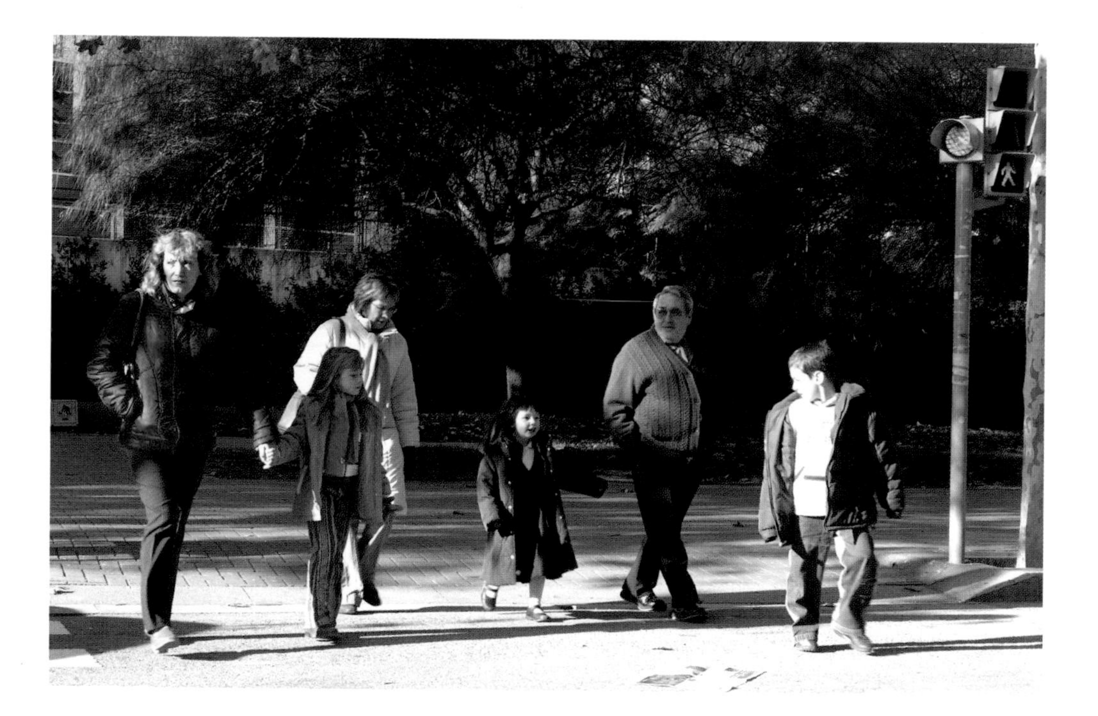

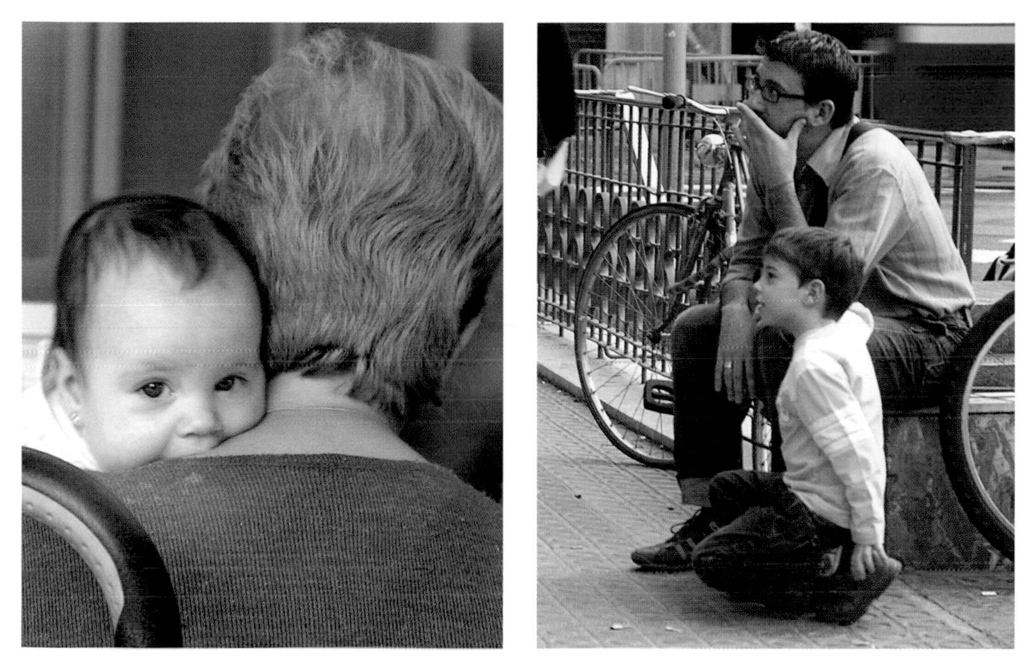

The functions of the eye are similar to those of a camera. After capturing an image, it sends the information to the brain via the optic nerve. The eyes do not understand what they are seeing, just as a camera cannot understand the picture it is taking; the image has no meaning until it is developed. Similarly, the images captured by the eyes are useless until they are interpreted by the brain.

The dyslexic child

• A simple definition of dyslexia is difficulty in learning to read experienced by children with a normal IQ, with no sign of any other physical or psychological problems that might explain this difficulty.

• A dyslexic child has great difficulty in distinguishing letters or groups of letters, as well as their order and rhythm within a word and/or sentence, and so she has serious problems with learning how to read and has an academic level significantly lower than that of her classmates and peers.

• Dyslexia affects all aspects of a child's life, as her behavior will be affected by her communication difficulties. Such children generally have problems with writing as well, and every task requires a supreme effort.

• Once visual, auditory, and neurological defects have been ruled out, the causes of dyslexia basically revolve around:

– A poor cerebral lateralization that makes it difficult to orientate letters correctly, which causes confusion, typified by inversions or omissions.

– Spatial and temporal disorientation.

– Problems with perception.

changes in psychomotricity (coordination, balance, etc.).

– Emotional disorders.

• It is very important to detect this problem early on – in the pre-school phase, or in the first 2 years of primary school – and call on the services of a child psychologist to provide individual reading tuition. It is essential to establish the root cause of dyslexia, in order to act swiftly and appropriately to prevent the problem from affecting a child's subsequent academic studies.

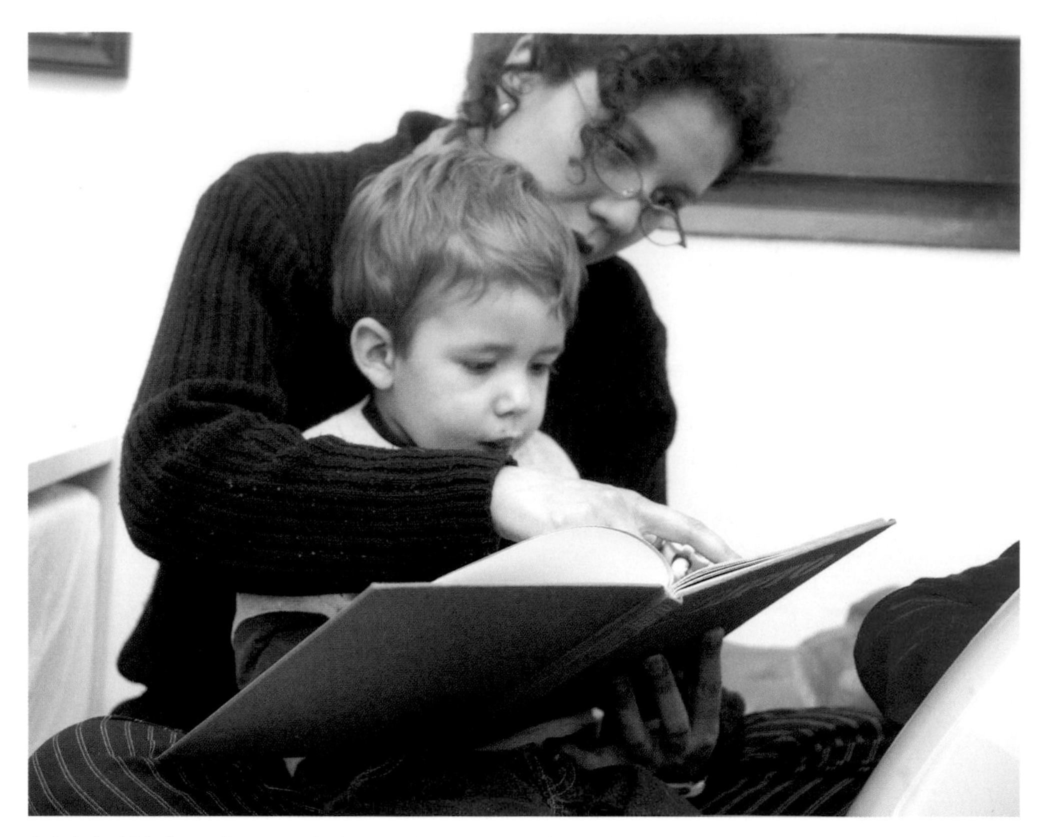

A dyslexic child often writes letters backward or in the wrong order. It is important to detect this problem early. The prognosis will depend on the age at which the dyslexia is diagnosed, as well as the support of parents and the presence of emotional or behavioral disorders. The prospects for improvement are better if the child goes to a good school and follows a specific program as soon as the problem is detected.

Disgrafia

This is a specific writing disorder. Children with disgrafia have a significantly lower academic level than expected. It manifests itself through the inversion of syllables, omission of letters, mirrored writing, inappropriate separations or continuity, etc. It is closely linked to reading disorders such as dyslexia.

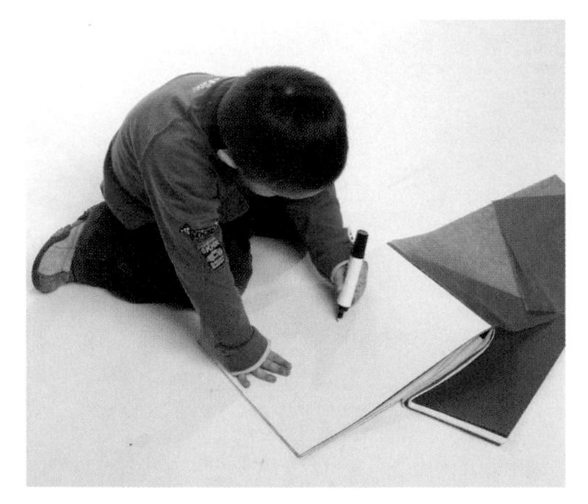

In some cases, a close study of the family circle is required to find out why an older child or adolescent is afraid to go to school. Such youngsters generally suffer from a more deep-rooted disorder, which requires intensive treatment. Their irrational fear of leaving the house and their parents can be treated successfully, however, if the appropriate professional help is solicited.

problems at school (II)

Attention deficit hyperactivity disorder (ADHD) is a mental health problem most common in childhood, affecting 3–5 percent of children of school age, predominantly boys. Children with this disorder are often incapable of paying attention to a specific task for any length of time, and they are usually hyperactive or restless, as well as disorganized and impulsive. Such children sometimes obtain poor results at school and are slow to develop social skills. In some cases, lack of concentration is the most noticeable factor; in others, it is hyperactivity that is most striking.

Symptoms of ADHD

• Children with ADHD may understand what they are being asked to do, but they are not always capable of fulfilling their objectives because they are impulsive, easily distracted, and lacking in focus. They are often unable to sit still or pay attention at school.

• Boys are 3 times more affected by this disorder than girls, although the reason for this difference is not clear.

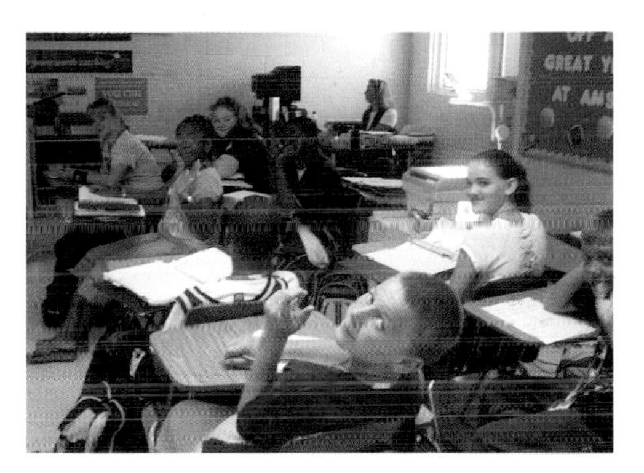

Hyperactivity and impulsiveness often form part of ADHD, although not in every case.

Indicators of ADHD

- Loss of equipment at school
- Forgetting to hand in work
- Problems with finishing work at school and at home
- Difficulty in paying attention
- Difficulty in listening attentively
- Problems with obeying a series of instructions
- Lack of attention to detail
- Brusque treatment of other people

The term "attention deficient hyperactivity order" was coined in 1994 by the American Psychiatry Association. Three subtypes have been defined:

• The attention deficit subtype, whose symptoms include:

– Inability to pay attention to details or a tendency to make careless errors in schoolwork and other activities.

– Difficulty in maintaining prolonged concentration in class or in games.

– Problems with listening.

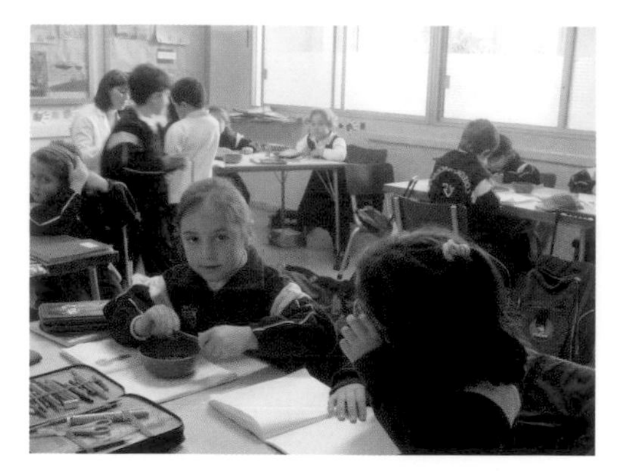

Children with ADHD are often considered dunces, but it is important for parents and teachers to delve into the root causes for habitual absentmindedness and loss of objects.

– Difficulty in following instructions.
– Problems in organizing activities.
– Avoidance and dislike of tasks that require mental effort.
– Tendency to lose toys, books, schoolwork, etc.
– Tendency to be easily distracted.
– Absentmindedness in everyday tasks.
• Hyperactive-impulsive subtype, whose symptoms include:
– Restlessness.
– Difficulty in sitting still.
– Excessive running and climbing.
– Difficulty in playing in silence.
– Sense of always being busy.
– Talking excessively.
– Difficulty in waiting in line or speaking in turn.
– Recklessness and a tendency to interrupt.
• Combined subtype. A child's behavior embraces both the other subtypes, although hyperactivity may or may not be present.

A diagnosis of ADHD should be investigated if the warning signs are seen in a child under the age of 7 over a period of 6 months. A child's behavior has to have a negative effect on at least 2 aspects of his life (e.g. his school or nursery, home, or friendships) before ADHD can be diagnosed.

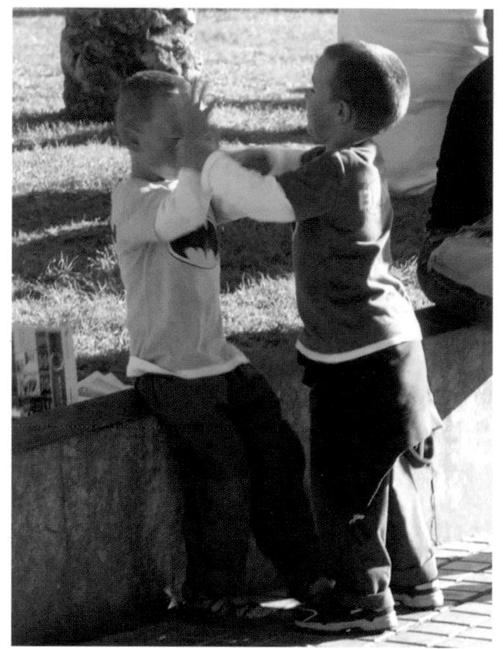

Hyperactivity and impulsiveness dominate in subtype 2 of ADHD.

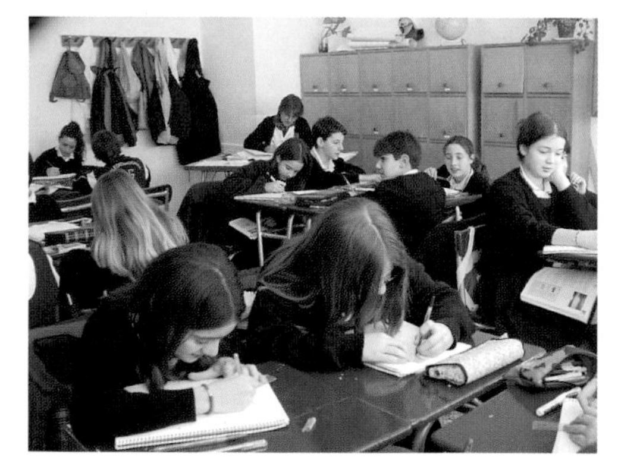

This subtype is dominated by behavior typical of lack of attention.

Compared with healthy girls, those with ADHD obtain lower marks in IQ tests and school exams,. as well as having more family problems and a greater propensity to depression and even attacks of anxiety or panic. They are more likely to take drugs or drink alcohol than boys who are not affected by this disorder.

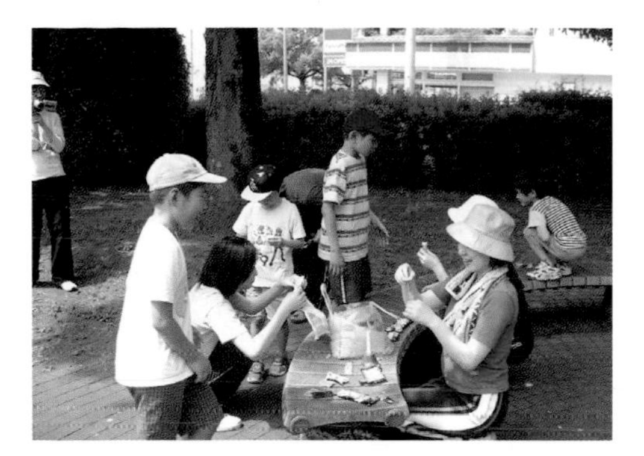

Although the cause of ADHD cannot be identified with certainty, it has been discovered that certain areas of the brain (frontal lobes and basal areas) are 5% to 10% smaller in children suffering from ADHD.

Causes of ADHD

ADHD has biological origins that have yet to be clearly defined. Although none of the causes of ADHD has been fully identified, current research is focusing on possible connections with genetics and the environment. Some studies have demonstrated that some children have a genetic predisposition to ADHD, as it is more common in children with a family history of the disorder. Other recent research has linked smoking and other substance abuse to the development of ADHD.

Hyperactivity and lack of control over impulses can be a result of stress in the home environment. Children who have lived through their parents' divorce, moved house, changed school, or experienced other significant upheavals in their lives, can present more impulsive behavior than usual and appear to be absentminded and distracted. These traits can be wrongly interpreted as symptoms of ADHD, so it is very important to rule out emotional factors before arriving at a diagnosis of ADHD.

Coexistence of ADHD and other disorders

• Almost half the children who suffer from ADHD also have an oppositional defiance disorder, characterized by obstinacy, an explosive temper, and a conflictive attitude.

• Mood swings such as bouts of depression are often found in children with ADHD, who feel inept, socially isolated, and frustrated by their failures at school. Small gestures of support in the social and academic fields can provide enormous relief in the midst of such depressions.

All children have occasional difficulty in paying attention or sitting still, but these behavioral defects occur more often in children with ADHD, and the impact is more disturbing for the people around them.

• Some children can suffer from mood swings unrelated to ADHD that may require psychotherapy and even medication.

• Many children with ADHD also suffer from learning difficulties, such as problems with foreign languages, math, reading, and writing (the last 2 being the most common).

Treatment of ADHD

• **Medication.** The most frequently used medicines are psycho-stimulants (methylfenidate, dextroamphetamine, etc.). Unfortunately, the effects of

Frontal and basal areas of the brain

Children with ADHD seem to have slightly reduced frontal and basal areas of the brain, although it is not known for certain whether it is this factor that accounts for the incidence of the disorder.

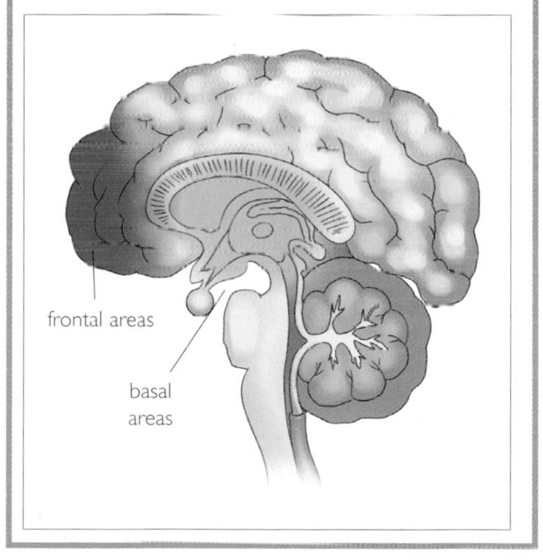

Although ADHD is not strictly classified as a learning disorder, it undermines a child or adolescent's concentration and can prejudice his school results.

these drugs are short-lasting and so several doses have to be taken every day, although new drugs that can be taken every 12 hours are now available. These types of drugs has side effects that include loss of appetite, irritability, and insomnia.

• **Behavioral therapy.** This includes instructions to parents and teachers about the optimal organization of the child's environment, and clear, concise explanations and instructions to the child, along with praise for good behavior.

The best results in the treatment of ADHD are achieved by combining medication with behavioral therapy.

How to help a child with ADHD

- Make changes to his environment to minimize distractions. It is not appropriate for a child with ADHD to sit round a table or with a group in a classroom, as he will find more to distract him than if he is seated alone but in a row. Talk to his teacher about strategies for making him create less disturbance in the classroom.
- Give clear instructions. Ask your child's teacher to both oblige him to note down the tasks he has been set and to make sure that they have been performed satisfactorily. Both you and the teacher need to be concise when you give your child problems, and write them down if they are complicated or involve several steps.
- Focus on his successes. Create a feedback system (such as a blackboard listing achievements) to highlight his positive results and congratulate him on his progress, even when this is less than expected. A daily list issued by his teacher, detailing any behavioral and academic attainments, can also serve as a yardstick for him.
- Help him to be organized. Encourage him to make daily lists and to check them before leaving school. This will enable him to bring home all the books and materials he needs to do his homework.
- Encourage the child to control his impulses and ask the teacher to praise good behavior. Congratulating a child for raising his hand before speaking in class can greatly help to quell disorder in a classroom.
- Encourage him to perform tasks that he enjoys or easily masters, and give him his feedback in private. Do not ask him to perform very difficult tasks in front of other people.
- Ask his teacher or psychologist to help draw up behavior programs that can help solve specific problems in the classroom.
- Encourage active learning. Teach your child to underline important passages as he reads and to take notes in class. Urge him to read aloud at home if he has problems with fluency and comprehension.

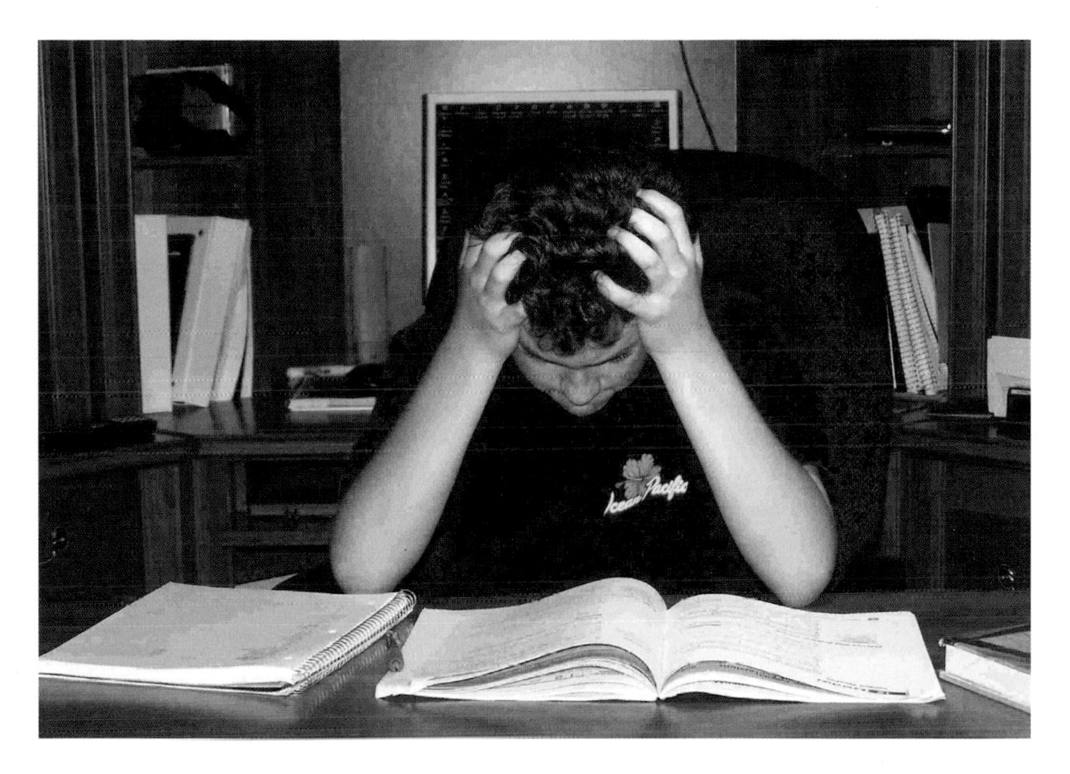

GENERIC DISORDER	SPECIFIC DISORDER	MORE SPECIFIC DISORDERS
Disorders starting in infancy, childhood, or adolescence	Learning disorders	• Reading disorder • Calculation disorder • Writing disorder • Miscellaneous learning disorder
	Communication disorders	• Expressive language disorder • Mixed expressive-receptive language disorder • Phonological disorder • Stammering
	Attention deficit and conflictive behavior disorders	• Attention deficit disorder with hyperactivity • Unspecified attention deficit disorder with hyperactivity • Dysocial disorder • Negativist defiance disorder • Miscellaneous conflictive behavior disorder
	Other disorders	• Disorders related to anxiety over separation

children with speech difficulties

Many children suffer from speech difficulties that prevent them from feeling comfortable or making friends at school, and this can mark them for life. The solution is to give this problem the attention it deserves and avert any long-term speech difficulties before it is too late. Except in the case of a physical speech impediment, language difficulties are generally problems that can – and should – be resolved and, of course, prevented. It is estimated that 1 in every 5 children aged between 2 and 5 has a speech difficulty, but not all children who speak badly are affected by them.

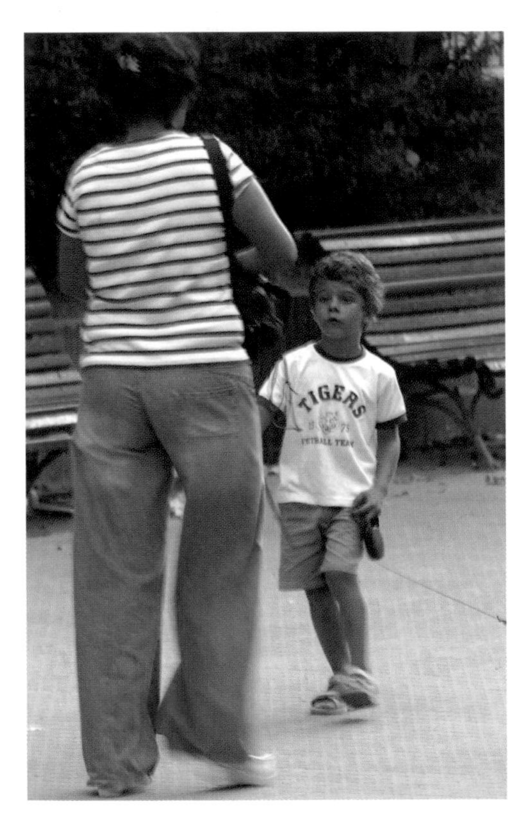

Speech difficulties

Stammering

• About 1% of children suffer from this problem, which consists of the unvarying repetition of a syllable or the inability to pronounce blocks of words starting with a plosive consonant (b, d, g, k, p, t).

• Stammering creates tension, and demands great effort for speaking, and suggests a blockage caused by anxiety or great emotion. Many children with stammers also have other symptoms of anxiety such as tics and grimaces, which can make it even more difficult for them to articulate

It is common for a child to repeat certain syllables mechanically up to the age of 3 or 4. In normal conditions, this occurs because he has still not completely developed his language skills and tends to repeat syllables while he is thinking of the word he wants to say. The persistence of this habit at a later age might arouse suspicion of a stammer.

Stammering

This is one of the most common speech difficulties. It usually appears between the ages of 3 and 4, but this may not be a permanent problem (as it is in adults), but merely forms part of one of the child's developmental phases. If it is given undue importance, the child can become inhibited and avoid talking so as not to make any mistakes. Professional help will be required if the problem persists beyond the age of 4.

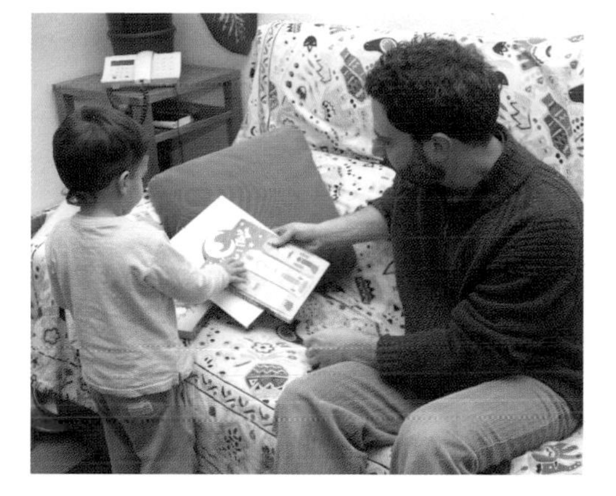

According to some experts, stammering is an expression of problems in the mother–child relationship. Most speech pathologists take this view, and so encourage the child's mother to play a leading role in his re-education process.

Dyslalia

This is one of the most common speech disorders found in children but in most cases it is not approached with sufficient seriousness. It consists of mispronouncing one or more sounds, which can make a child's speech incomprehensible as a result. For example, when a child aged over 4 says led instead of red, or when he misses out a certain sound, as when he says pate instead of plate.

correctly.

• Helping a child to overcome stammering involves tackling the underlying cause, and in many cases this requires psychotherapy.

• The ideal age for treating childhood speech difficulties is under 4 or 5, in the pre-school phase. The sooner parents think positively about treatment, the better the results will be, as it is easier to eradicate or overcome a problem at this stage of a child's development, as the neuro-physiological and psychological mechanisms that serve as a base for the acquisition and development of verbal language are still flexible.

• The guidelines given to the parents of children with speech disorders tend to focus on the following aspects:

– Monitoring and correction of the child's speech.

– Restoration of his self-confidence.

– Strengthening the child's emotional stability.

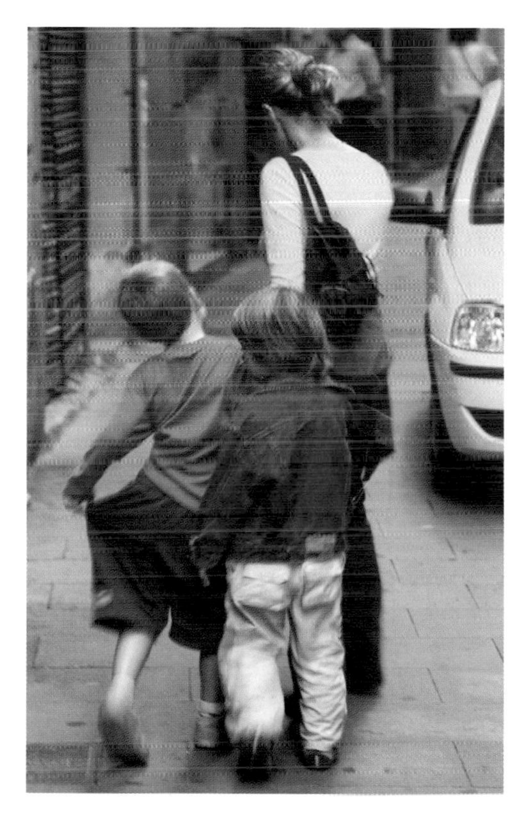

Starting school or the birth of a younger sibling can give rise to a stammer; in these cases, the internal conflict probably existed beforehand and the conflict surfaces when the child is faced with a challenging situation.

– Teaching hygiene and health habits.

• All these aspects need to be handled with understanding and affection by the child's parents, to create a supportive and reassuring environment that will help him overcome the problem.

Tips for parents of children with speech difficulties

• Avoid tension or anxiety at home, as these can make children feel insecure.

• Accept that your child is either right- or left-handed, without intervening.

• When he starts to stutter, be gentle and help him conquer his language difficulty. Never shout or act in an authoritarian manner when you correct him.

• When he starts to talk, it is important that he can make himself understood. His mistakes should not be repeated, especially by his parents.

• Try to talk to him concisely and clearly, so that he has clear sound/speech models. Comment on what your child is saying, trying to incorporate the words he is mispronouncing so that he can hear them uttered correctly.

• If the speech defect is very marked, it is a good idea to stimulate your child with activities that develop psychomotor skills, such as manual tasks. You can also encourage him to sing children's songs, so that he has positive experiences with speech, as singing uses different neuro-physiological mechanisms than talking; you will find that his stammering disappears when he sings, and maybe even when he does imitations or talks to himself.

• Avoid any abrupt changes to your child's lifestyle. It is unwise, for example, to send him to school when he has started to stammer or develop a speech defect, or to change his school once he is starting to adapt.

• Choose quiet places for family outings and vacations, free of commotion and factors that could make your child nervous or insecure.

• Both parents should work together to establish jointly agreed disciplinary and education rules, acting consistently and in coordination to ensure that they do not contradict each other in their instructions to their child. They should also make sure that no outside influences like uncles or grandparents destabilize the child.

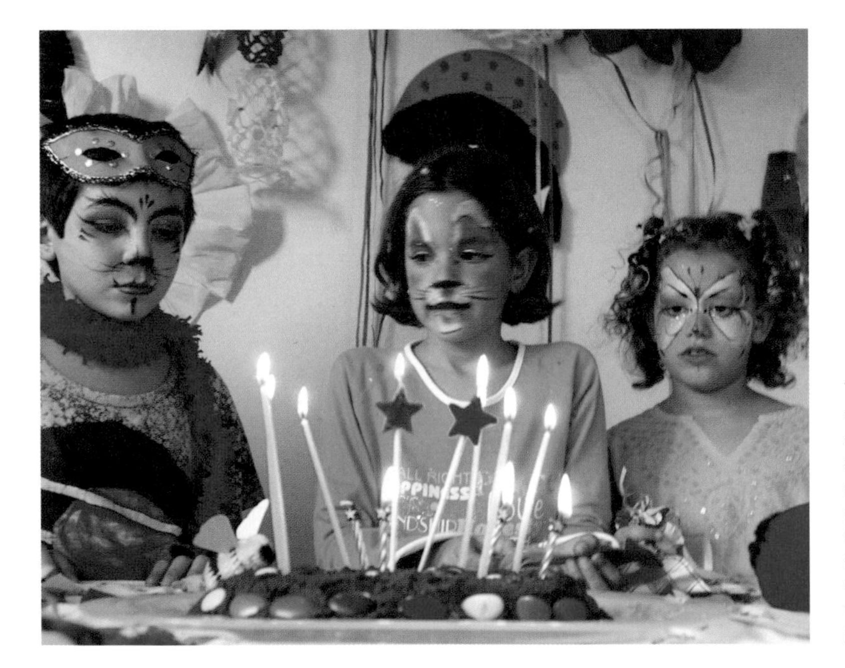

Try to avoid situations where a stammering child is left with little adult supervision. Older children at a party or a playground might make fun of a younger child's speech difficulty with disastrous results; in this respect, it is better to protect the child.

children with special needs: the gifted child

Recognizing a gifted child can prove difficult for parents, although they will immediately see that their child is very bright and does things that are highly unusual for his age. If he has not yet started school, take him to a specialist for an examination; if he is already at school, seek advice from his teachers.

How to identify a gifted child

A definitive identification of a gifted child is only possible with the guidance of a professional specialist, but there are some general characteristics that may indicate to their parents that they have a gifted child:

- He sleeps little.
- He learns to read very quickly.
- He says his first word at the age of 6 months.
- He says his first sentence at the age of 12 months.
- He can hold a conversation between the ages of 18 and 24 months, using a vocabulary that is highly sophisticated for his age.
- He learns the alphabet and counts up to 10 at the age of two and a half.
- He resolves simple problems of addition and subtraction at the age of 3.
- He asks about words he does not know from the age of 3.
- He asks exploratory questions at an early age.
- He has a great creative capacity.
- He shows great sensitivity to the world around him.
- He is concerned about issues of justice and morality.
- He is energetic and self-confident.
- He is very observant and open to unusual situations.
- He is very critical of both himself and others.
- He has a great capacity for attention and concentration.
- He likes the company of older children.
- He has low self-esteem and a propensity for depression.
- He becomes bored in class, because his capacities go beyond conventional educational programs. His teachers find him difficult to motivate.
- He seems to be very absentminded.

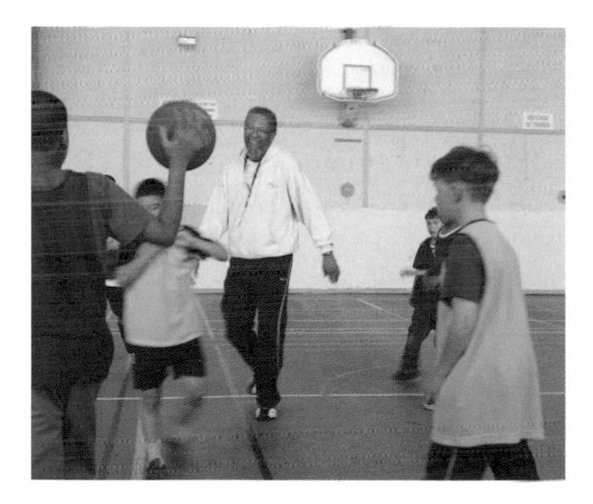

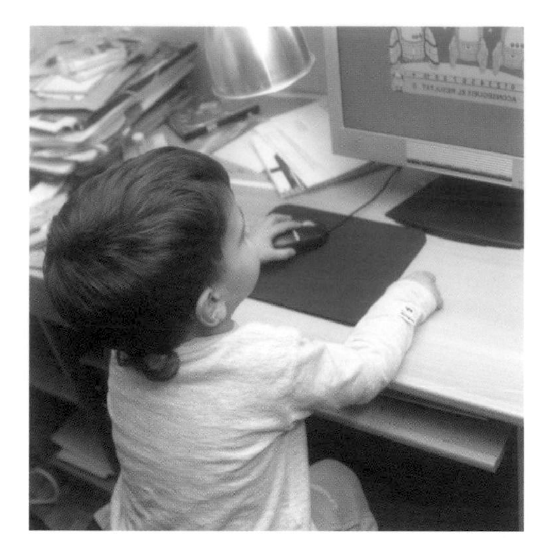

• His thinking is productive rather than reproductive, i.e. it is based on building ideas.

• He comes to feel misunderstood and strange.

• He is independent and introverted.

Experts stress the importance of observing children closely to assess their abilities and to determine whether they are gifted. If the education they receive is not suited to their needs, they become inactive, distracted, and ill-behaved. Teachers may even suspect that they have learning difficulties.

What should parents do?

If a child's parents observe that he has characteristics that could correspond to those of a gifted child, they should seek guidance from teachers or specialists. If it is confirmed that the child is indeed gifted, his parents should not panic, as they will receive all the advice they need. In any case, they have to continue working to further their child's development:

• By talking to him and playing with him. Chatting with him about everyday matters, encouraging him to express his opinion.

It is important to detect as soon as possible whether your child has an above-average IQ. Specialists recommend close observation of a child's behavior between the ages of 3 and 8, so that this attribute can be identified and appropriate action taken as a result.

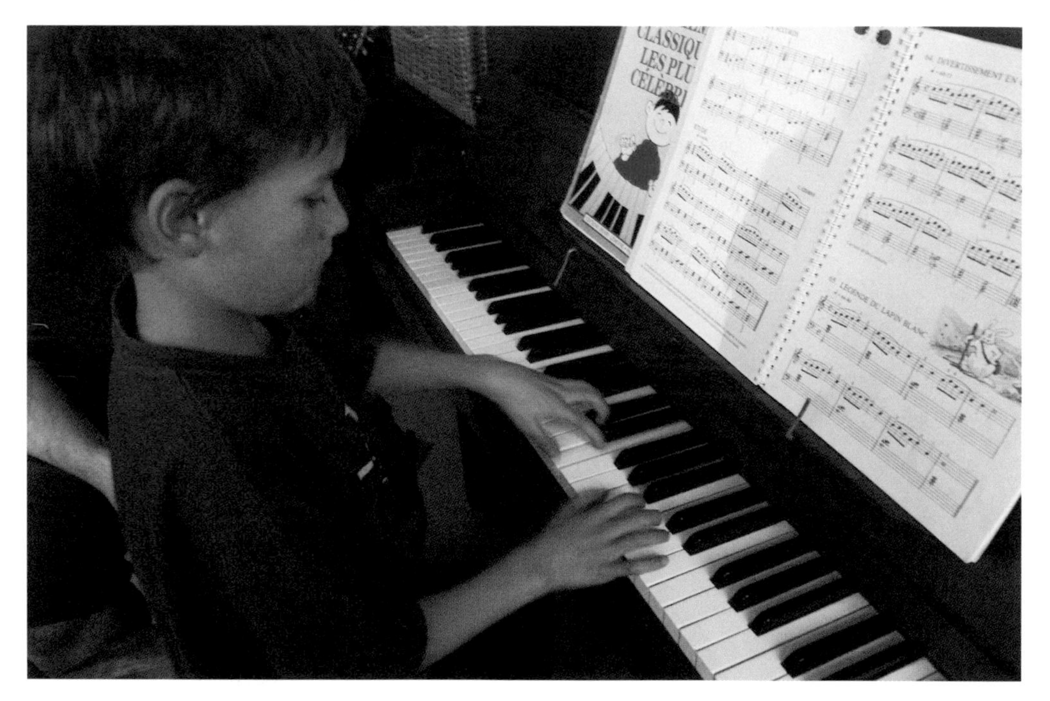

A gifted child may impress outsiders with his precociousness but the day-to-day reality is distinctly unromantic, as he is confronted by a host of difficulties. The intellectual development of these children is so fast that it is out of sync with other aspects of their personality; this means that their development on the emotional and social planes is different from that of other children. The pressures of their social setting can often make it hard for them to fit in.

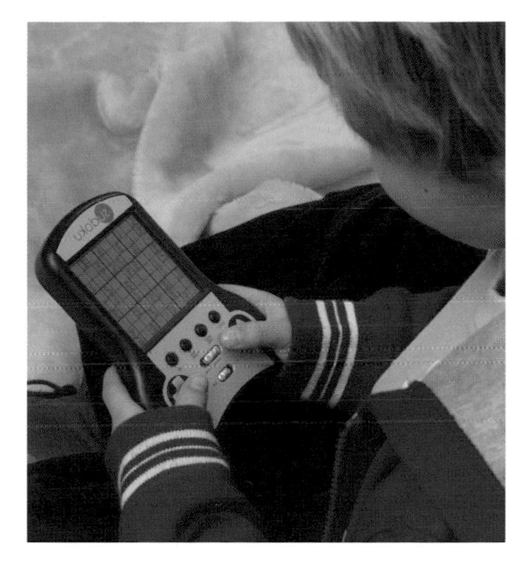

- By responding to his interest in science or the arts, and helping him to develop his abilities in these fields.
- By taking him to places where he can learn new things, such as museums, libraries, and community centers that organize activities.
- By stimulating him to prevent boredom setting in, and explaining to him that success is possible and will benefit him in the future.
- By creating a quiet atmosphere where he can read and study, and by helping him with his homework.
- By signing him up for activities outside school.

Should gifted children go to special schools?

Programs for gifted children have been severely criticized for their elitism but, although it is undoubtedly true that segregation is not recommendable, these children do nevertheless demand special attention.

Some experts recommend that gifted children go to a normal school but spend more time studying than the rest, following an enhanced curriculum. This method requires the child's teacher and family to work together to closely monitor progress.

Development of social skills

Some gifted children are excessively shy and have difficulty in communicating with other children or adults. The development of this communicative capacity can be reinforced at home, and parents can contribute by means of simple exercises:

- Making their child responsible for particular tasks when guests visit his home (i.e. answering the door, taking their coats, offering them something to eat or drink, etc.).

Some of these tasks can be rehearsed beforehand.

- Discussing what he needs to do to maintain friendships, and warning him of attitudes that could bring them to an end.
- Practicing activities like talking on the phone, pointing out other people's viewpoints, inviting a friend home, etc.

A gifted child can be further helped by encouraging him to:

- Develop hobbies. These are not only gratifying in themselves, but can also give him an opportunity to find friends who share his interests.
- Enroll in leisure groups in the local community (Boy Scouts, clubs, etc.) to provide him a valuable outlet for his energy, and an opportunity to interact with children of his own age.
- Participate in extracurricular activities at school, allowing him to spend time with children with common interests.
- Find a job or work as a volunteer in the local community (after school or at weekends), to enhance his social integration and raise his self-esteem

the adopted child

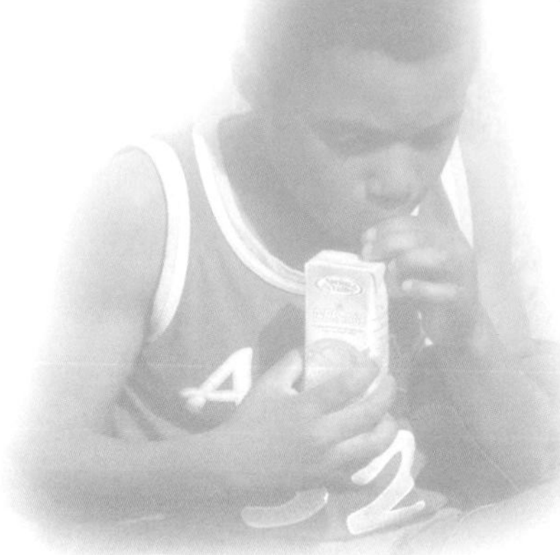

The adopted child

An adopted child's inalienable right

• An adopted child has a right to know the entire truth about his situation most appropriately, and most beneficially, from his adoptive parents. This will reinforce the child's trust in them and help to convey a positive message about adoption.

• A child may be overcome by anger and distrust if he finds out from another person, by accident or design, that he is not the biological child of his adoptive parents. He may come to interpret adoption as something shameful that has to be kept secret.

• All the experts are in agreement on this subject, although there is some disagreement about the best age to break the news. Some believe it is appropriate to do this when a child is 4 years old, as this will give him time to absorb the idea and come to terms with it at an early age; others are of the opinion that revelation at such an early age may cause confusion and recommend waiting until he is older.

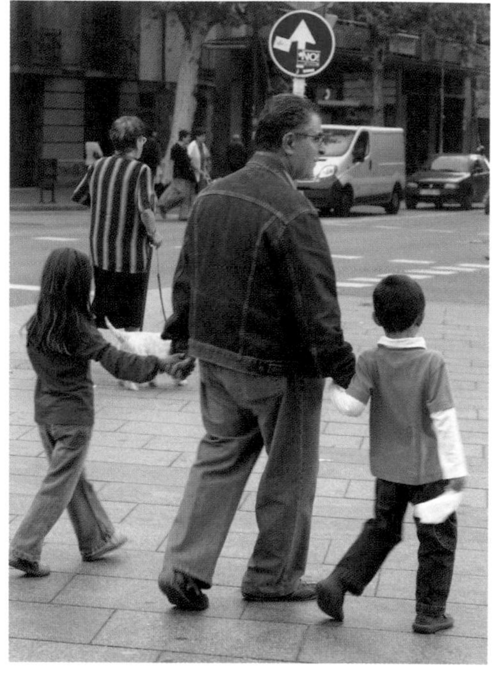

It is important for a child to know the exact circumstances of his adoption. Answer all his questions.

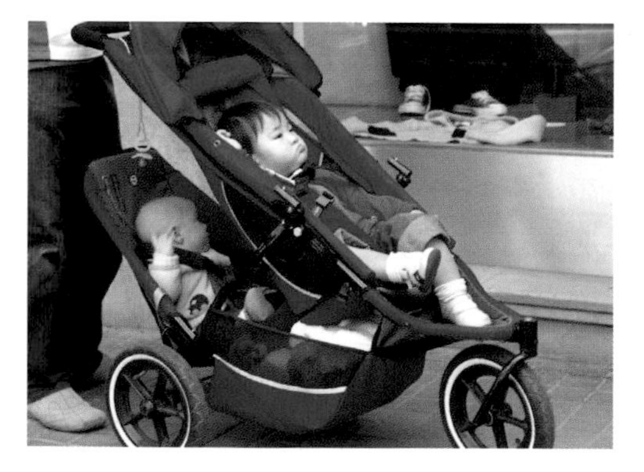

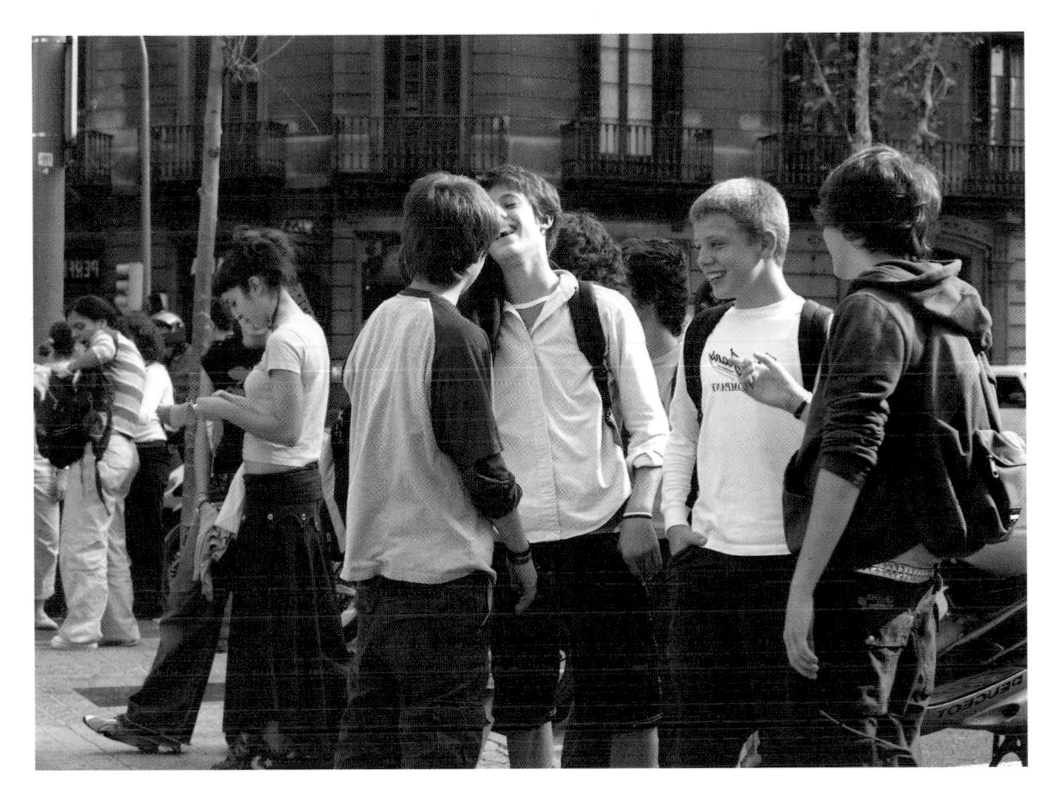

As all adolescents pass through a stage in which they are struggling to forge their identities, they ask themselves where they stand with their family, friends, and other people. It is reasonable for an adopted child to have a marked interest in his biological parents during this phase. This curiosity is common, and it does not mean that he is rejecting his adoptive parents.

• It is also important to use the word adoption naturally and in a positive sense, so that the child is accustomed to hearing it used without any embarrassment. Specialists advise parents to use it when they feel physically and above all emotionally close to him (at bath time, when held in their arms, etc.). It is vital to find the right moment, depending on the age of the child.

The child's adaptation to his new family

The adaptation process basically depends on the child's age when he is adopted; the younger the child, the easier it is. In all cases, however, it will pass through the following phases:

• An initial phase of anxiety, which may be marked by frequent crying, nervousness, insomnia, and even loss of appetite. A sense of abandonment produces anger and pain in a child aged over 2. To help him assimilate the transition, offer him repeated physical contact (hugs and caresses, demonstrations of affection) to make him feel safe and wanted in his new house.

• A phase of adaptation and the development of mutual understanding. The child will test the limits of what he can and cannot do, and he will learn what he can expect of other people. Both adoptive parents and the child will still be prone to anxiety and the child will probably cry for long spells. It is important to bear in mind that this reaction is not directed at the adoptive family but rather is a consequence of his previous history. His new parents must gently but firmly establish the parameters that he in fact craves, even when he is apparently being rebellious.

Normal reactions to learning about adoption

• Children can react in a number of ways to the news that they are adopted, depending on their age and degree of maturity. Some children refuse to accept the fact and escape into fantasy, such as

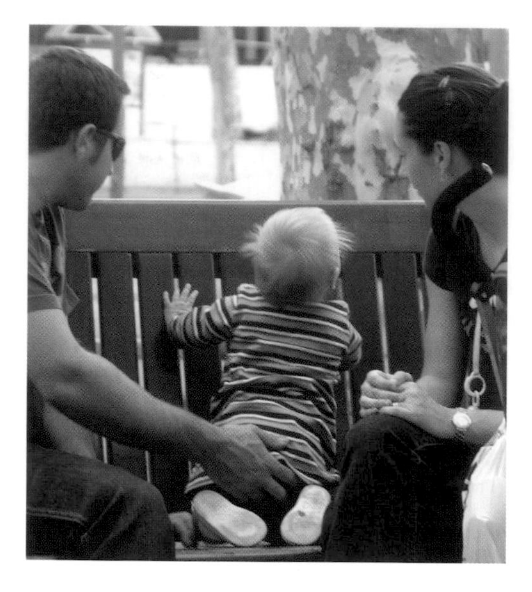

An adopted child can develop various emotional and behavioral problems. These can be the result of the insecurities and issues related to adoption, but they may have absolutely no connection. If his parents are worried, they should seek professional health. A psychologist or psychiatrist specializing in young people can help both the child and his parents.

the belief that they were only told that were adopted because they are naughty. If parents talk frankly about adoption and present it as something positive, their child is less likely to become victim to such worries.

Identity of the biological parents

If an adopted child wants to know who his biological parents are, he should be allowed to express this desire and be assured that he will be given help to find them when he is older, if he still wants to do so. He should not be pushed, but neither should he be obstructed. In the case of adolescents, parents can reply that it is natural that they have this wish and tactfully and sincerely offer them support and all the information available about their natural family (this will vary according to the legislation prevailing in the country in question). In many cases, adopted children eventually begin to see for themselves the difficulties and legal issues involved in this quest.

Some feelings that can be particularly marked in an adopted child

- Fear of being abandoned once again by his new family.
- Distrust of adults (as they have abandoned and failed him). Much love and patience will be required to regain his trust, as the child will constantly put adults to the test, to see if they really care about him. It is in these crucial moments that adoptive parents must not let him down but continue to show their unconditional love. This does not mean approving of everything he does but rather confirming their love for him even when his conduct is inappropriate.
- A feeling that nothing ever lasts, as he has never known stability (the child's age at adoption will make a difference to the degree of this problem).
- Experiences of separation, loss, and abandonment, which will inevitably be repeated to a greater and lesser extent throughout his life, will affect him particularly strongly.
- He may be highly sensitive and reluctant to start relationships based on trust, until his experience convinces him to take the plunge.

sex education

Sexuality is as natural to human beings as eating, sleeping and walking. As part of a child's education it should be approached naturally and honestly, and with understanding. Infant sexuality is one of the means by which a child develops his personality, emotions, and relationships.

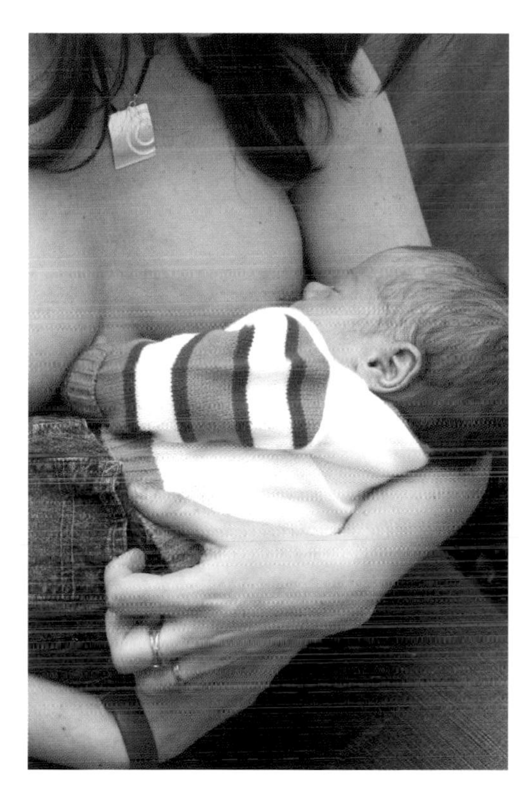

Children are interested in sexuality long before they reach the stage of asking questions about it. They are interested by the sight of their father or mother in the bathtub or of him caressing her belly when she is pregnant, and by the physical differences between themselves and their brother or sister.

Sexuality is part of everyday family life

Actions as banal as changing diapers, breast-feeding, and giving a baby a bath mark the start of his emotional and sexual education.

• Apart from biological and genetic conditioning, the choice of a name, a particular color of clothes, or a certain type of toy, form part of a child's early identification of gender. However strange it may seem, parents are continually educating their children sexually through their verbal and body language, their attitudes and values, and the roles they play in the home.

If sexuality is seen as a phenomenon far more wide-ranging than genitality – although this is a part of sexuality – it is easier to understand its importance and pervasive presence right from birth.

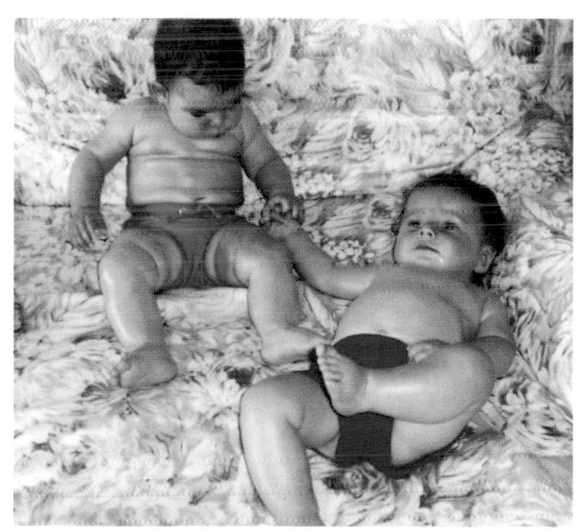

The main aim of sex education is to learn to call things by their names, in appropriate language adapted to a child's psychology, without indulging in any excess. Children nowadays receive all kinds of information, particularly via the media. When they ask questions, they are generally looking to their parents for confirmation or clarification of something they have learnt elsewhere. Any attempt to deceive them would only be counterproductive.

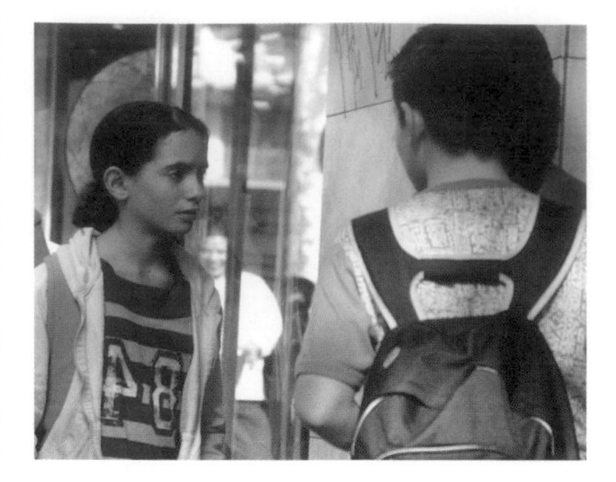

• For this reason, the greater the parents' awareness in this respect, the better they will prepare their child for the challenges and choices that he will face in the future. The family environment from a child's birth will help determine to what extent he will have a healthy and positive attitude to sexuality and love.

When parents take note of questions and answer them affectionately, sincerely, and simply, they are laying the foundations for a solid sexual education.

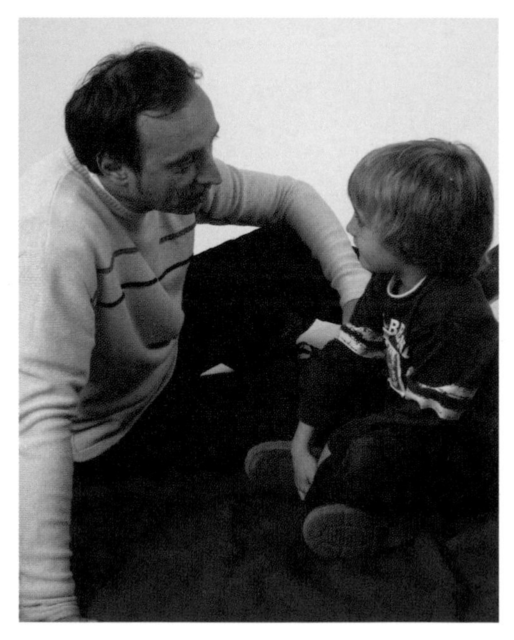

• Everyday situations can be used by parents to educate their child about anatomy, reproduction, and childbirth. They will not only be imparting information but also demonstrating to their child their willingness to talk to him about sex. This will establish a relaxed atmosphere of trust, in which the child will feel free to ask his parents for information about sex in the future.

Calling things by their names

• Many studies have demonstrated the value of teaching children the correct names for the sexual parts of their bodies. When parents use incorrect terms, diminutives, or euphemisms, they transmit the message that these body parts are in some way different and bad, because they cannot be mentioned openly. This can lead to children being ashamed of their genitals. Apart from encouraging a positive sexual attitude, knowing how to call things by name can be of crucial importance in cases of child abuse.

• Masturbation is a normal part of growing up, provided it does not become obsessive and hinder the course of other normal activities. Most experts agree that it is a healthy expression of sexuality, at any age. Parents' reaction to their children playing with their genitals is of great significance. Punishing or scolding a child or removing his hand conveys the idea that his genitals are bad and that touching them is a dirty action, and so makes him feel ashamed and guilty.

When parents refuse to be limited by society's expectations of the respective roles of a boy or girl, their children's personalities will be enriched.

Gender-based functions and identity

Some of the following ideas may be useful in broadening children's minds about what is expected of them:

- Share household chores.
- Encourage them to play with whatever toys they want and participate in games that deviate from traditional gender roles.
- Read them books presenting a variety of different behavior models, in which both men and women deviate from traditional stereotypes.
- Pay attention to language to avoid setting limits on male/female roles. Say both "he" and "she" when referring to professions considered typically masculine. Although this may be very difficult at first, it is extremely important.

• The time for starting up a dialogue arrives far earlier than many parents think. In the complex world of today, children deserve guidance and an education that has been well thought out from birth, though it is never too late to start. Although a child's parents are never his exclusive sexual educators, they can be, and generally are, his first and most important ones.

Children are very curious about the anatomy of not only their own body but also of the people around them. They are fascinated by bodily functions and the differences between the sexes. This interest can manifest itself in various ways: by playing at doctors, wanting to see their mother or father in the bath, touching their genitals, and comparing their body with that of other children (particularly of the opposite sex). A girl begins to wonder what happened to her penis, while a boy wants to know why his mother has breasts. Such questions provide opportunities to talk about sexuality, growth, and development. Remember that children are only seeking essential information and deserve simple, direct, and honest answers.

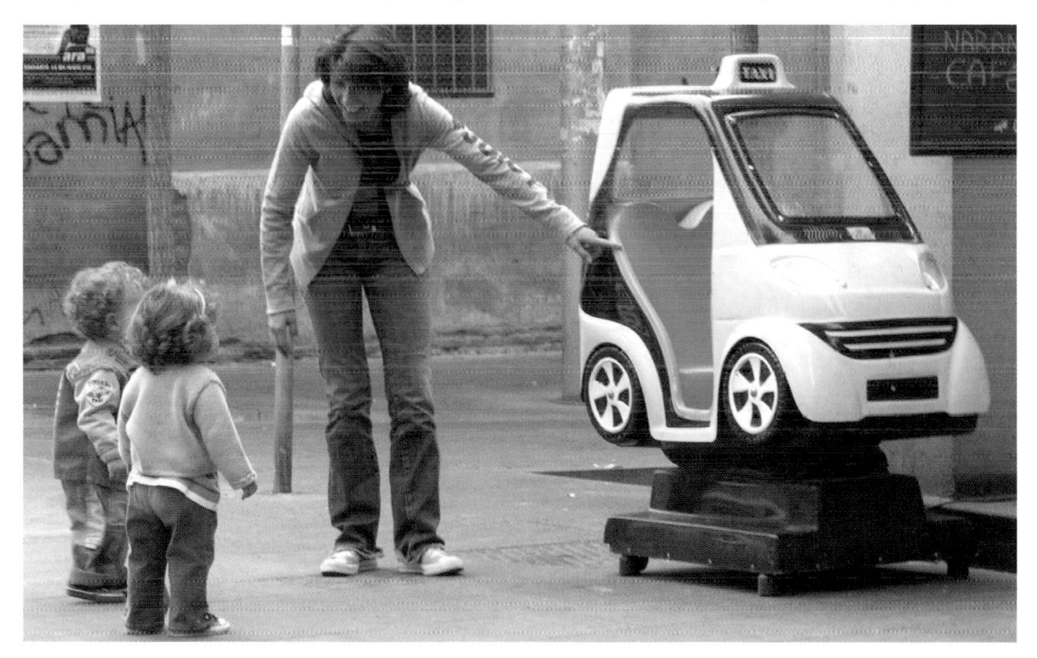

child abuse

Physical violence is not the only form of child abuse. Abandonment and emotional or sexual aggression also fall under this category. The statistics tell an alarming story; it is estimated that hundreds and thousands of children have suffered from abuse at the hands of their parents or relatives, and thousands have died as a result. Those who survive are marked by the emotional trauma, long after the physical wounds have healed. Immediate recognition and treatment of these situations are essential if their long-term effects are to be minimized.

Child abuse

The signs of child abuse

• Victims of child abuse, can have difficulties in establishing close relationships and trusting in other people when they are adults. They are also more likely to take drugs and suffer from anxiety, depression, medical disorders, and problems at home or at school. If a child does not get appropriate help, the consequences of abuse may haunt him throughout the rest of his life.

• Some signs of an abused child:

– Low self-esteem

– Fear of sexual relationships or, in contrast, an obsession with sex.

– Fear of starting new activities.

– Inability to love, trust, or depend on other people.

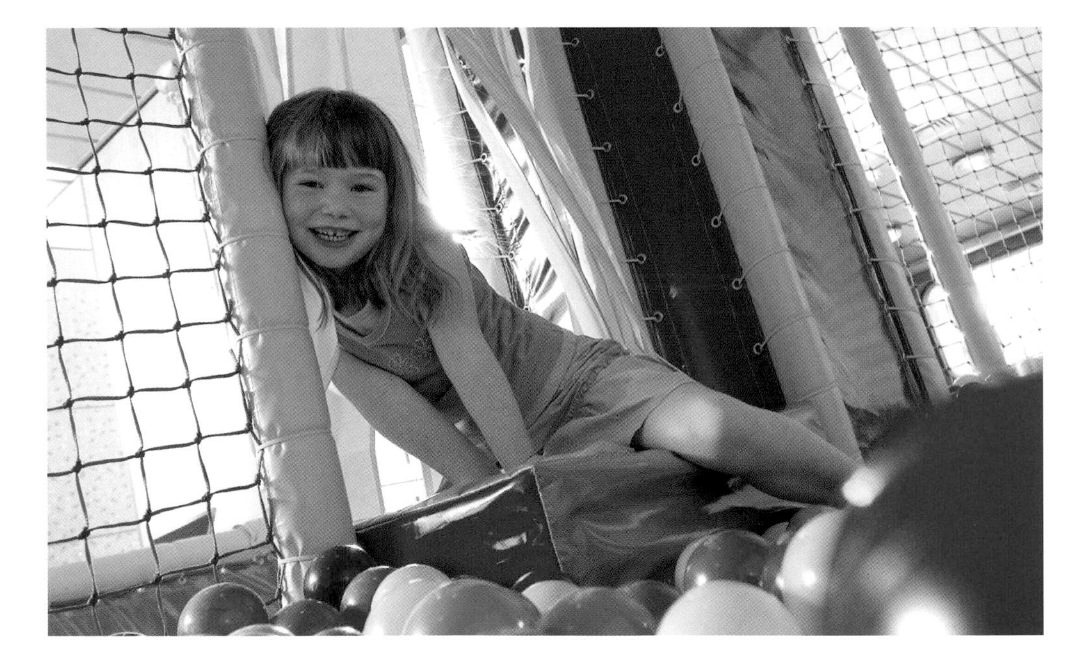

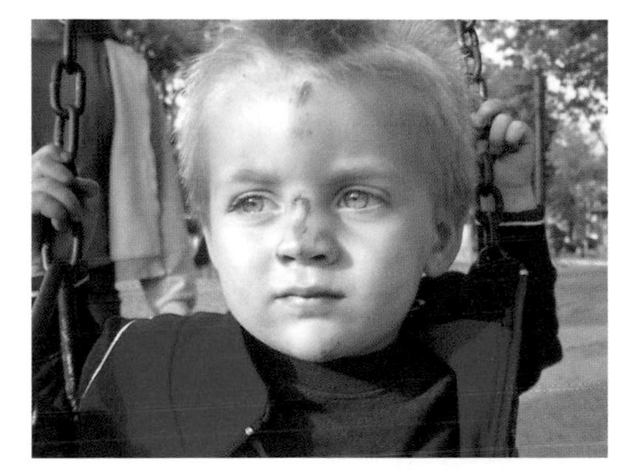

Apart from the physical injuries observed in a battered child, there is emotional and psychological damage, which often only becomes evident in adolescence or even later, when these children turn into adults who abuse their own children or other youngsters.

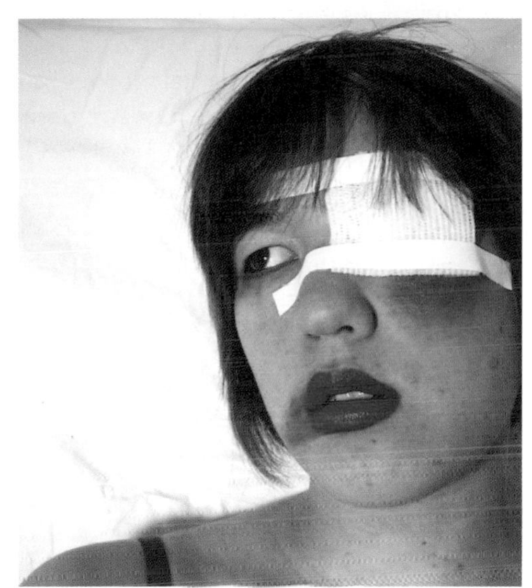

– Anxiety and fear.

– Aggressive behavior, disciplinary problems, and academic failure or other problems at school.

– Problems with the law

– Feelings of sadness or other symptoms of depression.

– Quick-temperedness

– Flashbacks of past experiences and nightmares.

– Self-destructive behavior or self-inflicted abuse, suicidal tendencies, and drug or alcohol abuse.

Sexual abuse of young children

• Sexual abuse of children can occur within a family (at the hands of a father, stepfather, brother, or other relative) or outside it (a friend, babysitter, neighbor, teacher, or stranger).

• No young child is psychologically prepared to confront sexual stimulation. Even children of 2 or 3 who have yet to assimilate any sense of sex as something dirty will have problems coping, as a result of their inability to handle excessive stimulation.

• Children aged 5 years or more who know and love the abuser feel caught between their affection or loyalty and the knowledge that what they are experiencing is harmful.

• Some children who have been victims of sexual abuse have difficulty in establishing relationships with other people that are not based on sex.

• There are often no signs of physical abuse on a child, or only ones that can be detected by a doctor

• Behavior that might be evident in children who are suffering, or have suffered from sexual abuse:

– Excessive interest in sex, or complete avoidance of the subject.

– Refusal to go to school.

– Delinquency.

– Difficulty in going to sleep, nightmares.

– Withdrawal and secrecy.

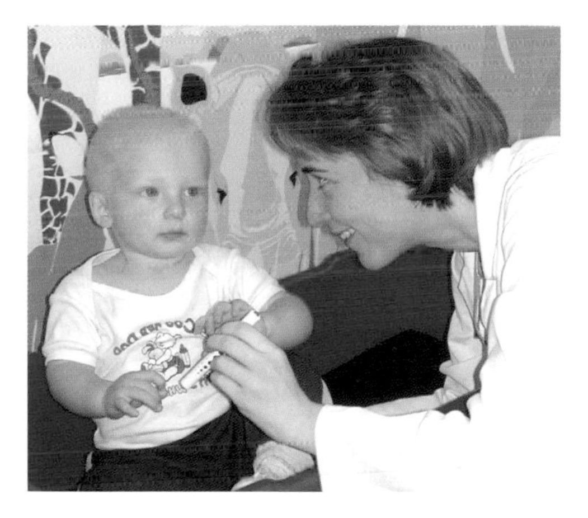

Prompt detection of child abuse and providing appropriate care are important in preventing long-term damage. The right professional help will enable an abused child to recover his self-confidence and trust in other people.

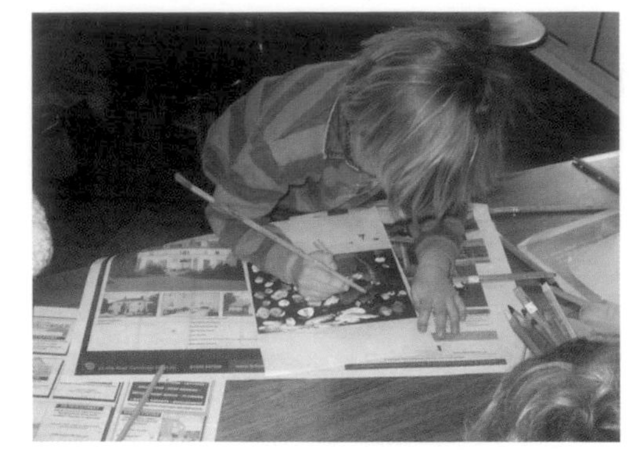

Abused children and their families need professional help and guidance. Psychiatrists who specialize in these problems can help children recover their self-esteem, overcome their feelings of guilt, and start the process of getting over the trauma. Such treatment normally reduces the risk of a child having serious problems as an adult.

– Depression or isolation from friends and relatives.

– Evidence of sexual abuse or harassment in their drawings, playing, or fantasies.

– Seductive behavior.

– Excessive aggressiveness.

– Declarations that their body is dirty or damaged.

– Suicidal behavior.

– Fear of something bad in their genitals.

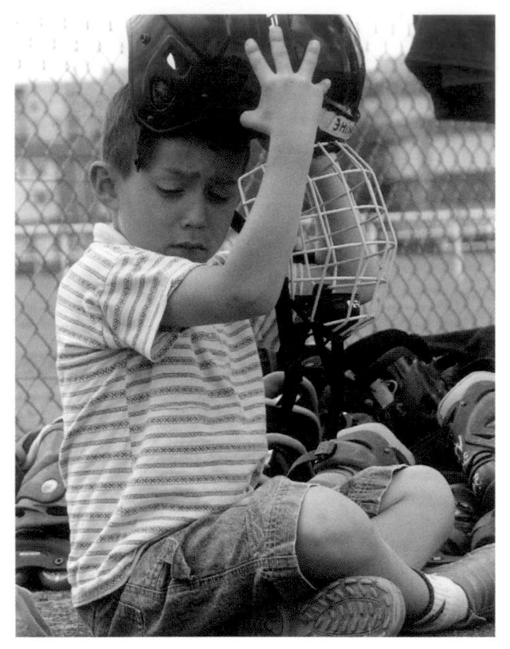

Preventive measures for parents

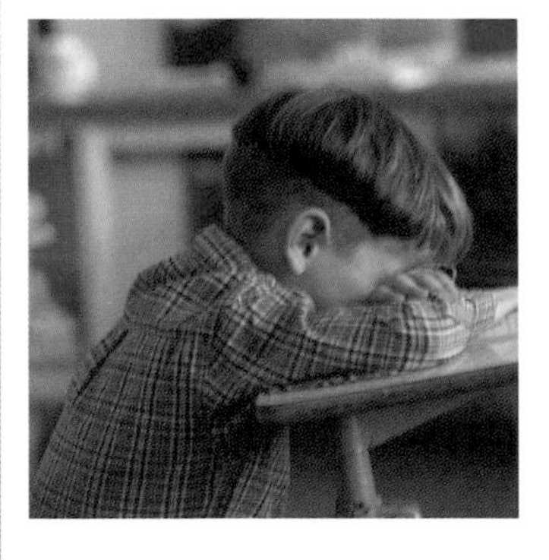

- Teach your child not to go anywhere with strangers if he is alone or out of your sight, nor to accept presents from them.
- Teach your child to say NO to anybody who tries to touch his body in an abnormal manner or do things that make him feel uncomfortable.
- Ask them to inform you immediately if they have any experience of this nature, stressing that they are not responsible or to blame, and that they will not be punished and can totally trust in their parents.
- Teach your child that respect does not mean blind obedience to adults and authority figures, so that he does not have to do absolutely everything that, for example, a teacher or babysitter may tell him to do.
- Encourage professional programs for the prevention of child abuse within the local education system.

drugs in childhood and adolescence

In recent years children have started drinking and smoking at an increasingly young age, although problems with addictive substances are more commonly found in adolescence. The process of forging one's own identity, of reaching maturity, and acquiring self-confidence inevitably involves a certain degree of distancing from the family circle. This process makes young people vulnerable to addiction, especially if a child has a weak personality that requires an extra backup to face the demands of growing up and going out into the world.

Drugs in childhood and adolescence

Drugs in themselves are not the problem: it is an individual who turns certain substances into drugs by establishing a relationship with them and developing patterns of use or abuse. Dependence results from the interaction between consumption and factors intrinsic to the consumer and his social environment

The search for new and risky sensations, self-doubt, and the need to belong to a group are some of the factors that often expose an adolescent to substance abuse and subsequent addiction.

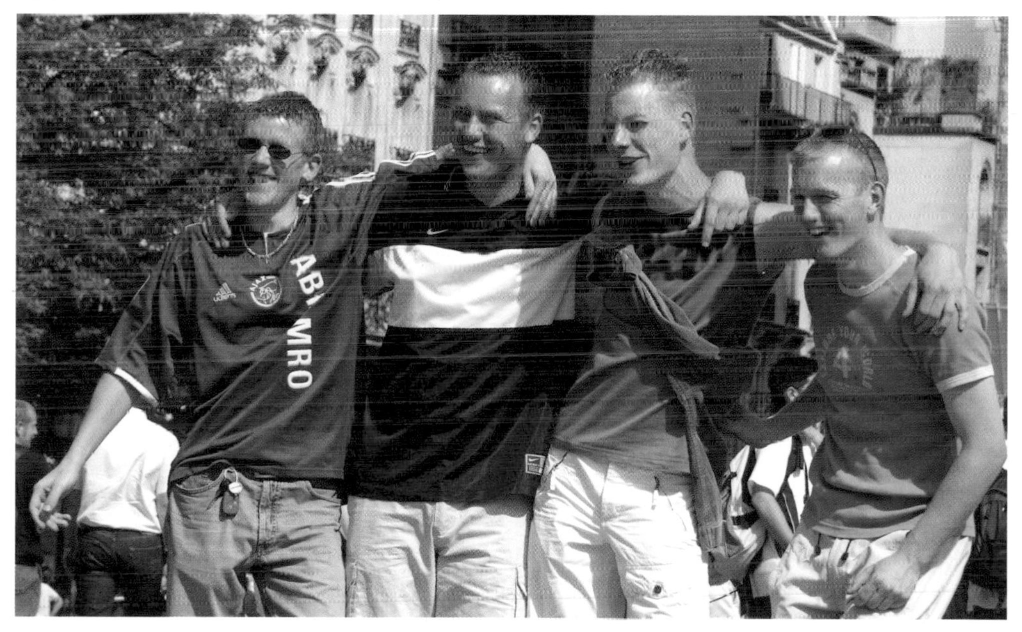

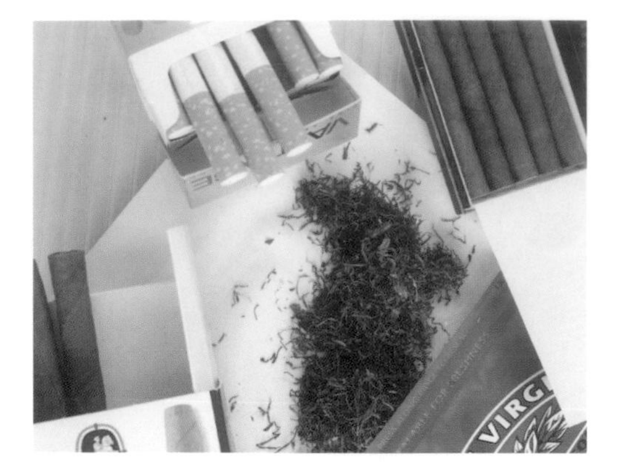

Peer pressure and the impact of advertising are key factors in young people's consumption of – and subsequent addiction to – legally permitted drugs.

Young people who are unable to bear frustration or suffering, whether on account of their own personality traits or their upbringing, are more strongly affected by the emotional conflicts typical of their age and are more liable to take refuge in the illusory relief offered by drugs.

Young people and alcohol

The drug that is currently causing the most social and health problems is undoubtedly alcohol, even though other drugs attract more attention and may seem more alarming.

Most young people who drink do so not only for pleasure but for many other reasons that can be grouped as follows:

- The need to feel good and at ease, or being more capable of relating with other people.
- Social pressure, either from friends or as a result of being bombarded by advertising and the media.

Youngsters also try alcohol out of curiosity, and are spurred on by the urge to experience something that is talked about so much and has an allure of danger.

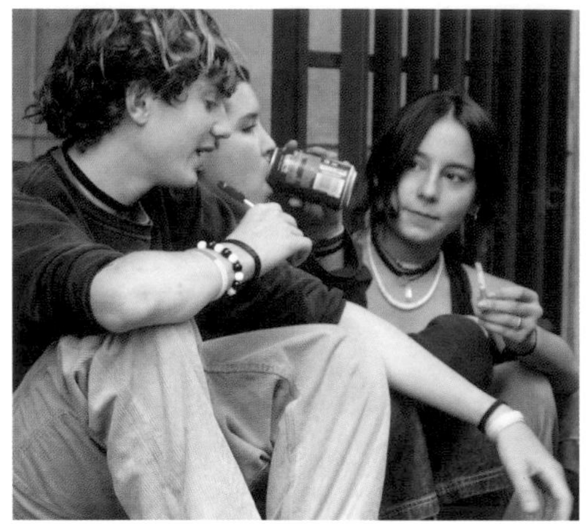

Alcohol can also be used to ease contact and communication in sexual relationships, even though, it really has the exact opposite effect.

Another of alcohol's attractions for young people is that it offers a gateway to the world of adults, whose attitudes are taken as reference points in many everyday situations.

The problems associated with alcohol always impinge on the health field and, although most young people are unaware of the medium- and long-term consequences, many are affected by various short-term consequences, such as personality disorders and, obviously, the high incidence of traffic accidents related to excessive consumption of alcohol.

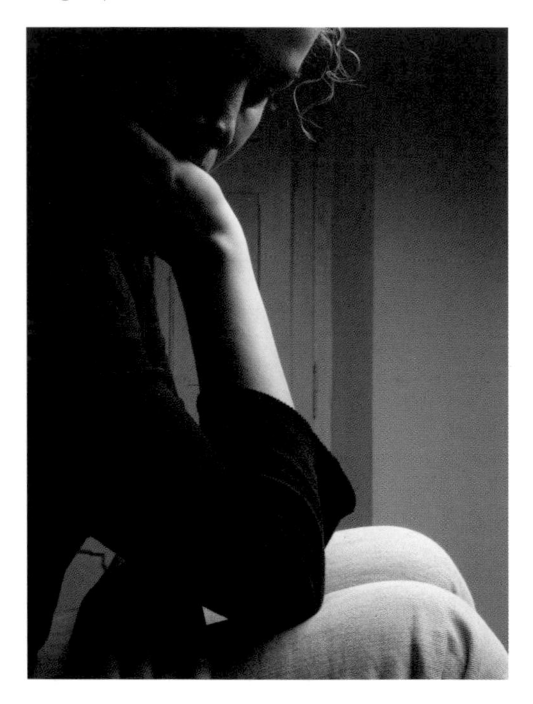

An adolescent is not conscious of the long-term risk of excessive alcohol consumption; more serious than this, however, is the lack of awareness of the associated risks such as traffic accidents, violent behavior, and involvement in crime.

Addictions unconnected with drugs can also be a cause for concern. Apart from the effects of the addictions themselves, having an addiction can be an indication that something is going wrong. Whenever a person – adolescent or otherwise – is compulsively glued to a cell phone or the Internet, then this might be a problem. The compulsion is a manifestation of the anxiety that is at the root of all addictions.

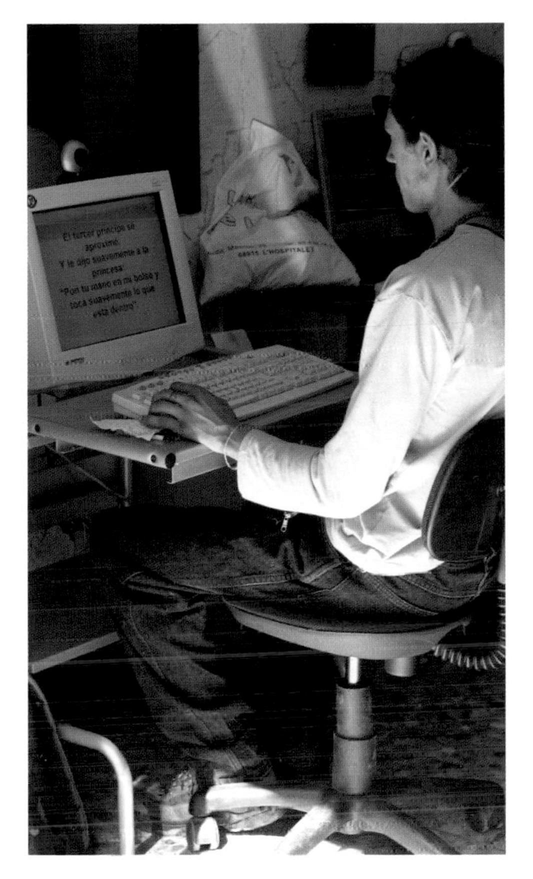

According to recent studies, young people who start to smoke marihuana before the age of 17 are 2–4 times more likely to develop addictions to other drugs (primarily cocaine and stimulants, then hallucinogens and, finally, heroin and other opiates) and display much higher levels of alcoholism in comparison to their peers who do not smoke, or first tried it at a later age.

Drugs and adolescence

The reasons that lead adolescents to take drugs and possibly become addicted are the same as those listed above for alcohol, as these apply to all situations involving dependent behavior:

Psychoactive chemical substances can be grouped in accordance with their effects:

- Depressant effects on the central nervous system (CNS). Drugs such as opiates (heroin, morphine, methadone), tranquilizers (valium, transilium), and hypnotics (barbiturates) impede the functioning of the brain.
- Stimulant effects on the CNS. Drugs that accelerate the functioning of the brain are divided into major (amphetamines, cocaine) and minor stimulants (nicotine).
- Altering effects on the CNS. Some drugs alter the functioning of the brain, giving rise to distortions of perception and hallucinations. The substances that produce these effects are hallucinogens (LSD), derivatives of cannabis (marihuana, hashish), inhalants (acetones, benzenes), and designer drugs like Ecstasy.

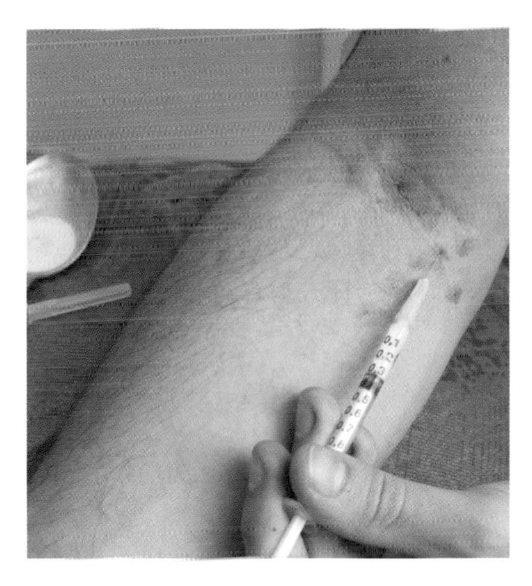

The consumption of marihuana can be the first step toward a subsequent addiction to harder drugs like cocaine, heroin, or designer drugs.

first aid in the home

Unexpected situations such as an accident or the sudden onset of sickness are frequent occurrences when children are around, and they can prove particularly upsetting or dramatic to anybody unaware of the basic initial measures required. This does not involve medical expertise, and, if you do not know exactly what to do, it is better not to take any steps that could harm a child, but instead stay calm and call an emergency service.

Basic principles of first aid

What not to do

1. Do not remain passive if you are sure what needs to be done.

2. Do not move an injured person before professional help arrives.

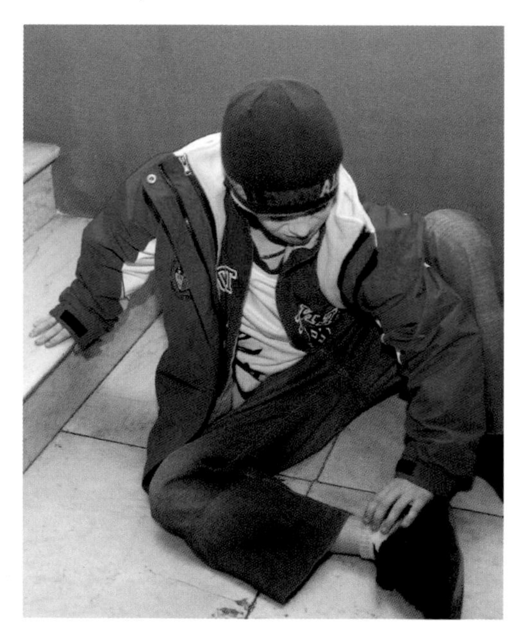

3. Do not touch any wound with your hands or mouth, or with any unsterilized object. Do not blow on wounds.

4. Do not wash wounds that are deep or caused by exposed fractures.

5. Do not clean wounds inward; always clean them outward.

6. Do not touch or try to dissolve clotted blood.

7. Do not try to sew up a wound.

8. Do not put cotton wool or sticking plaster directly on to wounds or burns.

9. Do not brusquely remove the gauze covering a wound.

10. Do not apply bandages that are damp or excessively loose or tight.

What to do

- Act confidently.
- Keep calm, so that you can act quickly and decisively.

It is not advisable to move a child with an injury or if there is any suspicion of a fracture, as this could make the injury worse or cause additional damage. In all cases, an emergency service must be called as quickly as possible. If the child is conscious, try to calm her down by conveying confidence and serenity.

First-aid techniques are primarily designed to save lives, but they also prevent complications and further injury, as well as making it possible to transfer an afflicted person to a health center, if the situation so requires.

A basic but reliable grasp of first-aid measures, along with a practical home kit, can mean the difference between life and death, or between the stabilization and aggravation of a sudden injury.

• Do not panic, so that you can instil calm in the injured child and do what you need to do with efficiency.

• Do not leave the child alone while you request any assistance you may require.

• Separate curious bystanders or anybody else whose presence is unwarranted, in order to avoid unsettling the injured child.

• Give priority to life-threatening events, such as hemorrhages, lack of pulse or breathing, poisoning, concussion and/or shock.

• Examine the child: check whether she has a pulse; whether she is breathing, and how; whether her nose or mouth are obstructed by secretions, the tongue, or any foreign bodies; and whether there is any bleeding or convulsions. If she is

The first-aid kit

It is important for every home to have a first-aid kit so that initial emergency measures can be implemented at once. Ready-prepared first-aid kits are available, but you can also assemble one yourself if you are aware of its indispensable components:

- Cotton wool.
- Sterile gauze.
- Sticking plasters.
- Surgical bandages.
- Antiseptics or disinfectants (alcohol, hydrogen peroxide and a povidone iodine solution like Betadine, as well as an antiseptic cream like Batricin).
- Scissors and tweezers (these must be washed and sterilized after use, so that they are in the appropriate condition the next time they are needed).
- Thermometer.
- Aspirin, paracetamol, or ibuprofen (for both adults and children) for fever and/or aches.
- Eardrops. Ask your doctor about the appropriate dosage and administration method.
- Cough mixture (for both adults and children).
- Anti-inflammatory creams, for burns and wounds.
- Astringent eye drops and, possibly, antibiotics for the eyes.
- Hydrocortisone cream, for insect bites and local inflammation.
- Rubber gloves, preferably sterile and of the right size (several pairs).

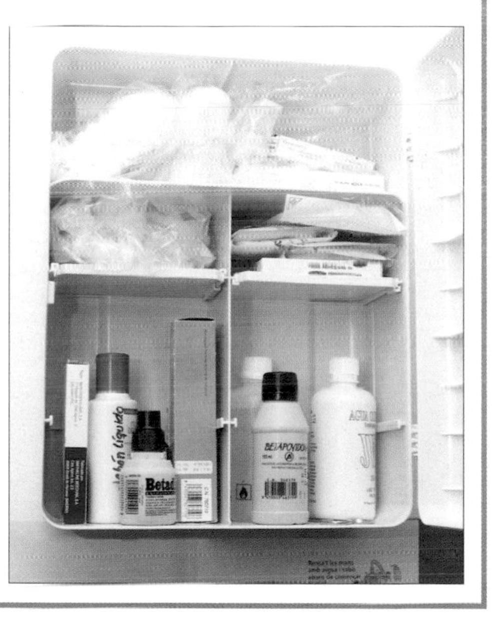

Medicines should be correctly labeled and have their expiration dates clearly visible. They also require specific conditions for optimal storage. Most medicines need a cool, dry environment, away from direct light. Liquid products are most convenient if they come in plastic containers. You should keep the fact sheet accompanying each medicine, as this allows you to know about any possible adverse reactions or contraindications. A domestic first-aid kit must be kept in its own special place – never under lock and key, but always out of reach of children.

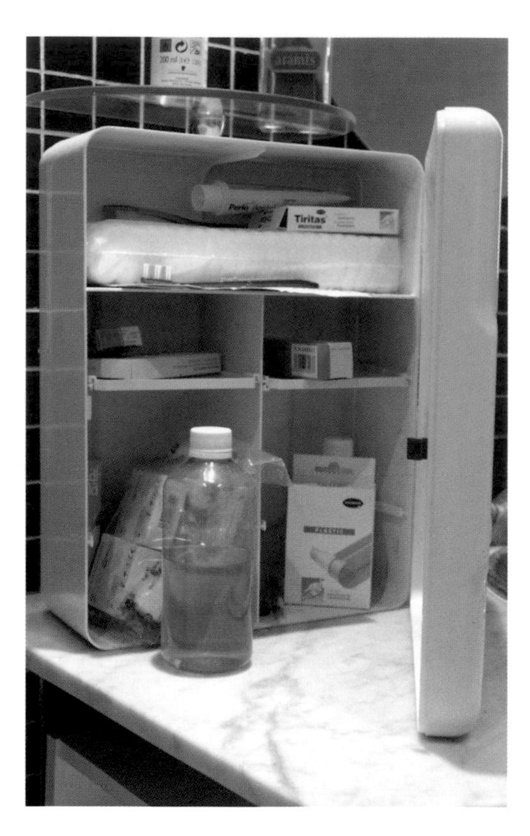

conscious, ask her to describe any pain she might be experiencing.

- Keep the child warm, but do not give her any stimulating or alcoholic drinks. Make her as comfortable as possible, without moving her – particularly if you suspect a fracture.
- Try to check any bleeding.
- Maintain the child's breathing.
- Inspire confidence. Use your common sense.
- Do not overreact.

Remember that a first-aid kit needs to be constantly replenished to ensure that none of its contents pass their expiration date. It is therefore necessary to check it at least once a month and verify that nothing is missing, and to replace any expired medicines.

Possible extras...

- If any member of the family suffers from a food allergy or has an allergic reaction to insect bites, it is advisable to keep at hand a syringe loaded with half a cubic cm of adrenalin, or an injectable cortisone derivative recommended by a doctor. In these cases, the doctor will advise you on the administration of such medicines.
- Other medicines that are useful to have readily available include: anti-histamines, anti-diarrhea drugs, and any product required by a family for specific complaints (especially diabetes, asthma, laryngitis, and convulsions) that has been previously prescribed by your doctor.

prevention of accidents in the home

A child spends many hours of her day at home, and it is therefore a place with a potential to produce an accident of some kind. Although all the members of a family could be involved in an accident, children suffer their consequences most frequently, as their ignorance and carelessness make them particularly vulnerable and defenseless.

Prevention of accidents in the home

Various studies have shown that the most common causes of domestic accidents involving children are, in descending order: falls, poisoning, allergies and contamination, burns, fires and explosions, electrocution, suffocation, and knocks. Although the risks of an accident can never be entirely eliminated, it is possible to minimize them, once a series of preventive measures are taken.

Preventing falls

- Keep the floor free of obstacles.
- Make sure the floor is not slippery.
- Use non-slip mats or adhesive stickers in the bathtub.
- Staircases should have barriers at each end to block the path of a small child, as well as handrails.
- Protect windows less than one yard from the floor with bars, grilles, etc.
- Fix bookcases securely to the wall.
- Do not allow your child to climb or stand on the furniture.

Preventing injuries

- As far as possible, keep any objects with a point or sharp cutting edge (knives, blades of a fan, blenders, razor blades, pins and needles, scissors, etc.) out of the reach of children.

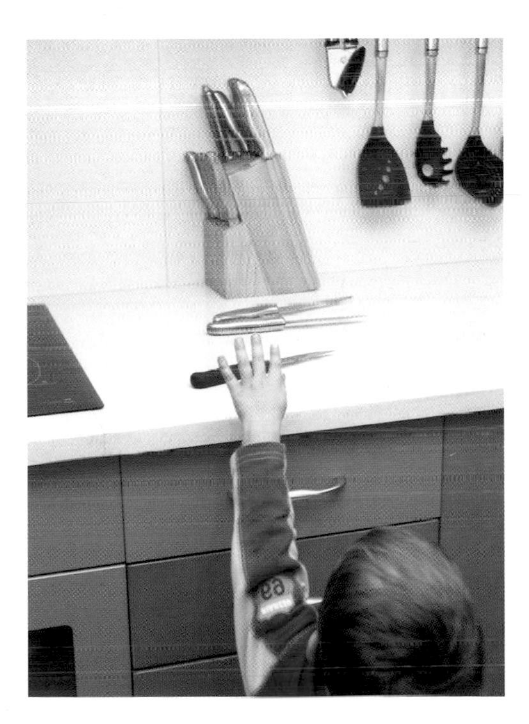

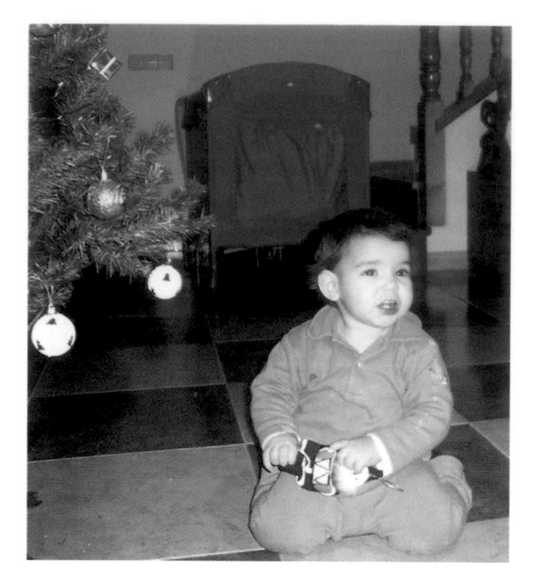

• Keep all tools in their appropriate packaging, with their points or cutting edges facing inward.

• Throw away any glasses, plates, or other crockery that are broken or have damaged edges.

• Keep prickly plants in visible places, out of reach of children.

Preventing a child from getting stuck or trapped

• When children are near doors, windows, or balconies, make sure that that their hands are not near the joins.

• Give your child clear reasons, expressed in comprehensible language, why she should only use an elevator in the company of an adult.

• Put children at the back of elevators that lack a double door or may not comply with safety regulations (especially in places where safety standards are not guaranteed).

Preventing poisoning, allergies, and contamination

• Put the first-aid kit, other medicines, insecticides, and cleaning and gardening products in a safe place, out of reach of children. Be aware of a child's ability (and inclination) to climb on to furniture to grasp something that has aroused her curiosity.

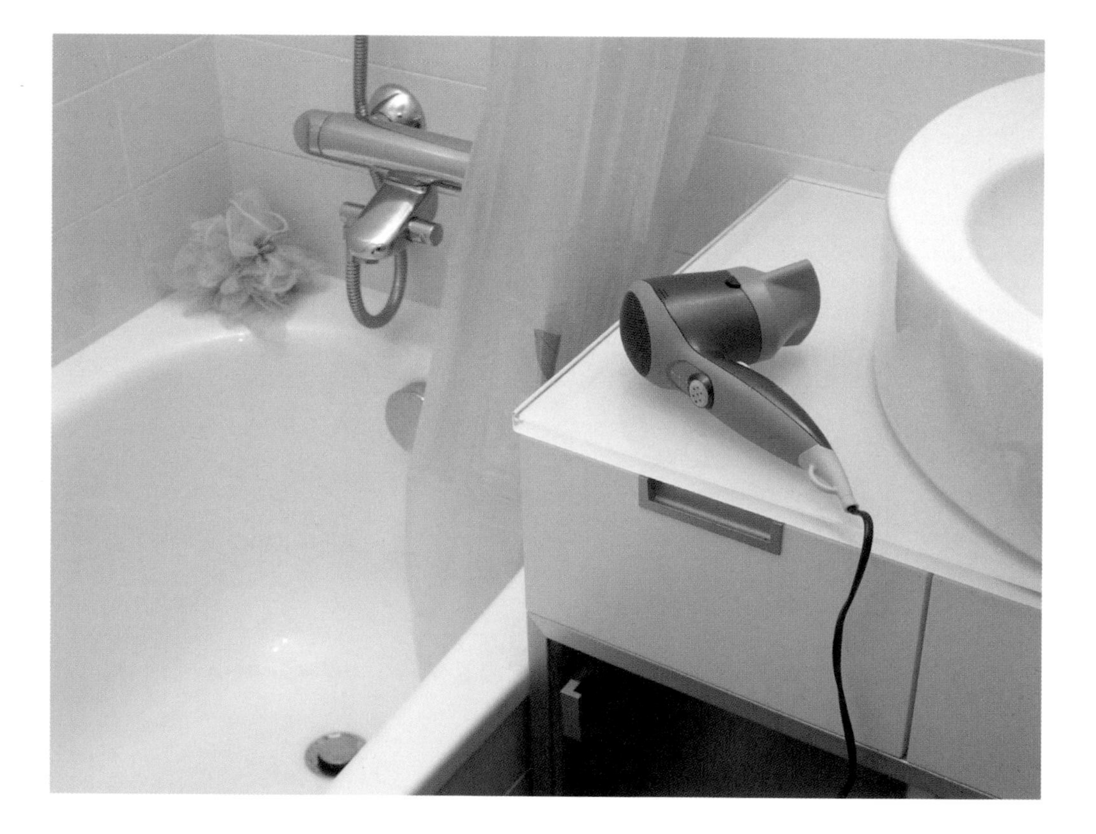

• Do not store different types of products in the same place (e.g. foodstuffs with bathroom items, toxic cleaning products, etc.).

• Do not linger in rooms treated with insecticides; leave a safe interval before you go back in, in accordance with the manufacturer's recommendations.

• Do not remain in rooms that have been freshly painted, or contain a recently varnished item, until the smell of solvents completely disappears.

• Avoid using stoves or heaters – or any other type of heating that is not totally innocuous in bedrooms.

• Turn off the gas supply when it is not in use (particularly at night) and keep children out of reach of gas bottles.

• Do not keep any plants that may be harmful if they come into contact with (or are eaten by) a child.

Preventing burns

• Avoid splashing hot liquids of any kind while you are cooking; cover your pans and keep watch of everything on the cooker at all times.

• The handles of frying pans and other kitchen utensils should not stick out in front of the cooker. Make sure that a child does not try to reach them by climbing on to a piece of furniture.

• Keep children away from the cooking and ironing area.

• Place hot objects or any live flames out of reach of children.

• Do not allow children to play with matches or lighters, or have access to any inflammable substance (whether liquid or aerosol).

Preventing fires and/or explosions

• If you are going out, do not leave food cooking on a burner and do not leave any high-consumption electrical devices switched on.

• Clean the filters of the hood over your stove on a regular basis.

• Make sure there are no drafts in your home that could blow out a flame, whether on the stove or any another device, particularly if it is unattended.

• Check your chimney, boiler, and heating equipment regularly.

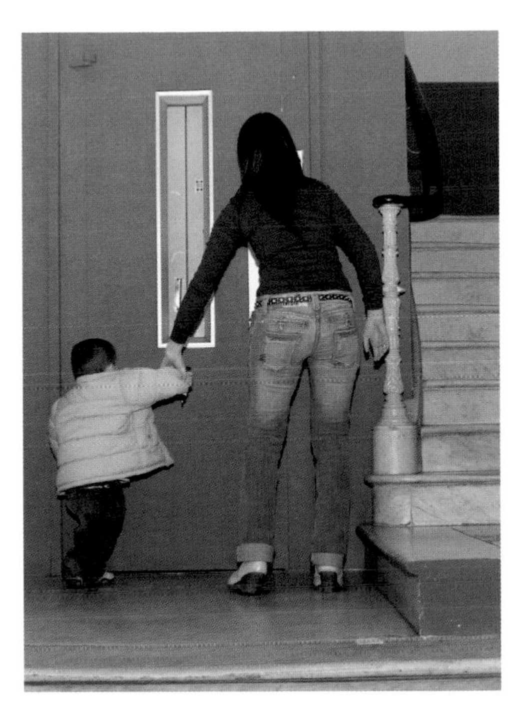

Preventing accidents with electricity

• Do not use any electrical devices or sockets that are wet, and do not plug in any such devices in rooms containing moisture, such as the bathroom.

• Avoid using or touching electrical devices with bare feet, even when the floor is dry.

• Make sure that sockets, electric stoves, and other devices are well away from children, especially in the bathroom (at least one yard from the bathtub, in case of splashing).

• Use specially designed, childproof safety sockets.

• Disconnect the main electricity supply whenever you are adjusting the wiring – no matter how quick and simple the operation.

injuries from falls or bumps

When a child starts to crawl and, shortly afterward, take her first steps, falls and bumps will become a constant feature of her life. As they are so frequent, they are a cause for concern for parents, who are sometimes unable to appreciate the extent of their impact and the occasional need for urgent treatment. The most common complaints in this respect include bruising, sprains, fractures, and dislocations. To limit the possibility of such serious situations, it is vital to place protective padding on the corners and edges of furniture, as well as non-slip mats in the bathroom.

Injuries from falls or bumps

Bruising

• A bruise affects the soft tissues, skin, and muscles; it can be caused by falling or being crushed or hit – for example, a bump in the eye or a knock in the face, chest, ribs, backs, genitals, limbs, etc.

• Bruising can be recognized by the following signs:

– A hemorrhage under the skin, with dark, irregular edges, whose color changes over the course of a few days as a result of the metabolization of the blood trapped inside.

– Swelling of the affected area.

The main aims of any treatment of bruising are to control any bleeding and prevent infections. Bleeding under the skin – the cause of the inflammation – requires the application of ice for around 10 minutes.

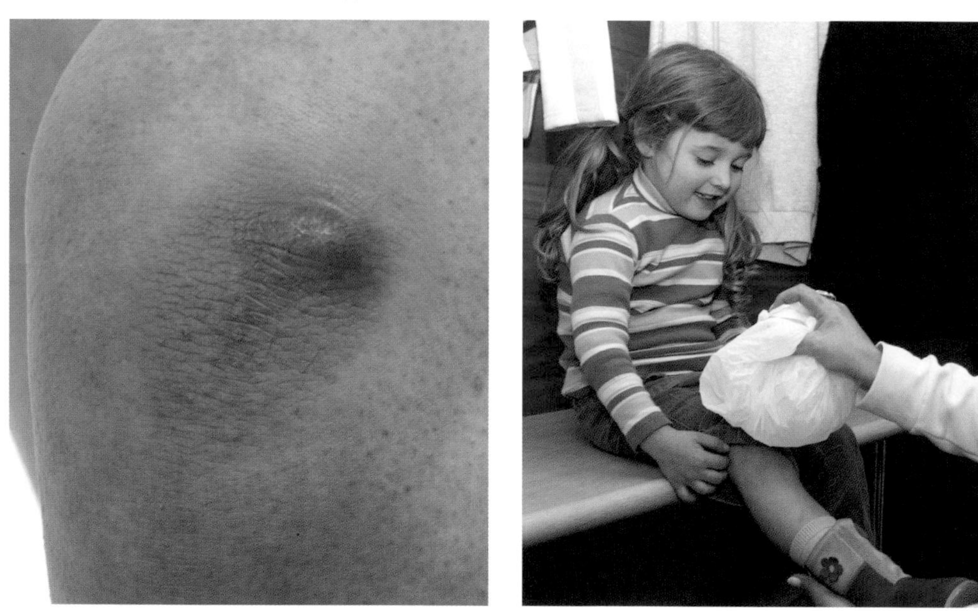

Some symptoms of a sprain

- Pain, especially with movement.
- Swelling of the joint and surrounding tissues.
- Difficulty in moving the joint.
- Pale skin (sometimes).

Attending to a sprain

- First, try to relieve the pain with a painkiller or analgesic (paracetamol, ibuprofen, etc.).
- Apply an ice bag to the site for at least 10 minutes.
- Do not move the affected joint or limb.
- Take the child to an emergency department so that the injury can be examined, diagnosed, and treated by professional specialists.
- If the sprain affects a joint in the leg, make sure the child does not put any weight on it when you take her to the doctor or emergency department.

– Pain.

– Possible presence of foreign bodies, such as splinters, dust, etc.

You must take the child to an emergency department:

• If she is in great pain or if there is considerable inflammation and she shows signs of infection, such as fever and reddening of the area around the bruise.

• If she is unable to move the affected area.

• If she suffers from diabetes, hemophilia and/or is taking aspirin or some other type of anticoagulant medication.

Sprains

• Sprains are classified as follows, depending on their severity:

Mild. The elongation of the fibers in the ligament causes only localized pain and slight inflammation.

Moderate. The fibers of the ligament are not only elongated but also partially broken, producing great pain and more inflammation.

Serious. The ligament is completely broken. There is usually less pain than in a moderate sprain, but the inflammation is greater.

Fractures

• A fracture is a loss of continuity in the surface of a bone, as a result of blows, exertions, or traction of an intensity that overwhelms the bone's natural elasticity.

• They can be:

– Closed or simple.

– Open or exposed.

• The main aim of the treatment of a fracture is to reduce the pain, prevent any greater complications, and control the bleeding, which can be internal (in a closed fracture) or external (in an open fracture). These objectives demand the following measures:

– Soothing the pain.

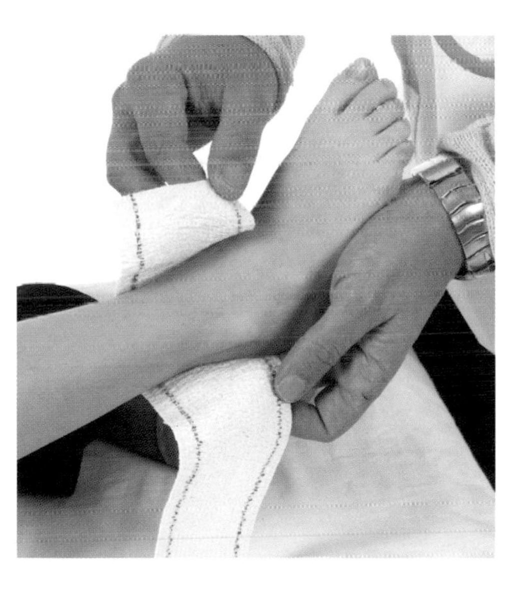

A sprain is a tearing of the ligaments, muscles, and/or joint tendons that occurs when the joint is forced beyond its normal range of mobility. It can sometimes be difficult to differentiate a sprain from a fracture. In such cases, an X-ray is used: a fracture will reveal a break or injury in a bone, while a sprain will show that the joint area is bigger than usual. The diagnosis of a sprain is basically clinical and requires the attention of a specialist.

Simple fracture

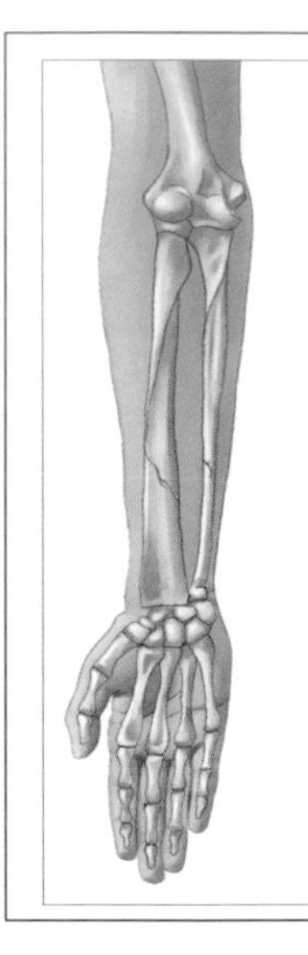

A simple or closed fracture is one that does not involve any injury to the skin around the affected area, and so the broken bone does not deviate from its normal position. It is characterized by intense pain, swelling, deformation (noticeable to the eye or touch), and functional impotence (impossibility of moving the affected area or limb).

Open fracture

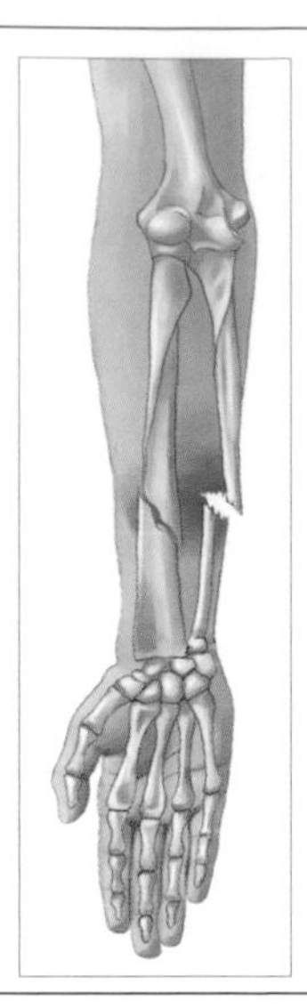

In an open or exposed fracture, one or both ends of the fractured bone damage and rupture the surrounding soft tissues and stick out of the skin. Its signs and symptoms are a bleeding wound, deformity noticeable to both the eye and the touch, intense pain at any attempt to move the limb, and functional impotence. This type of fracture is serious, as it can easily be infected.

– Applying pain relieflocally – for example, with an ice bag.

– Not moving the limb or affected area.

– Not immobilizing the limb with any bandages or splints.

• To move a child with a fracture, put pieces of wood or any other hard, stiff material under the affected area, so that she can support herself and find the position that causes her the least pain.

• If the fracture is exposed, it is important to control the bleeding by applying direct pressure to the wound for around 10 minutes. Cover the wound with a sterile gauze or dressing, held in place with adhesive tape.

• Always take a child with a fracture to an emergency department, to obtain a specialized assessment and treatment.

Dislocations

• A dislocation is an injury that affects a joint and the bone inside it; as a result, the bone is wholly or partially displaced from the joint. The areas most commonly affected are the shoulder, elbow, thumb, and/or jaw.

• The symptoms include:

– Intense pain.

– Deformity (especially when compared with the unaffected side).

Splints

A splint must be long enough to extend beyond the joint both above and below the fracture. Any material can be used, provided that it is sturdy: a broomstick or other piece of wood, a thin strip of metal, and even rolled-up newspapers or thick magazines. It is advisable to put pieces of cloth or another soft material between the fractured limb and the splint. Hold the splint in position with a bandage or strip of cloth, divided into at least 3 pieces.

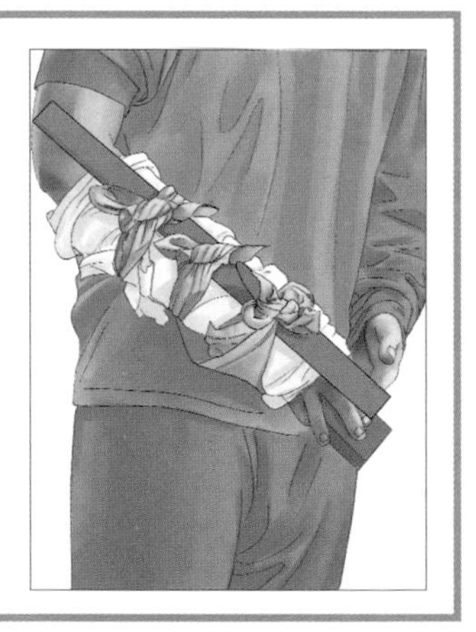

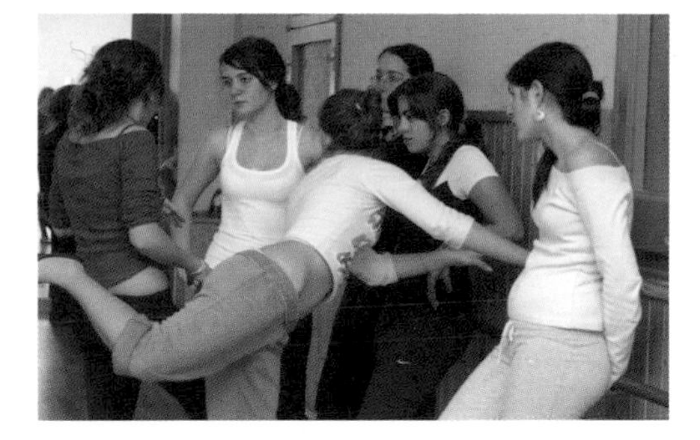

– Loss of mobility.

• As in the case of other injuries, the pain must be relieved and all complications averted.

– Apply cold to the site of the dislocation and, if possible, immobilize the whole area.

– Do not try to reinsert the bone into its original position.

– Always go to an emergency department, to receive a specialist's evaluation and treatment.

If a dislocation is suspected, no attempt should be made to put the bone back in its place. If possible, immobilize the joint and take the child to an emergency department.

Blows to the head

• Blows to the head can sometimes have serious consequences. As the skull is a rigid structure, it prevents any dilation of its contents; like all other body tissues, these tend to become inflamed when they are injured.

• Depending on the severity of this inflammation, the cerebral blood vessels can hemorrhage, increasing the pressure within the skull, as well as displacing and compressing the brain. This can give rise to various symptoms, most noticeably loss of consciousness.

• The most significant symptoms of skull injury demand emergency attention from a doctor. They can include:

– Loss of consciousness (this may only be fleeting).

– Disorientation regarding both time and space.

– Nausea, vomiting, and dizziness.

Periods of amnesia.

– Loss of strength in all the limbs.

– Changes in behavior or sensory sensations.

Injuries to the neck and spine

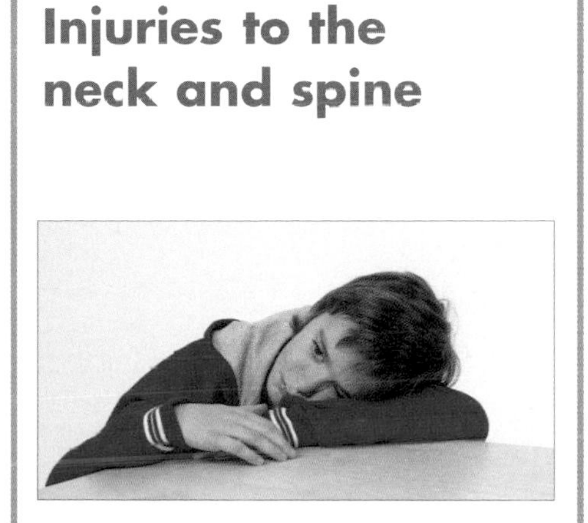

- Do not move the injured child until the appropriate assistance arrives on the scene (stretcher or ambulance).
- Call a doctor immediately.
- Move the child under the supervision of a doctor.
- Keep her calm and warm.
- Be prepared to use mouth-to-mouth resuscitation, if necessary.
- Do not move the child's head..

One or more of these symptoms in association with a skull injury requires an immediate visit to an emergency department. If a child's consciousness has changed and it is decided to take her directly to a health center, her cervical column must be protected by keeping her head immobilized

After a blow to the head, there may be signs such as headache, vomiting, and altered states of consciousness. The latter may manifest itself through a strange way of speaking, drowsiness, etc. Leaving a child to sleep after a blow to the head will not exacerbate the situation, but she should be observed and woken up from time to time to check her reactions. If she does not respond appropriately, she should be examined immediately by a doctor.

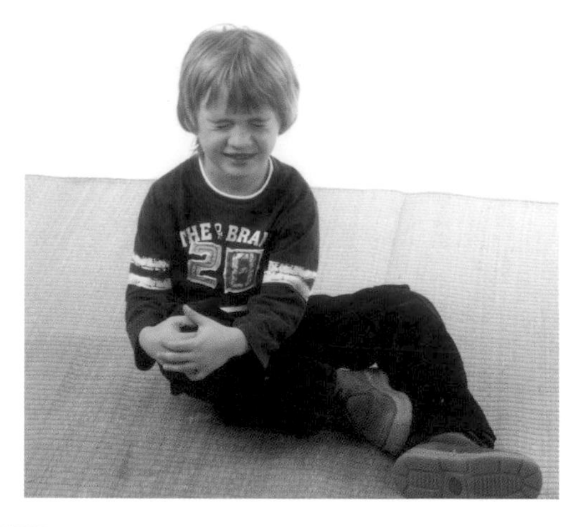

and aligned with her trunk. This can be achieved by placing cushions on both sides of her head, above her shoulders, or by using a couple of stiff objects that prevent her head from rolling. If a child is transported by car, it is advisable for her to be semi-upright, at an angle of 30°, rather than lying down.

Injuries from risky hobbies

- To avoid injury, it is very important to take protective measures, such as using helmets and pads for the knees and elbows, especially with skateboarding and rollerblading. Children should also be told to always choose a place free of cars to practice these sports.
- In the case of trampolines, it is vital that these are set in an area where the ground is not paved or very hard. The ideal solution is to place protective elements like mattresses around them, to break any falls. It should also be remembered that children should take it in turns to jump on a trampoline; if several children jump on it at the same time, they run the risk of bumping into each other and falling.

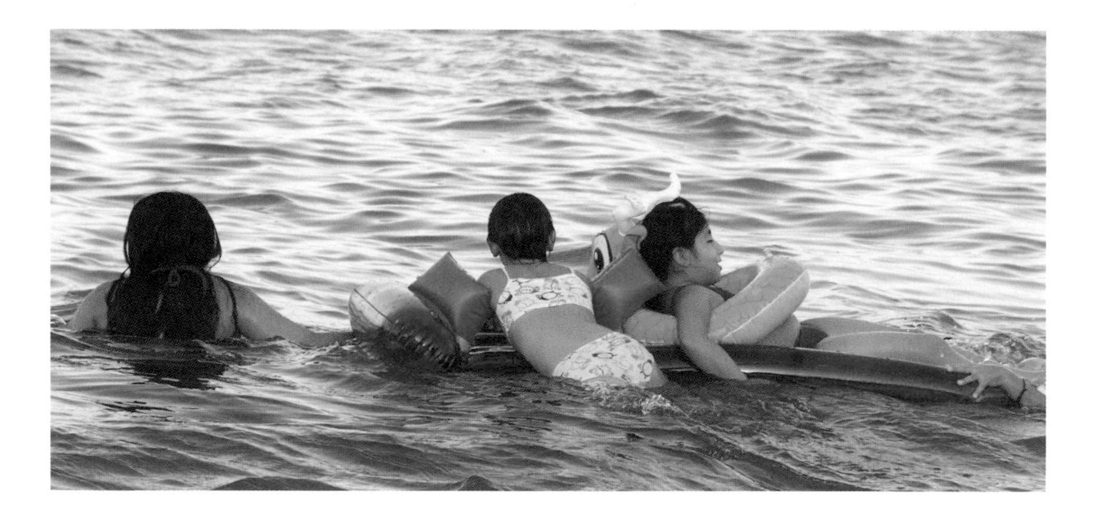

In recent years, there has been an increase in the incidence of injuries to the spine (particularly the cervical area) and the limbs (fractures and sprains) in children and adolescents, due to the practice of sports like skateboarding, rollerblading, and trampolining. Although these types of activity have positive benefits for a child's health (relief of stress, acquisition of agility, etc), there is a significant risk of fractures.

drowning

If a child is drowning, she has to be rescued immediately, otherwise in just a few minutes she could asphyxiate and die. A child can drown in as little as two inches of water _ so it is extremely important to keep close watch when she is near a swimming pool, a pond, a bathtub, or even a bucket of water.

Drowning in the home

Leaving aside accidents in swimming pools, about two-thirds of deaths by drowning in homes occur in the bathtub.

Buckets with a capacity of 3–6 gallons (10–20 liters), used constantly for everyday tasks, are a real danger for babies taking their first steps. Their high, straight sides and their stability make it almost impossible for young children to free themselves if they fall in.

Toilets are often not considered as risk areas for drowning, but accounts of children under 3 years of age falling head first into a toilet bowl are reasonably common.

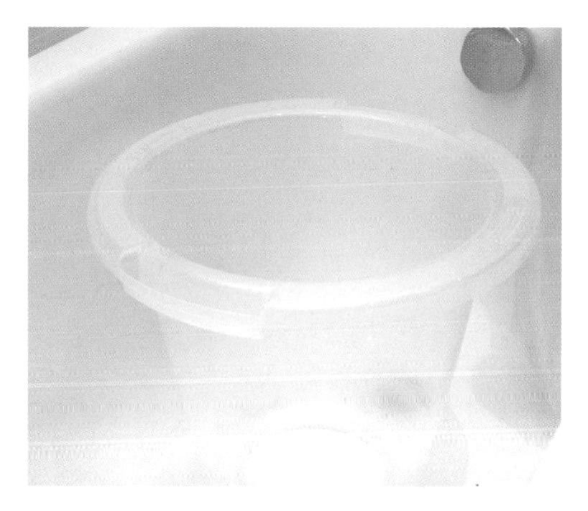

Drowning consists of death through asphyxia while underwater. It is vital that anybody who is rescued after having nearly drowned receives first aid and medical attention immediately.

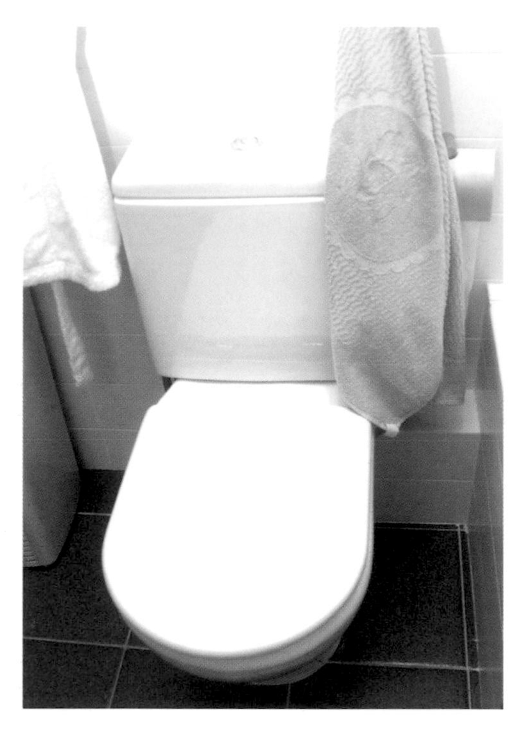

Jacuzzis and swimming pools also pose a threat. Safety covers and nets may not be sufficient to stop toddlers finding their way in, even when the cover is apparently in place; once a child has found her way underneath it, she is trapped in the water.

Chances of surviving submersion

• This basically depends on the circumstances of the rescue.

• The prognosis is poor when:

Asphyxia due to submersion

Submersion causes the lungs to suck in water, triggering a protective reflex that closes the airway (laryngeal spasm). This leads the victim to swallow large amounts of water, both voluntarily and involuntarily. If the submersion continues for a long time, there is a sharp drop in the oxygen levels in the body's organs (hypoxia), especially the brain. Hypoxia eventually causes the protective laryngeal spasms to stop, allowing water to enter the lungs, which aggravates the situation still further.

Prevention of drowning in the home

- Never leave a baby alone in a bathtub, even for a second, and make sure she is always within your reach.
- Never leave a small child alone in a bathtub or with a young sibling, even if she is using a bath seat designed for babies. Children can drown quickly and silently.
- Keep the toilet lid closed, and keep young children out of the bathroom when they cannot be supervised. Consider putting a lock on the bathroom door, out of reach of children.
- Be sure to empty any container holding liquid as soon as you have finished using it. Do not leave empty buckets in patios or gardens, as they can fill up with water and attract young children.
- Check regularly that safety covers and barriers for Jacuzzis and swimming pools are secure.
- Learn how to perform cardio-pulmonary resuscitation, as this can save lives in a situation in which every second counts.
- Cordon off swimming pools with a sturdy door and an appropriate barrier (minimum height of 5 ft (1.5 m) and a distance of 5 in (12 cm) or less between vertical bars). This measure alone has reduced the incidence of drowning by 50–70%.

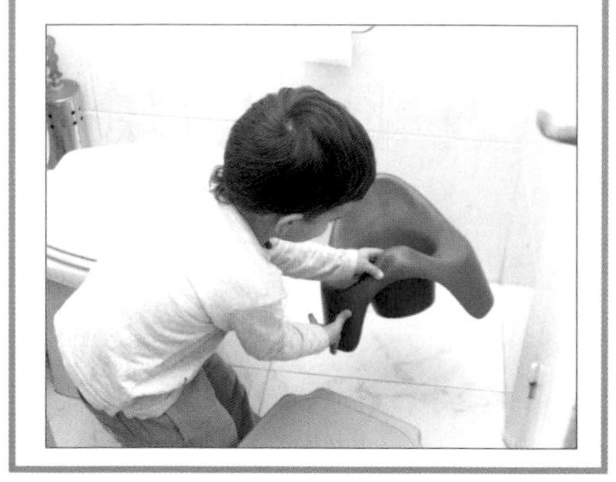

Emergency measures in cases of asphyxia through submersion

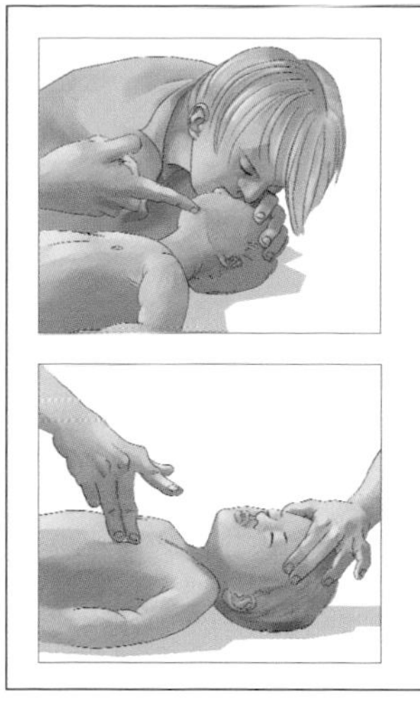

The most important measure to be taken in this situation is the immediate administration of basic cardiopulmonary resuscitation (mouth-to-mouth ventilation and, if necessary, cardiac massage).

1. Unblock the airway and keep it open.

2. Perform mouth-to-mouth ventilation. In the case of very small children, your mouth must cover both the mouth and the nose; in older children and adults, cover the victim's mouth with yours, and cover her nose with your hand.

3. Cardiac massage and ventilation, at a rate of 5 compressions for each ventilation, for all ages. Use the heel of your hand to massage an older child or adult, pushing down on the chest at the vertex of the sternum. The same technique is applied to babies of under a year, only with two fingers, as illustrated.

4. Ask for help and call an emergency service.

– The child is aged under 3 years.
– The submersion lasts for more than 5 minutes.
– Resuscitation techniques are not applied within 10 minutes after the child's rescue.
– The child is unconscious on arrival at the emergency department.

When 3 or more of these factors are present, the possibility of survival or absence of serious brain damage is less than 5%.

Submersion can easily turn into an exceptionally dangerous situation. A call for help or attendance from emergency services should never be delayed – the outcome can be decided in just a few minutes.

If it is not possible to keep an attentive watch over a child in a dangerous place (swimming pool, sea, etc.), then she should not be taken there – the risk is too high.

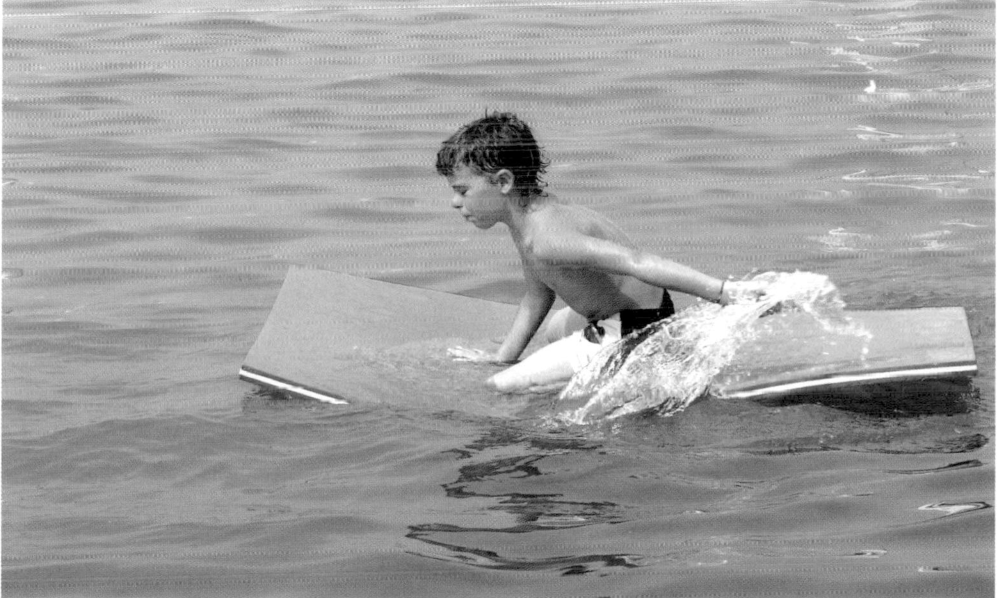

choking

When a child accidentally chokes, on food or anything else, her airways are obstructed, which causes a lack of oxygen in the lungs and brain. If this oxygen deficit lasts for more than 4 minutes, it can cause brain damage and even be fatal. It is important to be able to recognize when a child is choking and know what to do. The Heimlich maneuver, an emergency procedure designed to assist choking people, saves thousands of lives every year.

Choking

Symptoms of choking

- Partial obstruction. Painful throat and cough, noisy breathing, and difficulty in speaking.
- Total obstruction. Inability to breathe, paleness in the face followed by blueness, agitation, and loss of consciousness.

To avoid the danger of choking at the meal table, do not allow a child to play or make unnecessary movements.

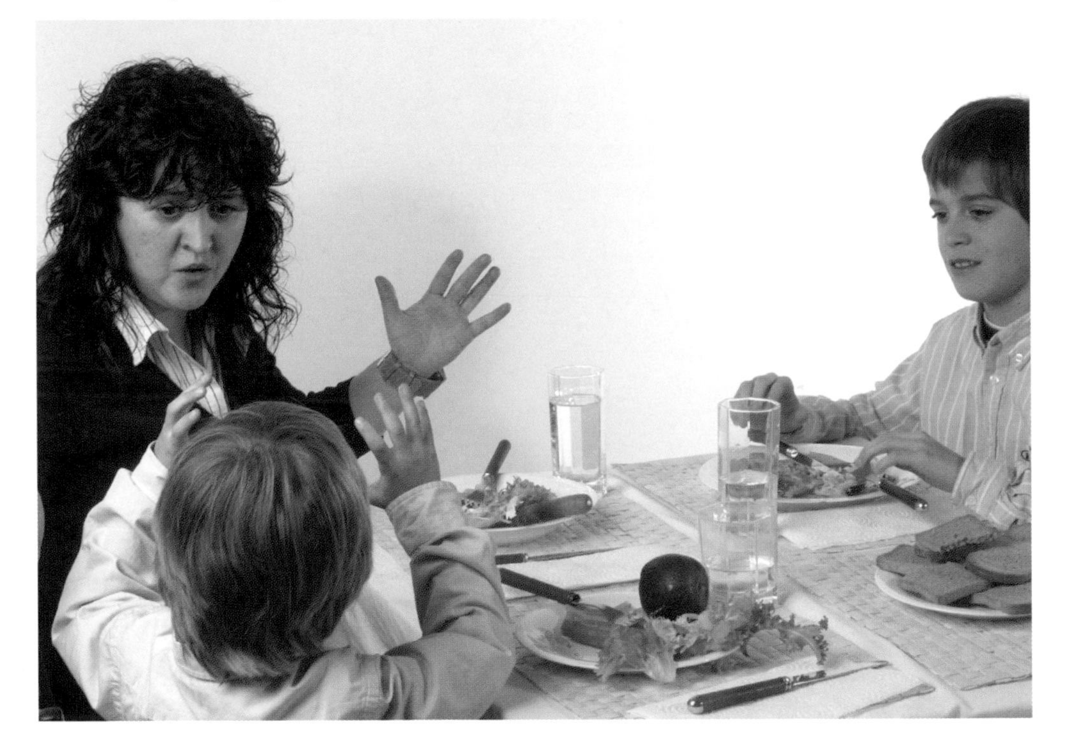

Heimlich maneuver

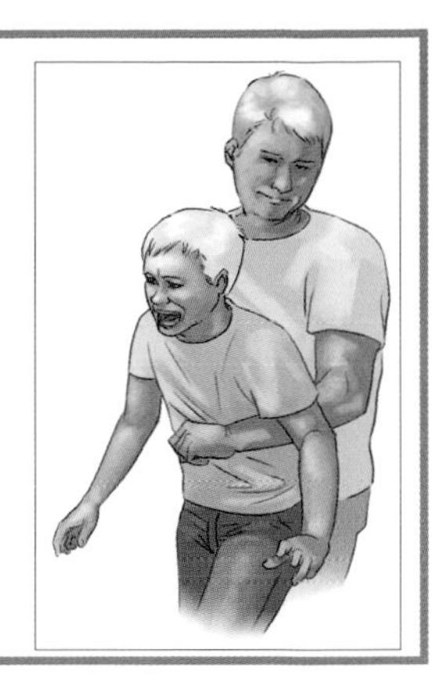

- The Heimlich maneuver involves lifting the diaphragm and forcing sufficient air out of the lungs to cause an artificial cough, thereby pushing air toward the trachea and expelling the obstruction through the throat and mouth.
- Although this maneuver is simple and effective, it can be painful and even cause injury. It should only be used in genuine emergencies, when it is clear that a person really is choking.

In cases of choking, one good strategy is to put a fist just above the person's navel while applying pressure to the abdomen.

Preventive measures

Choking can generally be avoided in babies and children if the following precautions are taken:

• All small objects and toys with small pieces should be kept away from children 3 years of age and under.

• Prevent a child from running, playing, or walking with food or toys in her mouth.

• Children aged under 4 years should not eat food that could easily stick in their throat, for example, sausage, walnuts, chunks of meat or cheese, grapes, hard or sticky candies, popcorn, or raw carrots.

• Keep watch over children when they are eating.

• Prevent children from giving dangerous foodstuffs or toys to their younger siblings.

First aid in small children

Techniques other than the Heimlich maneuver should be used on babies and small children.

Children under a year old

Perform the following maneuvers if the child is choking and cannot breathe, but do not use them if she is coughing, talking, or crying. In all cases, medical help must be urgently requested.

1. Place the child face down on your arm, supporting her head with your hand.

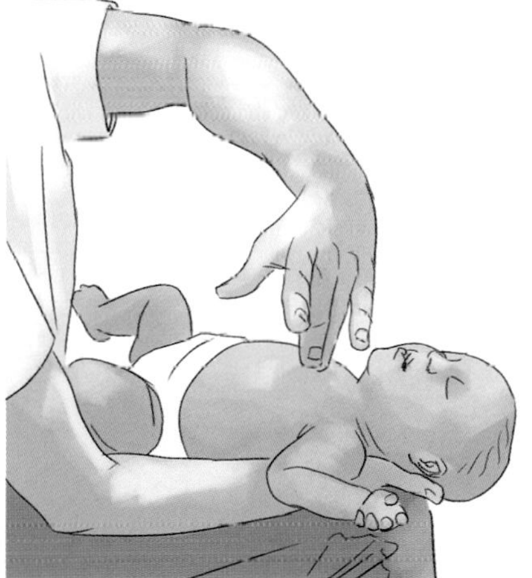

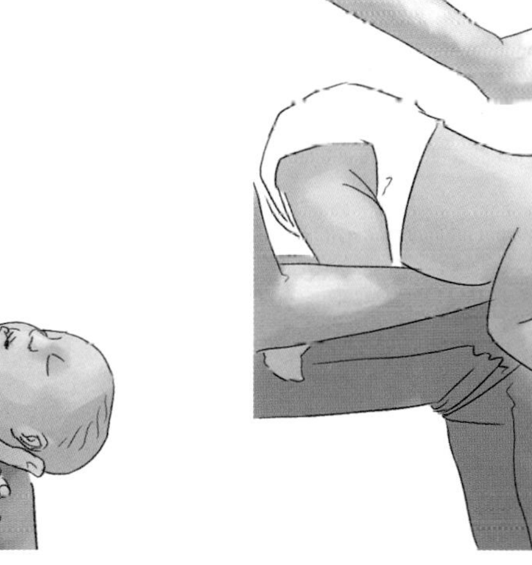

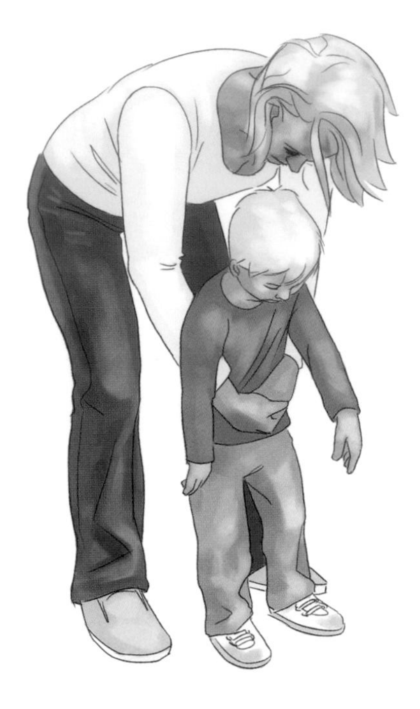

2. Strike her back between the scapulas 5 times with the heel of your hand.
3. Place her face up on your forearm.
4. Press your hand down 5 times near the center of the sternum.
5. Repeat the previous 4 steps until the child spits out the obstruction, starts to breathe, or loses consciousness.

If she does lose consciousness:

6. Open her mouth and lift up her tongue. If you see an obstruction, take it out with your finger.
7. Lean the child's head backward. Try to give her two breaths mouth to mouth.
8. Start performing cardio-pulmonary resuscitation if she does not respond to stimuli, is no longer breathing, or has no pulse. You should make sure that somebody has called the emergency services.

Children over a year old

Carry out the following maneuvers if a child is choking or cannot breathe. These maneuvers must not be performed, however, if she is coughing, talking, or crying, although medical help should still be summoned immediately.

1. Place the part of the fist comprising the thumb and forefinger in the middle of the abdomen, above the navel. Hold your fist with the other hand.
2. Press upward 5 times, quickly.
3. Repeat steps 1 and 2 until the child expels the obstruction, starts to breathe, or loses consciousness.
4. Start cardio-pulmonary resuscitation if the child does not respond to stimuli, is no longer breathing, or has no pulse.
5. Make sure that somebody has called the emergency services.

Although many parents' desire that their child should eat heartily to grow strong is an admirable one, never oblige your child to eat if she is not hungry. Excessive insistence can lead a child to struggle to avoid eating, and this can lead to choking.

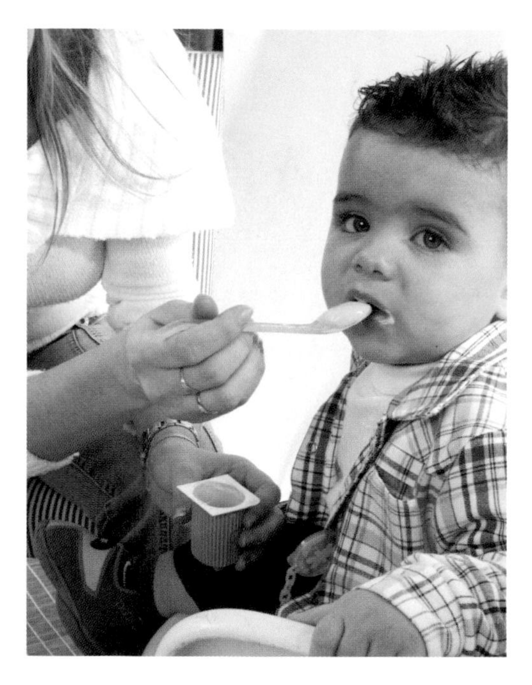

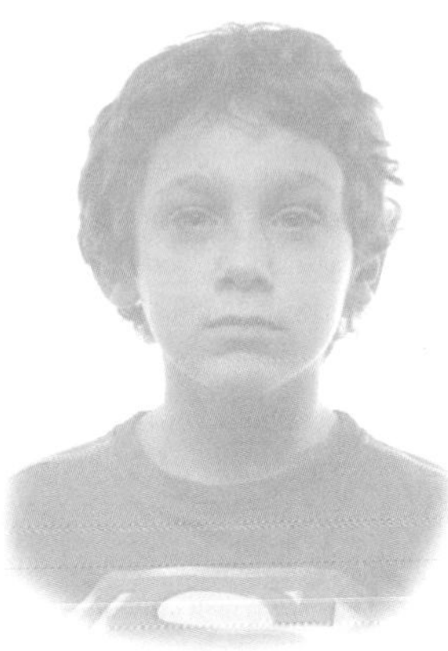

injuries from foreign bodies

Numerous substances and particles of many kinds are grouped together under the generic term foreign bodies. These can give rise to a variety of injuries in children. Although they are not life-threatening, they can be troublesome and, especially when sensitive areas like the eyes are affected, need urgent medical attention.

Foreign bodies in the eye

These can be pieces of dust; insects; particles of wood, metal, or glass; caustic or corrosive substances; folded contact lenses, eyelashes; textile fibers, etc. They can be on the surface of the eye or firmly embedded in it.

They make their presence known through redness, sensitivity to light, a painful, burning sensation, a watery eye, difficulty in keeping an eye open, etc.

Foreign bodies in the ears

When an insect is involved, the child will notice it moving around and buzzing inside her ear, as well as being in pain and having her hearing impaired. If the problem is a small object and the outer ear is not totally blocked, the symptoms can be negligible – mild irritation and slightly impaired hearing. In more serious cases, where the outer ear canal is injured or subsequently even infected, the pain and discomfort will be considerably greater.

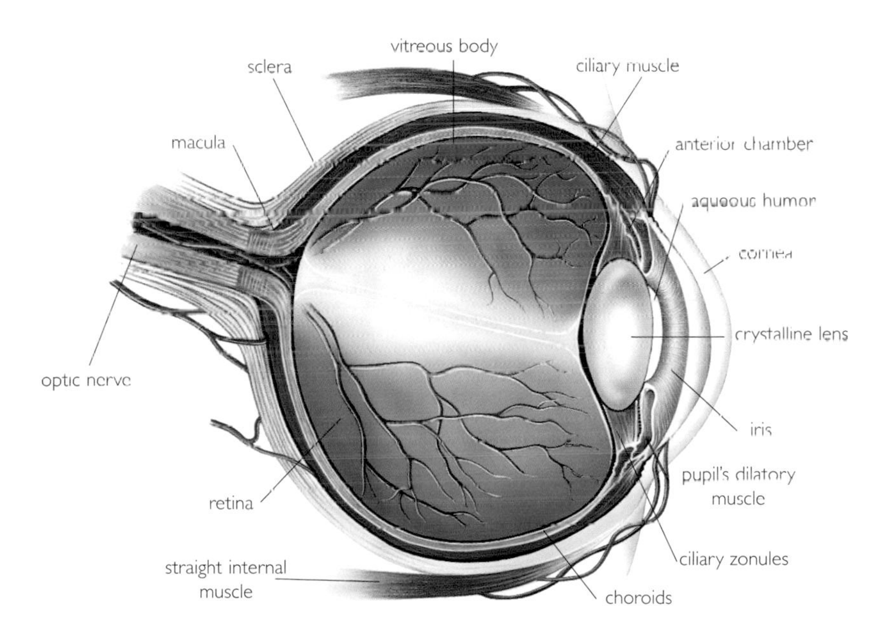

Foreign bodies can stick to the surface of the eyeball (cornea) or the top eyelid – causing irritation and damage to the cornea when blinking – Aor even penetrate the eye.

First-aid measures

- Wash your hands with soap and water.
- Seat the child in front of a light, with her head leaning backward.
- Position yourself next to the affected eye or behind the child.
- Gently separate her eyelids, then ask her to move her eye up and down and toward either side, to allow you to locate the foreign body.
- Once you have spotted the foreign body, try to remove it by washing the eye. Lean the child's head to one side and pour on water or saline solution, from the inner corner of the eye outward, using a syringe or jug, so that it can sweep the foreign body away.
- If this does not work, try to remove the foreign body with the damp tip of a handkerchief or moist cotton wool.
- You will have to turn up the eyelid if the foreign body is underneath it. If you do not manage to remove it, cover the eye with a dressing and take the child to the nearest health center.

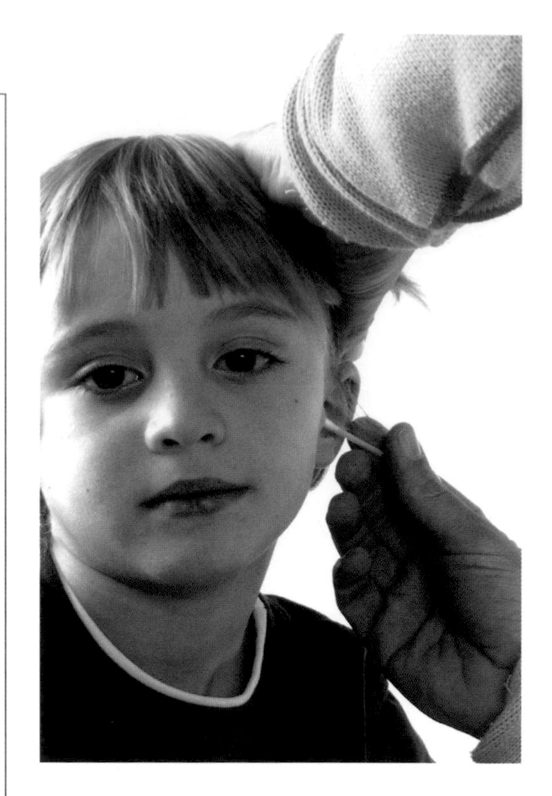

Under no circumstances should any instruments or cotton swabs be inserted into a child's ear, whether to clean it or to extract a foreign body from the hearing canal.

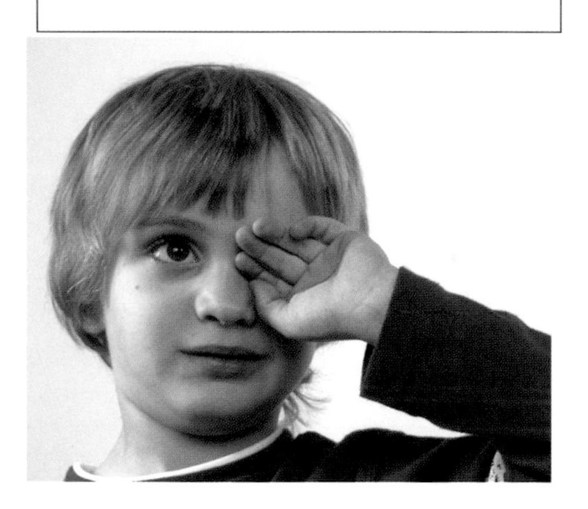

First-aid techniques

An insect in the ear

• Wash your hands with soap and water.

• Ask the child to sit down and tilt her head in the opposite direction from the affected ear.

• Apply 3 or 4 drops of warm oil.

• Wait for a couple of minutes until the insect dies, then tilt the child's head to the other side so that the oil can drain out by itself, bringing the insect with it.

• If the insect still fails to come out, you must take the child to the nearest health center. Do not try to remove the insect with any type of instrument.

An object in the ear

• Ask the child to sit down and tilt her head in the direction of the affected ear to see if the object falls out.

• If this does not work, do not use tweezers or any other implement to extract the object. Take the child to the nearest health center.

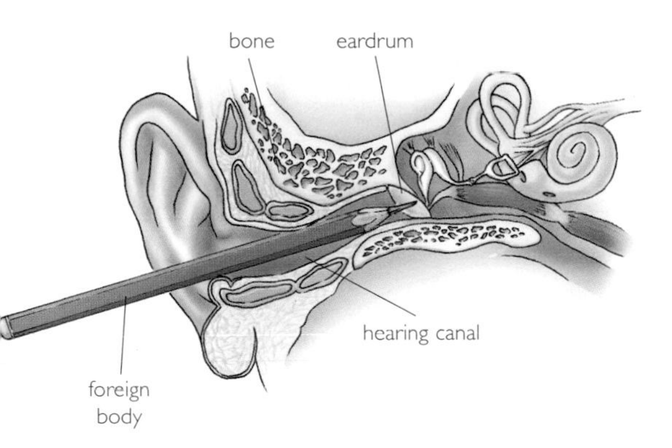

Foreign bodies of all types, including live insects, find their way into the ears of children fairly frequently.

Foreign bodies in the nose

When these are small and only affect one nostril they can often go unnoticed and not impair the child's breathing. This is a frequent occurrence in small children, the main culprits being breadcrumbs, pips from fruit, marbles, small balls, buttons, etc.

If the object is bigger it can cause breathing difficulties, pain, inflammation of the nasal mucous membranes, and, on occasions, a purulent, foul-smelling mucous secretion. If a small blood vessel is damaged along with the mucous membranes, there may be a nosebleed (epistaxis).

To deal with this problem, you must first ask the child what type of object has entered his nose; if it is a seed, you should seek medical help, as the nasal secretion will make it expand, and it will be very difficult to remove.

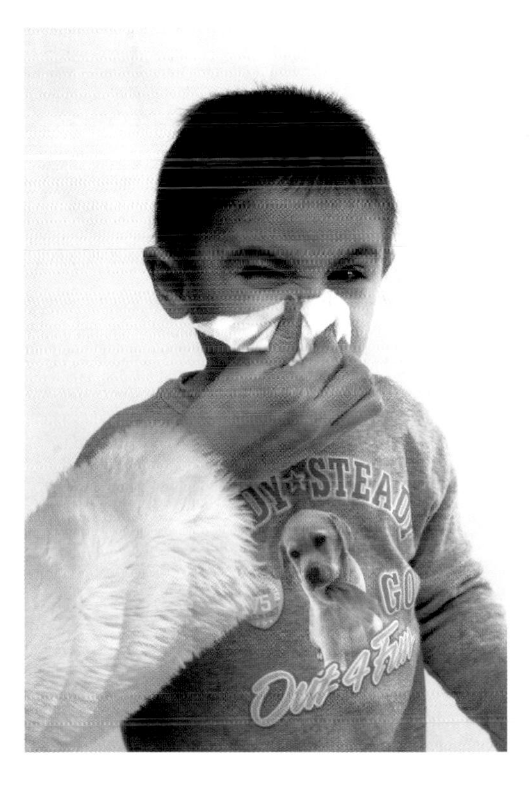

Foreign bodies in the skin.

Take the following steps in these cases:

- Wash your hands with soap and water.
- Sterilize the tips of a pair of tweezers with a flame.
- Wash the affected area with soap and water, then disinfect it with iodine.
- Grasp the splinter with the tweezers, as close as possible to the surface of the skin, and pull it outward, without changing its angle. Press the skin around the hole to make it bleed slightly.
- Disinfect the area again and cover it with a dressing.
- Consult a doctor about the need for any protection against tetanus.
- If the splinter does not come out easily or breaks, you should take the child to the nearest health center.

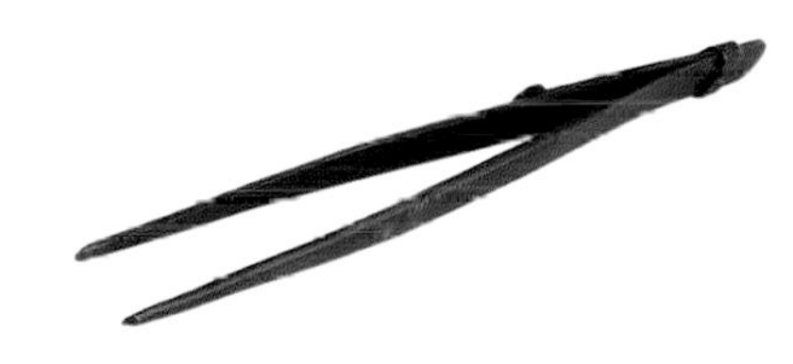

If a small object enters a child's nostril, try covering the other nostril with your fingers and tell him to blow his nose; the resulting air current should force the object out of the nose. If this does not work, you should take the child to the nearest health center.

burns

Burns are one of the main accidents experienced by children, both inside and outside the home; they often lead to complications that can affect a child for the rest of his life and they are also one of the most common causes of death in children. The seriousness of a burn depends on both its extension and its depth, as well as the characteristics of the structures affected. Various things can cause burns, these include sources of heat (fire, boiling water or other liquids, gas, steam, etc.),as well as sources of cold, certain chemical agents, electricity, and ultraviolet or other radiations.

Some points of interest

• Accidental or involuntary lesions are the main cause of fatality among children, adolescents, and young adults.

• Burns are the fourth most common cause of accidental deaths in children (traffic accidents are at the top of the list).

• Almost 75% of all burns that affect children are preventable.

• Babies just starting to walk and older children are the most vulnerable to scalding and burns.

• Of those children under the age of 4 years who are admitted to hospital for burn-related injuries, 65% suffer from scalding and 25% from contact with a heat source.

• Burns from hot faucet water cause more deaths and hospitalizations than those resulting from any other hot liquid.

First-aid measures

When a child has been burnt, the first steps to take are as follows:

• Place the burnt skin under a stream of cold water from the faucet.

• Remove any clothing covering it under this stream of water.

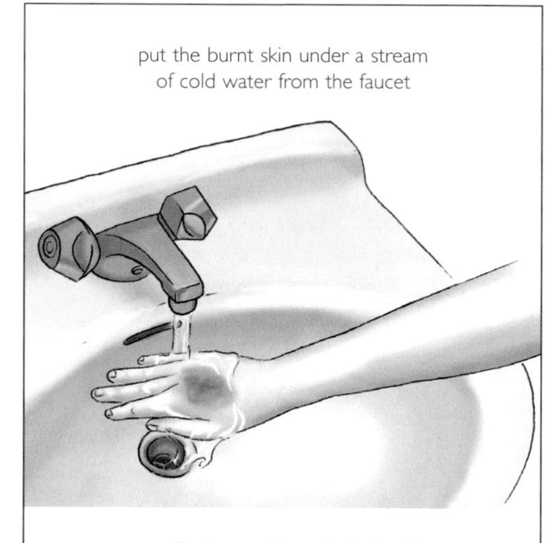

put the burnt skin under a stream of cold water from the faucet

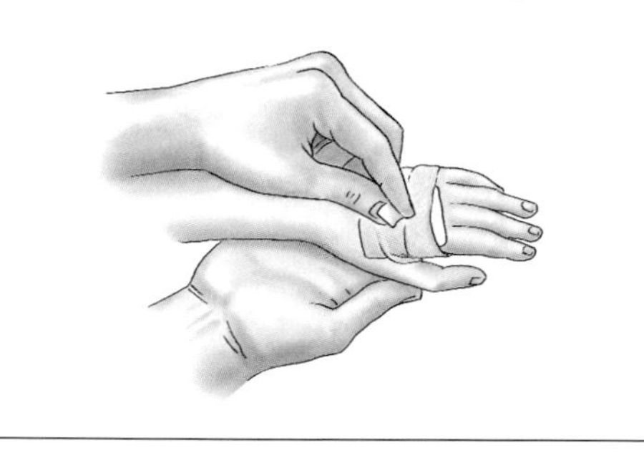

cover the burn with a sterile bandage

Burns classified according to depth

The depth of a burn determines its seriousness. First-degree burns affect the outer layer of the skin or epidermis and cause pain, red skin, and inflammation (erythema). Second-degree burns affect the epidermis and the inner layer of the skin or dermis, causing erythema and blisters. The damage from third-degree burns extends down to the hypodermis, causing destruction to not only the entire depth of the skin but also the nerves, leading to numbness.

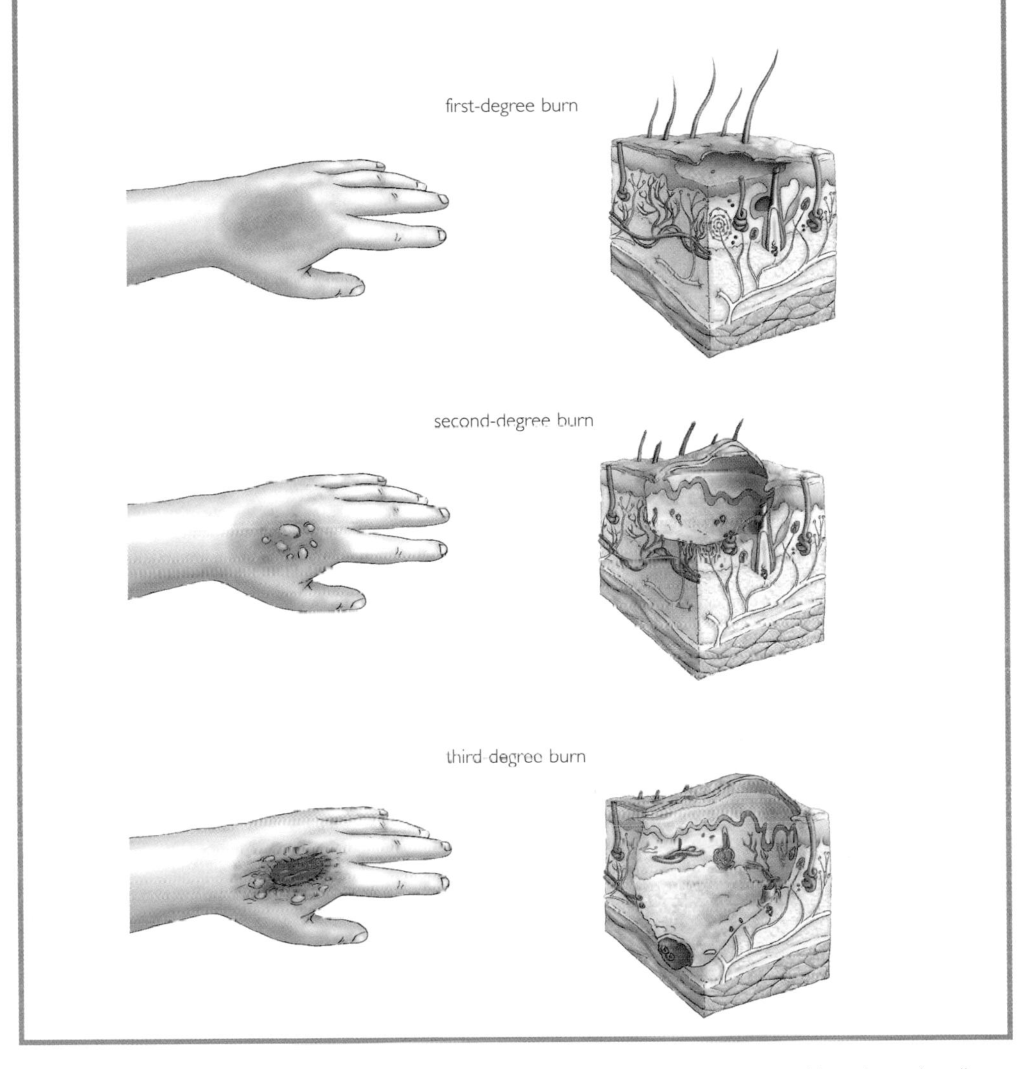

• Do not be alarmed if some skin comes off with the clothing. If the clothing is firmly stuck to the burnt area, cut off the parts that are free from the skin.

• Do not break any blisters that may form.

• Cover the burnt area with a clean, dry diaper or towel and take the child to the nearest emergency department or doctor.

• Do not apply any type of creams, disinfectants, or homemade remedies to the burn.

As with other health problems, prevention is the most important factor; in the case of burns, this means being fully informed. So, knowing what to do when a child is burnt is of primary importance for both his parents and other people responsible for looking after him.

MAIN CAUSES OF BURNS IN CHILDHOOD	
CAUSE	**INCIDENCE RATE**
Hot liquids: tea, milk, oil, water, food	59.6%
Hot objects: irons, stoves, ovens, teapots	27.7%
Fire, embers, ashes, matches	5.5%
Electricity	3%
Others: fireworks, balloons filled with gas, explosives, sun, chemical products	4.2%

Preventive measures

• Do not allow children to play or wander about in the kitchen while food is being cooked, the oven is switched on, or water or oil is boiling.

• Do not cook food with a baby in your arms.

• Keep children away from any object with an electric cable that they could grab: irons, kettles, etc.

• Mark out the area within which small children can play, using a playpen or safety doors, to prevent their curiosity from leading them to touch stoves, enter the kitchen, or grab any objects that could cause them harm.

• Do not put any stoves or other devices that produce direct heat near beds or curtains, to avoid starting a fire.

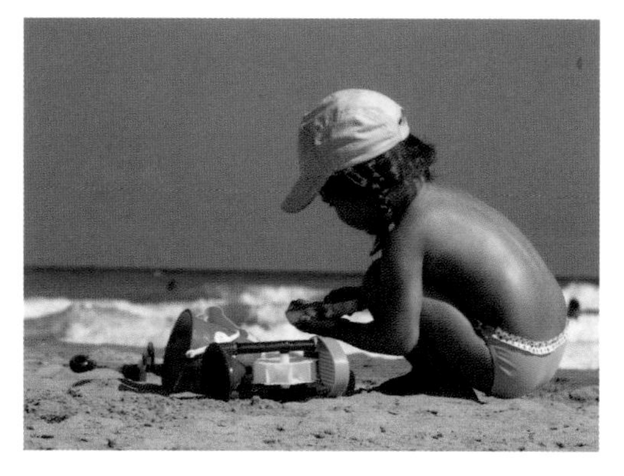

Small children should not be directly exposed to sunlight, as they do not adapt well to variations in temperature. At this age it is advisable not to overdo the use of sunscreen and instead opt for a parasol and clothing that protects the skin.

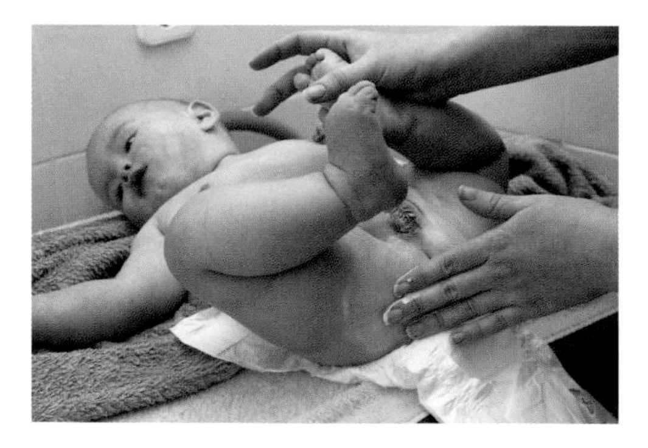

A child's skin should be protected in the summer with sun creams containing sunscreen with a protection factor of at least 30, and over 50 in the case of children with a pale, sensitive skin.

accidents caused by electricity

Electrocution or getting burns from an electric shock are relatively frequent occurrences in domestic settings _ and children are the most vulnerable, as they may play with electric devices, unaware of their inherent danger. Such devices sometimes also come into contact with a wet surface. It is vital to bear in mind that water and steam are highly efficient conductors of electricity and so a child can receive an electric shock through them. Electrocution is characterized by the presence of two burns on the body: one at the point where the current entered the body and another where it left. In between, the electric charge will burn all the tissues in its path, altering the composition and functioning of the organs involved, with sometimes fatal results.

Electrocution

If somebody receives an electric shock, you must never use the palm of the hand to check whether the electricity is still flowing (either in the victim or the apparatus in question). Aalways use the back of the hand. Otherwise, your hand will contract and clasp the victim or the electrical device, increasing the risk of receiving a shock yourself.

The nerves (responsible for transmitting electric signals), muscles, and blood vessels are all good conductors of electricity. In contrast, bones, tendons, and fat offer great resistance to the passage of electricity and tend to heat up and coagulate rather than pass on the current.

The skin constitutes the first line of resistance against the advance of an electrical current inside the body. Much of the energy is dissipated by the skin; this causes burning but can prevent more serious injuries deep inside the body.

Bearing in mind that the human body is a conductor of electricity, when an electrical current overcomes the resistance of the skin, it passes indiscriminately through the tissues, causing them

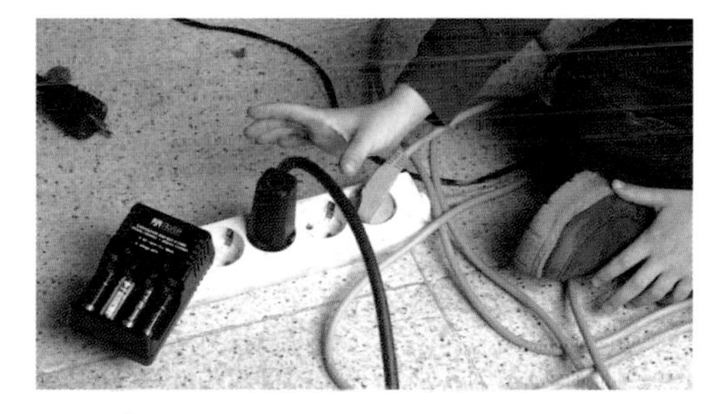

Some 60–70% of electrical lesions are caused by low-voltage currents, which are responsible for about half the total deaths from electrocution, and 1% of all deaths from household accidents. Over 20% of electrical lesions affect children. Small children explore everything with their mouth, so electrical burns are most commonly found in this area.

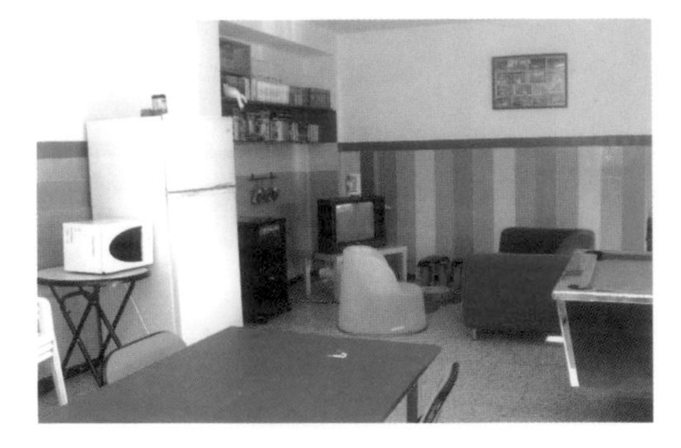

A domestic alternating current is 3 times more dangerous than a direct current (e.g. from batteries) of the same voltage, as it stimulates the muscle fibers 40–100 times per second, causing a tetanic muscular contraction. The hands are the part of the body that most commonly come into contact with sources of electricity and, as the flexor muscles of the hand and forearm are stronger than the extensor muscles, this tetanic contraction prevents the victim from voluntarily releasing the source of electricity, thereby prolonging the contact with the current.

damage, usually in an irregular manner, with untouched areas side by side with burnt tissues and lesions in structures apparently far removed from the point of contact.

Electrical current that passes through the heart or thorax can cause irregular muscle contractions of the heart (arrhythmias) and/or direct myocardial damage, with a subsequent mortality rate of 60%. A current that passes through the brain can cause a respiratory arrest, direct brain damage, and paralysis, with, once again, fatal consequences in many cases.

If a current passes through the eyes, it can cause cataracts. It can cause ventricular fibrilation (irregular and inefficient contractions of the heart) and/or respiratory failure more easily when it passes through the head or thorax than through the lower limbs.

The alarm signals in a victim of an electric shock are loss of consciousness, disorientation, sleepiness, muscle tremors, and burns that leave the skin and muscles very dark.

First-aid measures in cases of electrocution

1. Do not touch the victim directly while he is contact with the source of the electric shock, to avoid receiving a shock yourself.

2. If possible, turn off the electrical supply or remove the plug of the electrical device responsible for the shock from its socket with the help of a wooden stick.

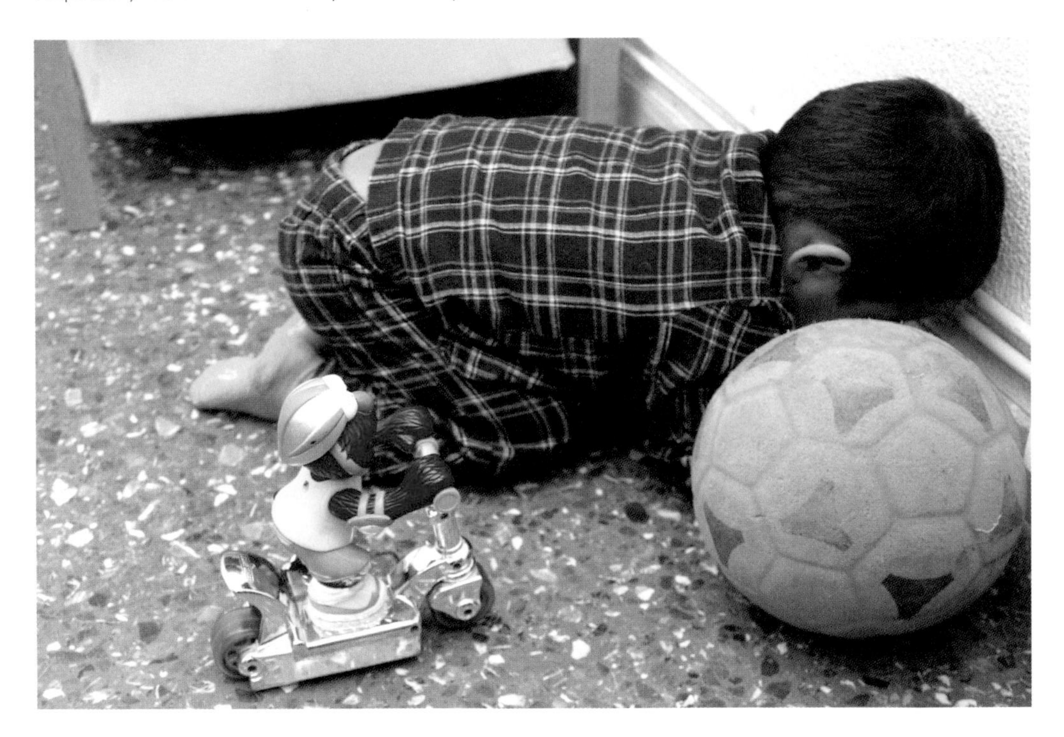

Symptoms

The symptoms most often provoked by electrocution are:

- At the point of contact: burns, muscle damage, vascular thrombosis, gangrene.
- In the rest of the body: cardiac arrest, asphyxia, internal burns, strong muscle contractions, brain and kidney damage.

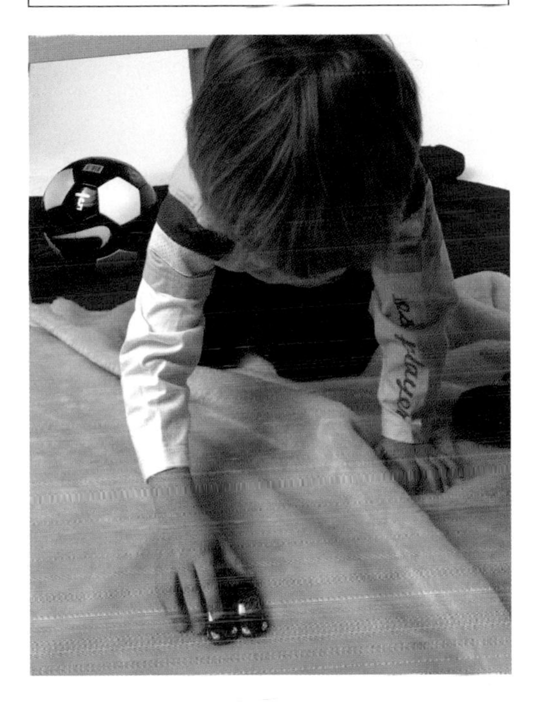

3. If the floor is wet, do not approach or step on it.
4. If the current cannot be disconnected, step on something dry (like a blanket, rubber mat, or newspaper) that cannot get wet and cannot conduct electricity. Never stand on metal.
5. If the cable attached to the source of the shock cannot be pulled out of its plug, try to pull the victim away by moving his feet with a wooden object or rope.
6. Once the victim has been separated from the electrical source and you are no longer at risk, check his breathing and pulse. If necessary, perform artificial respiration and re-establish his heartbeat.
7. Protect the burnt area with a clean cloth that does not stick to the skin, and take the victim straight to a hospital.

Preventing accidents caused by electricity

- Do not switch on electrical devices that are wet.
- Use deep sockets or rotating safety plugs that cannot be moved by children.
- If you are making any kind of electrical repair or adjustment, turn off the main supply, and check that there is no current.
- In the bathroom, keep all sockets, stoves, and other electrical devices out of arm's reach of children.
- Try not to use any electrical equipment while barefoot, even when the floor is dry.
- Place an earth conductor in all the bases of sockets. This conductor must be attached to the outer cases of all electrical devices that do not bear the symbol of double isolation.
- Check that the metal water pipes (hot and cold), bath and sink drains, etc, are connected to each other, as well as to earth by means of a conductor.

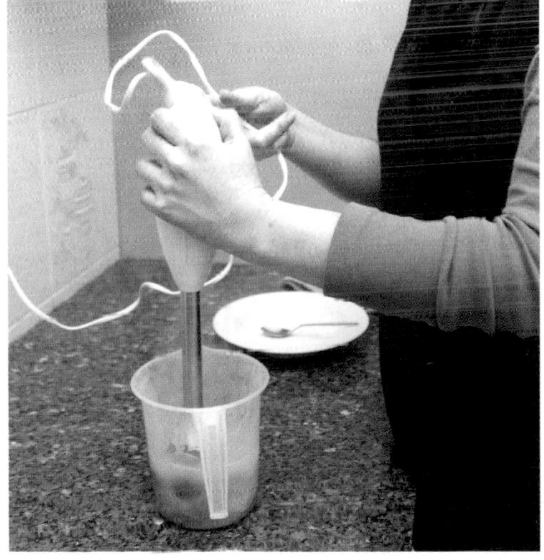

hemorrhages

A hemorrhage can be seen with the naked eye when blood leaves the body – from a wound or nosebleed, for example, or when it is expelled by vomiting or coughing. There are other circumstances, however, in which bleeding is not so evident, for example when it occurs inside various cavities in the body. This is known as an internal hemorrhage; examples of this include a cerebral hematoma and an abdominal hemorrhage. In these cases, an exact diagnosis can only be reached with the help of medical tests; a number of signs and symptoms can suggest the presence of an internal hemorrhage, however, and these should prompt appropriate action.

Types of hemorrhage

• Arterial hemorrhage: loss of blood through a rupture in the wall of one or more arteries; the blood is bright red and comes out in intermittent jets, following the rhythm of the cardiac pulsations.

Turn the wounded area upward and apply a compressive bandage. If blood continues to gush forth, cover the wound with a belt or elastic bandage, and tighten it until the flow of blood ceases. If the victim's transfer to an emergency department takes more than an hour, this improvised tourniquet must be loosened to allow irrigation to start up again, before tightening it again.

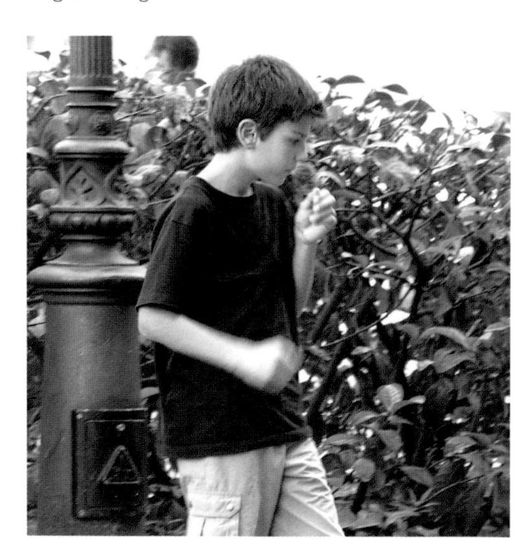

• **Venous hemorrhage:** loss of blood from the veins; the blood is darker and pours out in a continuous flow, sometimes profusely (particular if a major vein has been ruptured).

Apply a compressive bandage and, if a limb is affected, where possible raise it to the height of the heart, without removing the bandage. If the latter becomes soaked with blood, cover it with another dressing.

• **Capillary hemorrhage.** Loss of blood from the capillary vessels; the blood is a of similar color to the venous blood – the capillary vessels contain both arterial and venous blood – and runs slowly. It is usually seen in superficial wounds and is easier to control.

Blood carries oxygen, water, and nutrients around the body. If a child loses a significant amount it can be fatal, depending on his age. Wounds caused by cuts and grazes are rarely serious and can be treated at home, unless they become infected. Other types of wound can bleed copiously, however, leading to concussion, loss of consciousness, and, in serious cases, shock.

CHILDREN UP TO THE AGE OF 1 YEAR	CHILDREN AGED FROM 1–8 YEARS
Normal circulatory volume: 0.6 pint (300 milliliters)	Normal circulatory volume: 4–6 pints (2–3 liters)
Loss of blood capable of causing death: 0.05 pint (25 milliliters)	Loss of blood capable of causing death: 1 pint (500 milliliters)

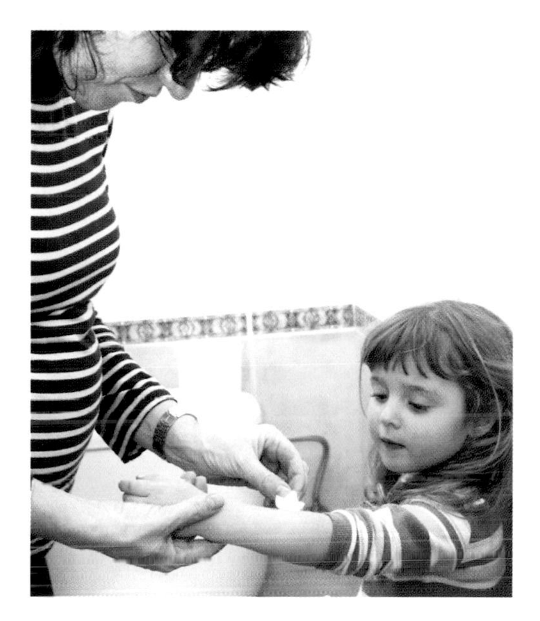

- **Internal hemorrhage**

Symptoms: cold, pale, sweaty skin, fast, short breaths, fast but weak pulse, and feelings of unease.

A victim of an internal hemorrhage can even lose consciousness: in these cases, lay him down, outstretched, and raise his legs. Check his breathing and pulse, then cover him with a blanket. Do not give him any kind of liquid. Request urgent help in transferring him to a health center.

First aid in cases of hemorrhage

1. Place a handkerchief or piece of clean cloth on the wound and press down firmly with your hand. If no cloth is available, try to close the wound with your fingers and cover it with your hand.
2. Apply pressure directly on to the wound, keeping the handkerchief or cloth firmly in place on the wound with a bandage improvised with a dish towel or tie.
3. Raise the affected area, provided there is no fracture.

Nosebleed (epistaxis)

- Seat the child with his head leaning forward above a receptacle. He must breathe through his mouth and avoid swallowing any blood.
- Compress the nose tightly for at least 10 minutes. If the bleeding does not stop, repeat this action for another 10 minutes.
- If the hemorrhage does not stop, gradually insert a piece of gauze (soaked in hydrogen peroxide or another substance that constricts blood vessels) into the nostril that is bleeding.
- Press ice against the bleeding nostril or neck (on the side or nape).
- If the nosebleed lasts for more than 30 minutes, take the child to the nearest health center.

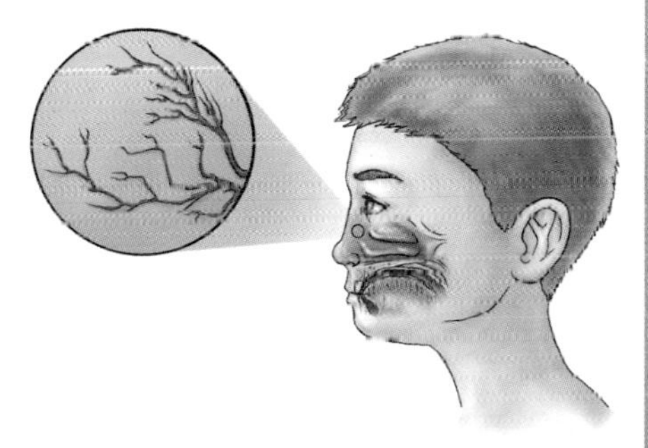

The nose has numerous blood vessels, including many small arterioles, and these can bleed easily. Nosebleeds are most common in winter, when heating may dry up the nasal membranes, giving rise to tiny scabs that become irritated and bleed when a child picks or blows his nose. Nosebleeds can sometimes be a sign of an underlying problem, such as a clotting disorder.

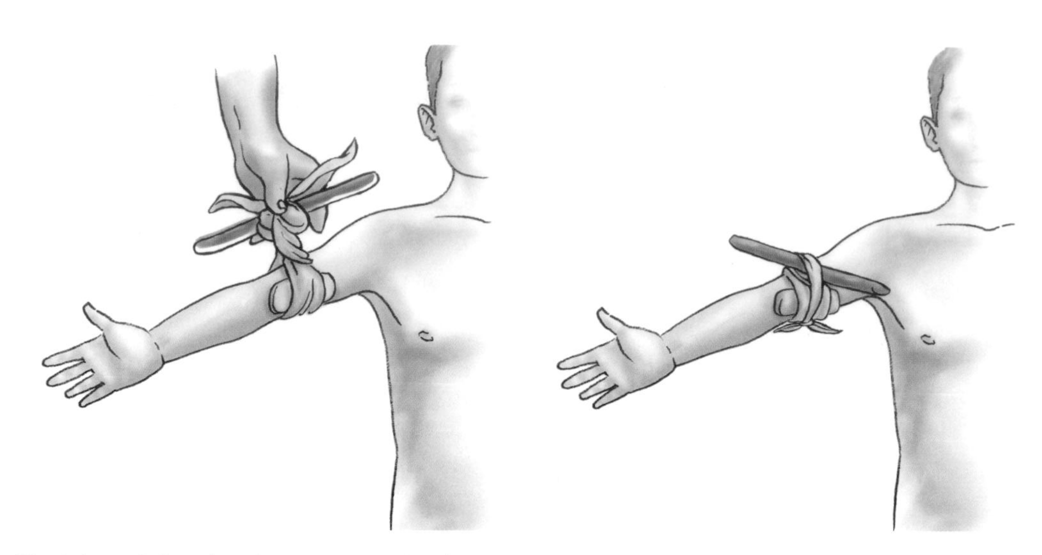

The circles mark the points where pressure needs to be applied to stem bleeding from the arms or legs.

4. Ask the child to lie down.

5. Call a doctor or emergency service.

6. Keep the child warm by covering him with a sheet or blanket and placing something underneath him, so that he is not lying on a cold or wet surface.

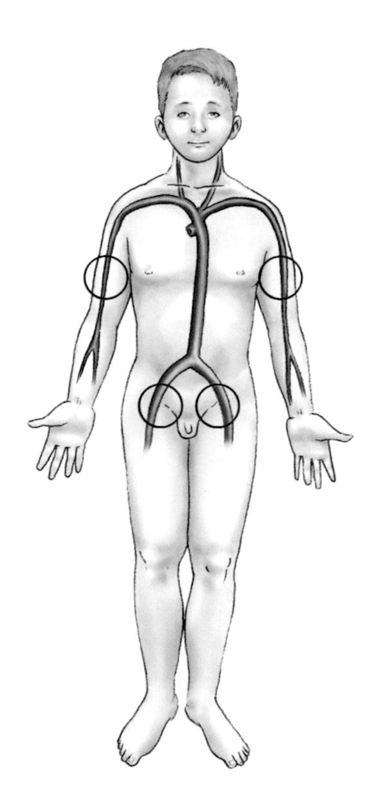

7. If he is conscious and can drink liquid, you can give him a little tea or water. If he is unconscious or is possibly suffering from an abdominal hemorrhage, he should not be given any liquid at all.

8. Use a tourniquet when a hemorrhage cannot be controlled on account of an accidental crushing, amputation, or laceration of a limb.

9. Any wide piece of strong fabric can be used as a tourniquet. Never use wire, cord, or any other such materials. Attach the tourniquet to the upper part of the limb, above the wound. Tie a knot, place a piece of wood on top of it and make another knot, then rotate the wood until the fabric is tight enough to stop the bleeding.

10. If help is slow in arriving, the tourniquet must be loosened every 20 minutes. If the bleeding has stopped, leave the tourniquet loose, but ready to apply again if the bleeding starts once more. Keep constant watch over the tourniquet until the child reaches a hospital.

When making a tourniquet, remember to use a wide piece of fabric, but never a wire or cord.

poisoning

As soon as a child begins to move about and explore his surroundings, he can gain access to a host of everyday household cleaning products, cosmetics and toiletries that can have a potentially toxic effect; as a result, poisoning is one of the most common causes of accidents in the home. A child can be poisoned by swallowing or inhaling a particular substance, or merely through contact with his skin, depending on the characteristics and active ingredients involved. This is not the same as an allergic reaction, which requires a specific predisposition on the part of the child, as the allergen in question is not inherently dangerous.

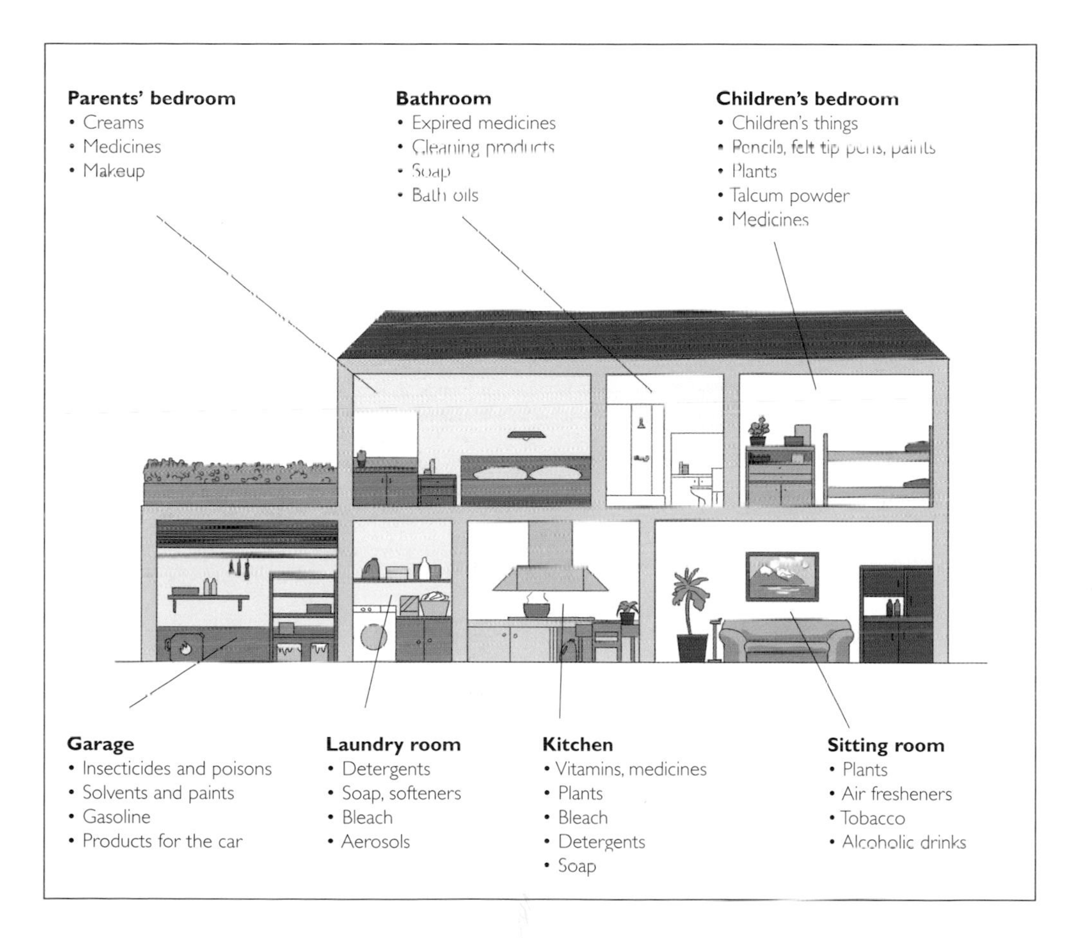

Poisoning

Potentially toxic products used around the house

• Several substances that are constantly found in a domestic setting can cause poisoning if they are handled inappropriately.These include hair dye, suntan lotion, aftershave, deodorant, and perfumes. They pose no problem when used for the purposes for which they were designed, but they can have toxic effects of varying severity, if young children swallow or inhale them, or even, in some cases, merely touch them.

• The illustration below features a series of potentially toxic everyday products and their usual location in the home.

Symptoms of poisoning

• The most frequent symptoms are generally vomiting, headache, abdominal pain, diarrhea, dizziness, red skin, sleepiness, and altered states of consciousness.

• These general signs are complemented by effects particular to the poisonous substance, especially in the case of medicines. Respiratory and cardiac disorders, blood clots, drops in blood pressure, and shock can combine with neurological symptoms and damage to vital organs to endanger a child's life if appropriate action is not taken in time.

The most frequent cause of poisoning (over 30%) is the accidental ingestion of medicines, followed by that of household products (25%), food, tobacco and liquor (12%), and chemical products.The most dangerous (and potentially fatal) medicines are tricyclic anti-depressants, antihistamines (prescribed for allergies), aspirin, benzodiazepines (for anxiety, depression, and various nervous disorders), and sympathicomimetics (for a wide range of pathologies). Poisoning from medicine is 3–5 times more common in children aged under 15 years (particularly in the 2–3 age range).

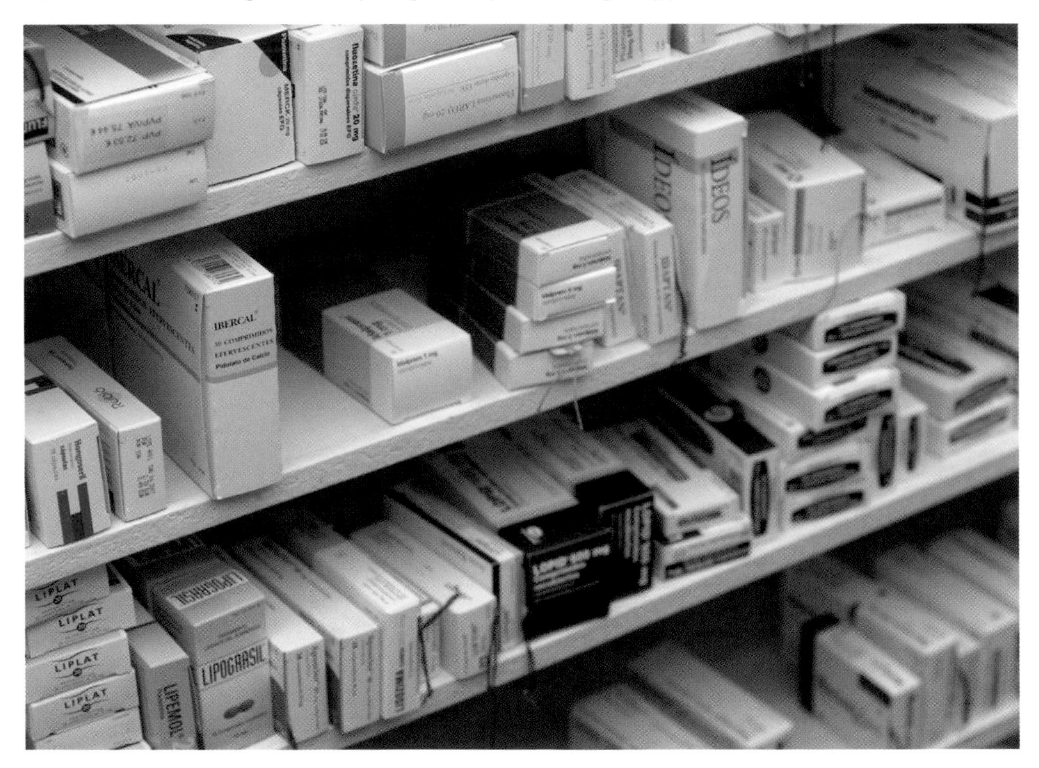

If a child swallows a cleaning product, the first thing to do is to look at the label, which should have an emergency telephone number. Call to ask for information before taking any action.

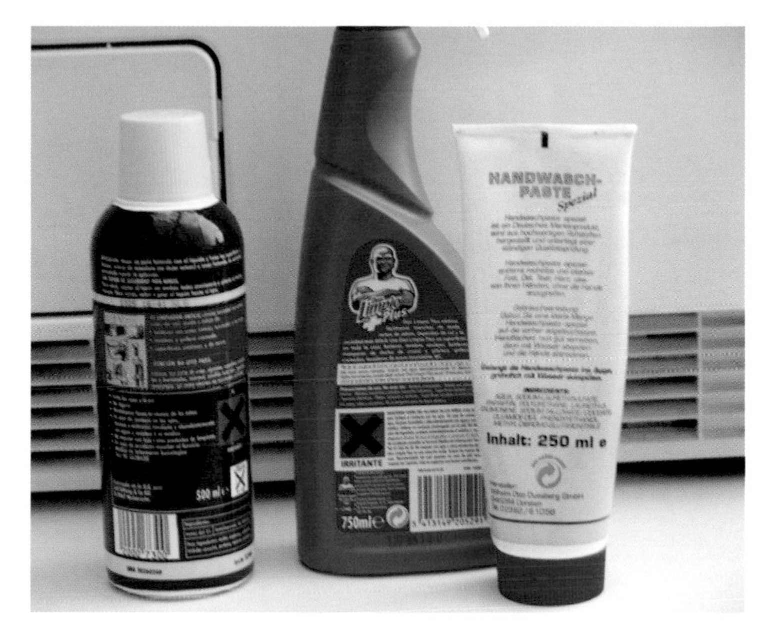

Emergency measures in cases of poisoning

- If a child shows signs of being poisoned, call an emergency service immediately.
- Once you have verified that a child has swallowed medicine, try to ascertain when this happened and the amount taken, on the basis of how much remains in the packaging. The emergency service will probably tell you to give the child a syrup designed to make him vomit on the way to hospital. If you have no such product available, you can give him water or milk, but nothing else.
- It is not advisable to induce vomiting by thrusting your fingers in his throat or pressing down on his abdomen.
- Do not induce vomiting if the child has swallowed caustic products or fuels like gasoline or paraffin, or if he is unconscious.
- If he has inhaled gas, take him away from the area, open the windows, and loosen his clothes.
- If he is not breathing, perform basic resuscitation techniques while on the way to an emergency department.
- Take him to the emergency department as soon as possible; remember to take the packaging of the medicines or substances that have caused the poisoning.

Prevention of poisoning

- Take special care when your child visits other people's houses.
- Do not take medicine in the presence of children.
- Do not tell a child about to take a medicine that it tastes like candy.
- Take great care when using heating equipment and gas-run devices.
- Teach your child not to eat plants or anything that could cause him harm.

allergic or anaphylactic shock, insect bites

An allergic or anaphylactic shock happens suddenly as a result of an allergic reaction; it can endanger a child's life in a matter of minutes. There can be a number of causes for this, such as a reaction to medicines, to a blood transfusion, to insect bites, to preservatives and food coloring, etc.

Clinical picture of an allergic shock

Preventing an allergic shock

• If the reaction was caused by a foodstuff, preservative, or additive, this allergen must be permanently eliminated from the child's diet.

• If the reaction was caused by a medicine, you should inform your doctor and avoid this medication (and all its derivatives). If possible, avoid injectable medicines and stick with oral ones. Do not give your child medicine without informing a doctor.

• Even if a child has no history of allergies, she must receive appropriate anti-allergic treatment every time she has a radiological study involving iodized contrast agents.

• If the reaction was caused by an insect bite, your child should try to avoid places with bees,

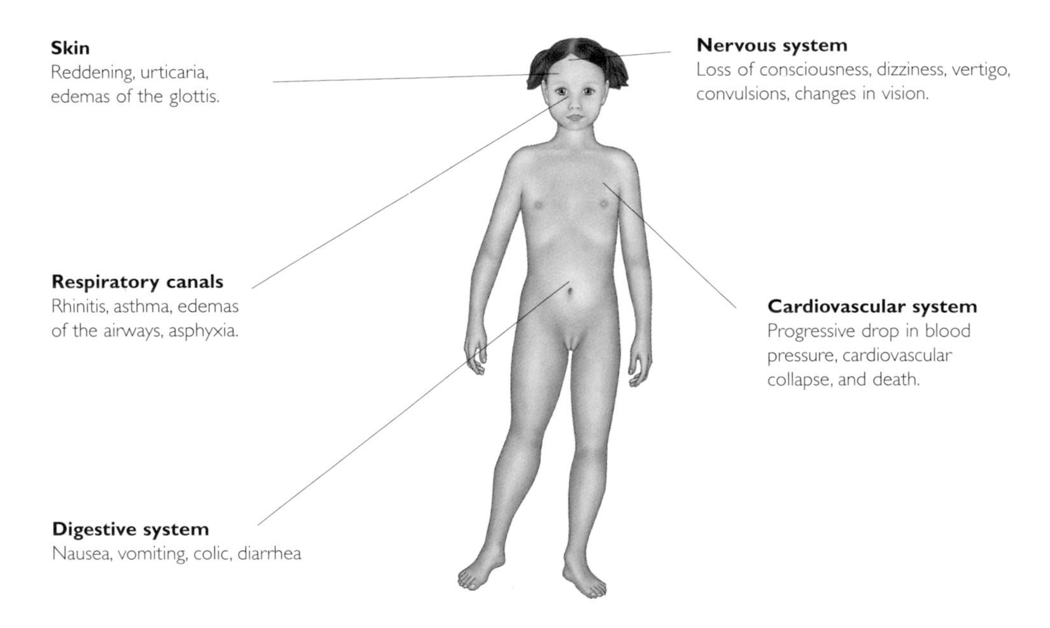

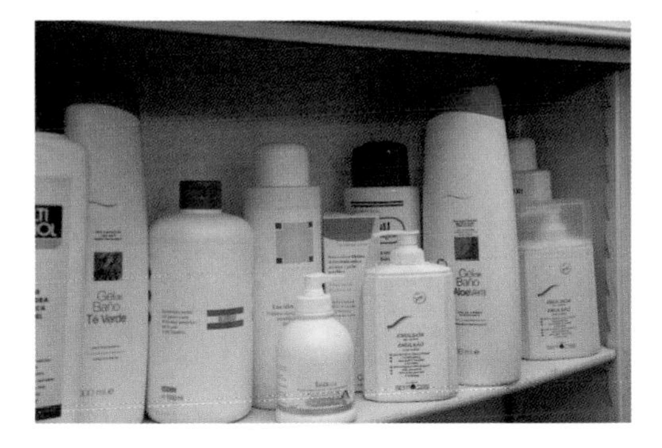

At every medical consultation, it is vital to inform the doctor of any allergy to medicines and ask that it is recorded in all medical and clinical records, particularly when a child is admitted to hospital.

wasps, or red ants (the main cause of anaphylactic reactions in children).

• Consult an allergy specialist to confirm the diagnosis, so that a reaction can be avoided in future; if this is not possible, find out which medication is most effective for treating an allergic shock and learn how to use it.

• Children at risk of a severe allergic reaction should have their own first aid kit and be trained to use it if medical assistance is not at hand.

• Access to a corticosteroid alone is not enough to prevent a new reaction. The correct implementation of resuscitation measures, along with the use of adrenalin and bronchodilators and a speedy transfer to an emergency department, may all be required to save a child's life.

Preventing insect bites

• Keep a child's body clean and free of sweat and perfumes, as strong smells attract insects.

• Dress her in clothes with subdued colors that cover her entire body. Make sure that she does not ride bikes or motorcycles.

• Before a child gets in a car, make sure that there are no insects inside, then close the windows. Wasps often get inside cars.

• Stay away from beehives or places where wasps can establish their nests, such as beams.

• Bees leave their sting in the skin, with a small sac containing venom. Do not press the skin to extract the sting – all you will do is inject more venom into the child's body. The sac should be removed with tweezers.

• If your child sits down in the open air, examine the area carefully beforehand and do not allow her to walk barefoot.

• Children at risk of an allergic reaction from an insect bite should take an emergency kit with them to places where they are likely to be vulnerable, and they should know how to take the appropriate medication.

Prevention in cases of allergy to medicines

- Medicines can cause adverse reactions that can be fatal in a susceptible person.
- It is very important to make a detailed record of the symptoms to help an allergy specialist arrive at a diagnosis, substitute the drug that causes an adverse reaction, and advise on how to avoid any more undesirable incidents in the future. For these purposes, the patient or doctor must:
  - Identify the medicine(s) taken before the allergic reaction.
  - Make a note of the symptoms and confirm the diagnosis with a specialist, in order to substitute the medicine in question and avoid future adverse reactions.
  - Identify the medicine causing the allergy.
  - Make the allergy to a medicine known at every medical consultation and request that this information is noted on every medical record or clinical history.

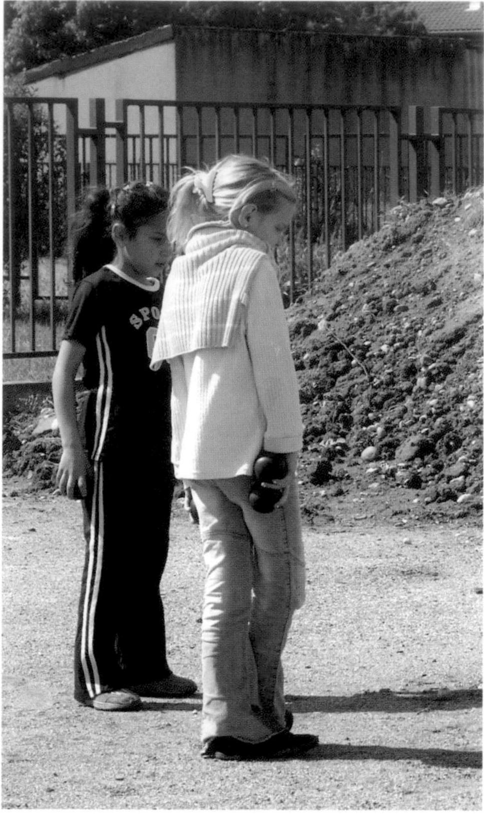

Take great care in cases of allergy to ant bites, as the main culprits are red ants, which are very small. They can be found on sidewalks and in open spaces, gardens, or areas around a house.

Restrict a child's outdoor activities in periods of greatest risk and avoid water, flowers, and trees bearing ripe fruit. Swimming pools attract bees and wasps in search of water to drink. Use insect repellents.

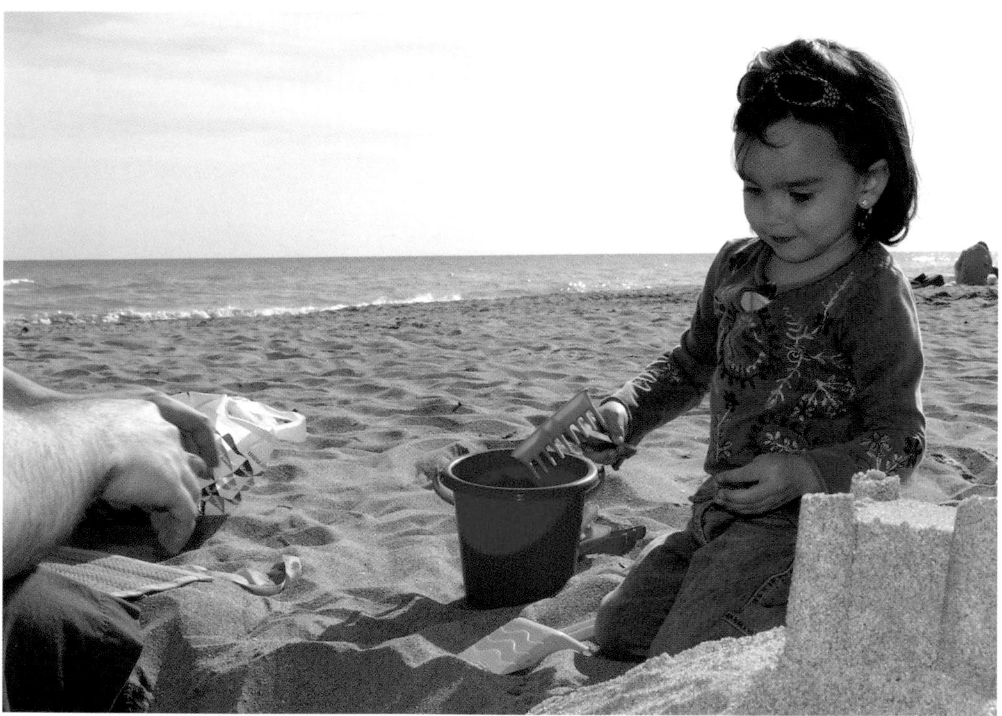

exercise, health and the personal development of children and adolescents

The benefits of physical activity are many: not only for physical and mental development but also social relationships. Regular physical activity combined with a balanced diet helps regulate body weight and prevents obesity (80 percent of obese adults were obese children), as well as degenerative diseases like arteriosclerosis, which is closely linked with cardiovascular diseases in adulthood.

Benefits of physical exercise during childhood

• Excercise contributes to a child's overall physical, mental, and emotional development.

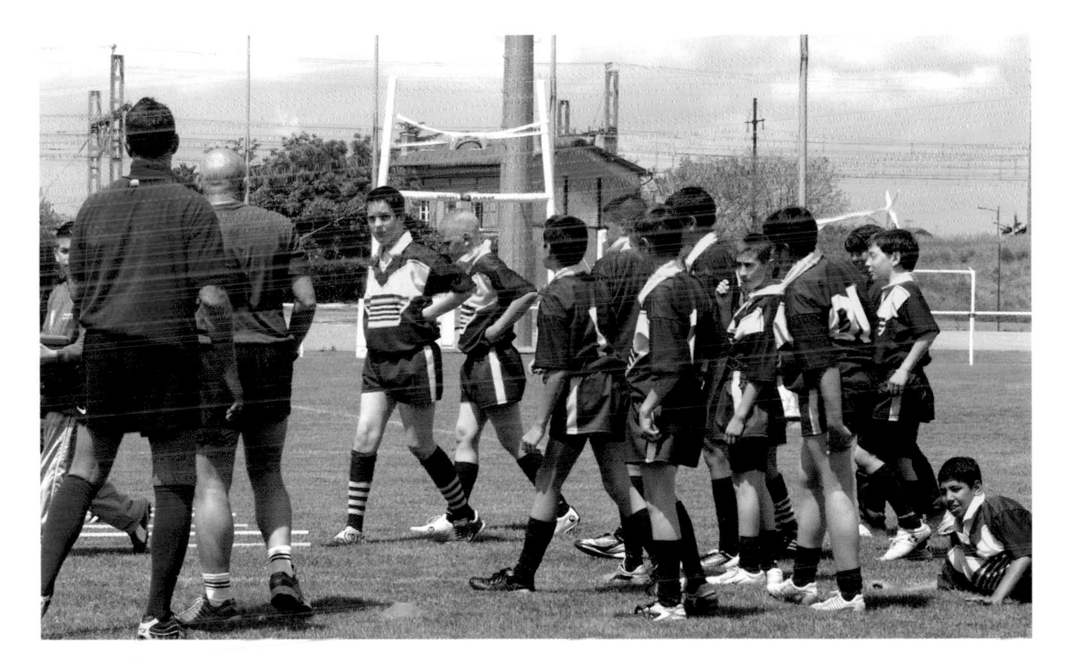

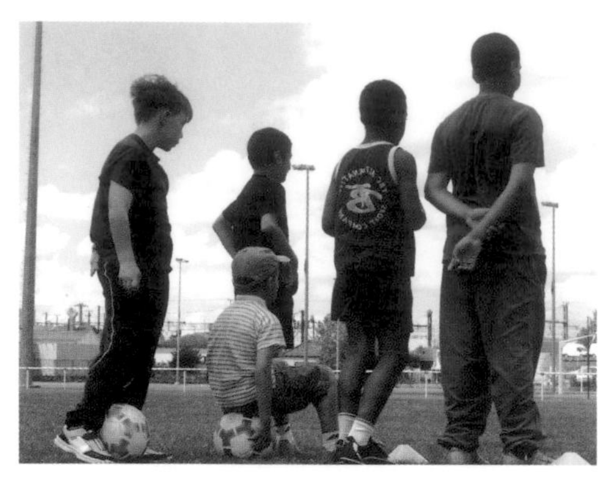

Sport is the most effective means of passing on to children skills, thought processes, values, knowledge, and comprehension that will hold them in good stead throughout their lives.

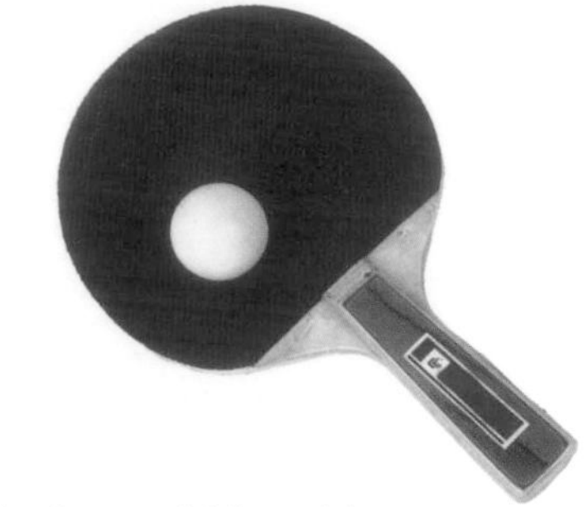

- It helps a child to become accustomed to physical activity and stimulates interest in caring for his health; this will be of fundamental importance in later life.
- It helps a child to respect his own body, and that of others.
- It strengthens a child's self-esteem.
- It develops a child's social awareness by preparing him for competitive situations and accustoming him to face both victory and defeat. It also stimulates the collaboration and sociability essential to being part of a group.
- It improves a child's health and prevents damage derived from a poor posture.
- It can positively affect a child's academic performance.
- It gives a child experience in structured activities, with clear and specific aims.
- It helps to develop abstract thought through concepts such as speed, distance, depth, strength, momentum, fair play, etc.
- It encourages a child's capacity for concentration and participative activity.

At this age, a child does not necessarity learn any specific sport, but he should be encouraged to enjoy giving free rein to his body movements.

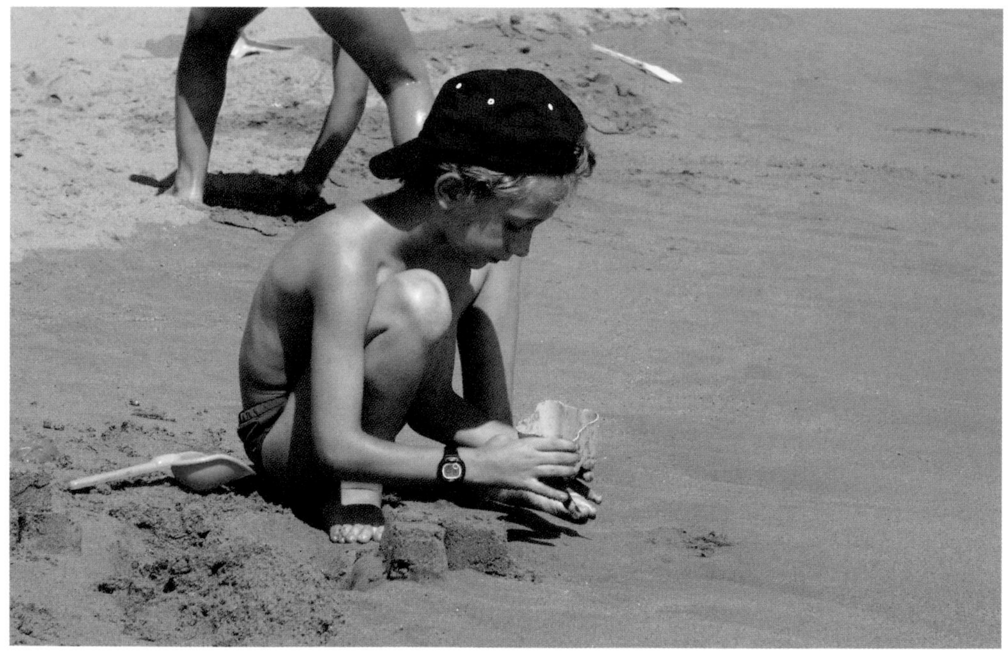

Importance of aerobic activities in infancy

Disciplines such as infant aerobics are focused on a child's body, sense of rhythm, and movements; they allow him to develop skills that will enrich his education as a whole through:

- Psychomotor development.
- Self-expression through body movements.
- Development of physical capacities. Aerobics improve a child's co ordination and posture, thereby enhancing his range of movement.
- Relationships with other children; aerobics as a means of social integration.
- Maintenance and improvement of health. Statistics indicate that half of today's children are overweight, and a considerable proportion of these are obese, because of a poor diet and a sedentary lifestyle. This not only has physical consequences but can also have psychological and social repercussions.
- Enjoyment of non-competitive exercise and recognition of its value as a leisure activity. A young child should feel free to participate in physical activity, whatever his ability.

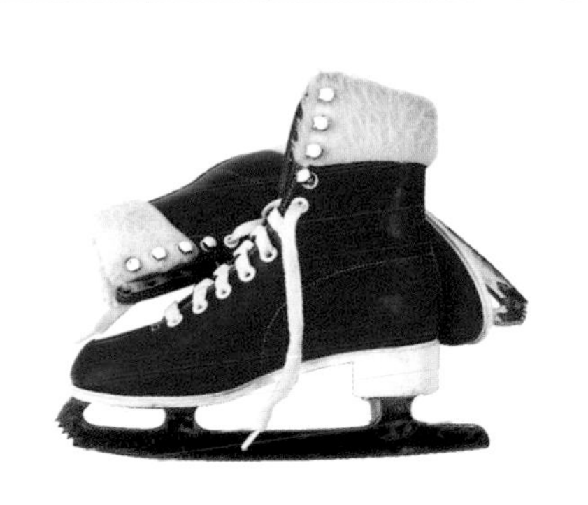

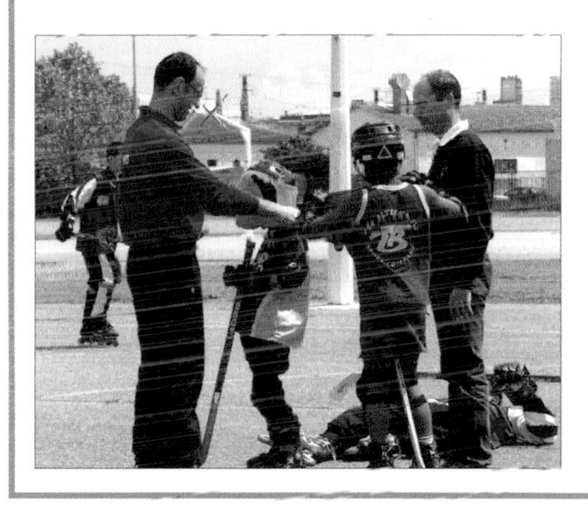

- Compensation for today's sedentary lifestyle resulting from excessive use of transport to get around, too much time spent in front of a television, console, computer, etc.
- Knowledge and respect for a child's own body. Every child can reach the level that his physical capabilities allow, without attempting to achieve impossible goals. It is important that he accepts himself as he is, feels good in his own body, and learns to control it efficiently.
- Self-awareness. Movement is a means to self-knowledge, as well as providing opportunities for exploring and understanding the immediate environment. By becoming aware of his body, a child also becomes aware of the world around him.
- Prevention of discrimination. Aerobics classes in young children help to challenge social preconceptions that associate rhythmical movement with girls and competition and shows of strength with boys. If an aerobics class is presented as a game that appeals to the interests of both girls and boys, it raises questions about these negative stereotypes.

Pre-sport games in children aged 4–7

Pre-sport games constitute the basis of a child's future sporting activities. These games involve an array of motor skills that can later be applicable to any sport he may play in the future, whether an individual or team sport, or a martial art.

Children use play as a form of expression, a path to learning, and a means of making friends. It is also an effective instrument for the development of

Prevention of drug abuse

There is evidence to show that youngsters who play sports have significantly lower rates of consumption of the 3 most popular drugs (tobacco, alcohol, and cannabis) than their more sedentary counterparts. The same is true of other drugs like cocaine, heroin, amphetamines, barbiturates, tranquillizers, etc.

It must be pointed out, however, that a child who, for example plays basketball but does not practice for more than a couple of hours a week, is probably little different from sedentary youngsters.

When it comes to preventing drug abuse, therefore, it is advisable to encourage children to commit themselves to a sport they enjoy from an early age.

The degree of contact with addictive substances has a close relationship with the type of sport played (less consumption in players of individual sports like athletics and swimming), with the starting age (less consumption in youngsters who begin playing a sport before the age of 14), and with the amount of time spent training (the more hours per week, the less contact with drugs).

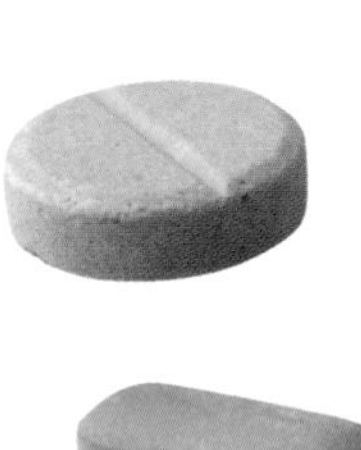

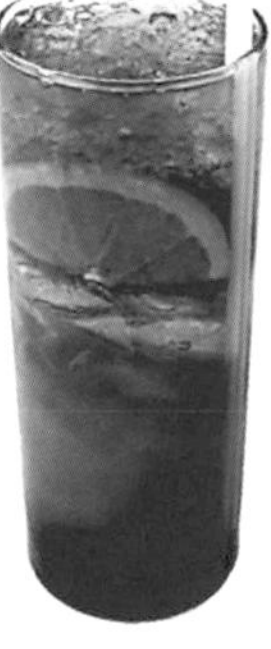

If a group of young people from 18–20 years of age who play sport 12 hours per week were to be studied, it would probably be the case that they have never had any contact with cocaine, hallucinogenic drugs, or cannabis, that they do not smoke or drink alcohol, or do so to a far lesser degree than young people of the same age and social background who do not play sport.

Parents should be aware that the seeds of heart diseases (hardened arteries, high blood pressure) and type-2 diabetes can be sown in childhood, although they generally manifest themselves later on in life.

thought structures. In short, it is an essential element in the organization, development, and confirmation of a child's personality.

In general terms, pre-sport games involve:

- Development of basic skills and dexterity:

– Moving about in all kinds of ways (backward, on hands and knees, squatting, on "3 legs" with another child, kicking balls with one foot only, on top of benches, etc.).

– Receiving and carrying objects (balls, hoops, cones, etc.) with one hand, both hands, on the stomach, on the back, with eyes shut, etc.

– Handling objects (large, small, with companions, etc.).

– Climbing (wall bars, piled-up mats, etc.).

– Jumping (with one leg, with both legs, forward, sideways, zigzag, etc.).

– Spinning (on a vertical axis, on a horizontal axis, with balls).

- Development of perceptive skills:

Perception of both stationary and moving objects.

– Perception of moving children and objects.

– Perception of trajectories of objects.

- Development of balance: dynamic and static situations, imbalance.

- Development of a sense of rhythm: controlling situations of acceleration and slowing down, as well as coordinating perceptions.

How much exercise is needed to prevent obesity in children?

The latest recommendations state that both children and adults should undertake at least 30 minutes of aerobic activity of moderate intensity most days, or, if possible, every day, of the week. This means any physical exercise (walking, jogging, swimming, cycling, etc.) performed at an intensity that makes the heart work within a range of pulsations between 55 and 85 percent of the maximum cardiac frequency.

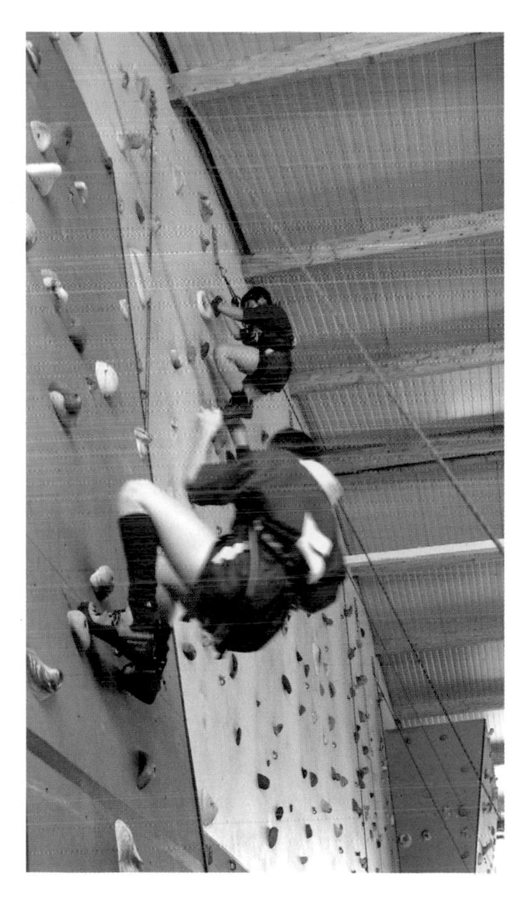

Unfortunately, it is not possible to know exactly how much daily physical activity provides protection against obesity. Children, like adults, put on weight when they consume more calories than they burn. An excessive consumption of junk food and sedentary leisure activities (watching television, playing with consoles and computers) are normally found in overweight children. In contrast, children with a greater commitment to sport have less body fat. Therefore, exercise is just as important in the fight against obesity as food intake.

Prevention of obesity and associated diseases

Various studies carried out on children and adolescents have revealed that:

- Arteriosclerosis can start to develop in the first years of a child's life.
- Obese and sedentary children will probably be obese and sedentary adults.
- The risk factors that contribute to the development of heart disease (obesity, smoking, sedentary lifestyle, high cholesterol levels, etc.) can also be identified in the early years of life.
- It is reasonable to suppose that a reduction in the incidence of these risk factors in childhood and adolescence, when the irreversible degenerative changes associated with heart disease have still not had time to develop, could lead to a considerable reduction in the high mortality rate from associated diseases.

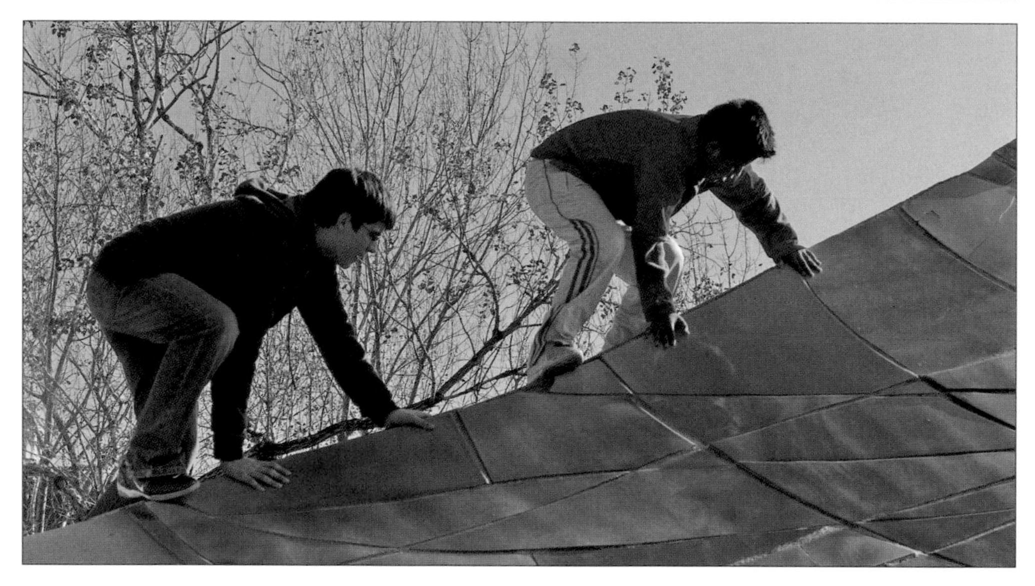

A healthy child needs to do more than walk on flat ground, as this will be insufficient for him to reach the desired cardiac frequency. This is not the case, however, when he walks on hilly terrain or goes climbing or hiking.

Type-2 diabetes is closely related to excess weight and generally emerges in the fourth decade of a person's life. The increase in the rates of childhood obesity in developed countries has meant, however, that in recent years it has been increasingly evident in children and adolescents.

Age (years)	Maximum cardiac frequency (CF) (beats/min)	55–85% of maximum CF (beat/min)
10	210	116–179
15	205	113–174

traveling and vacations with children

The arrival of vacation is one of the moments of the year most keenly anticipated by both parents and their children. When traveling with children, it is important to take into account that the journey will be much more relaxed and pleasurable if you take precautions that, while not guaranteeing the total absence of unexpected problems, can at least minimize the chances of them arising: the appropriate choice of destination, means of transport, accommodation, luggage, toys, and first-aid kit are all factors that need to be considered before setting off.

Vacations with children

Essential baggage

- When traveling with babies or children, some items are indispensable:
  - A baby's traveling crib.
  - A thermos flask (large or small, depending on the number of children traveling).
  - A heater for a baby's feeding bottle.
  - Sunhats.
  - Pacifiers.
  - A couple of each child's favorite toys.

Bath towels, soap, comb, hairbrush, moisturizing cream, sunscreen, diapers, moist wipes, plastic bags, and bibs.

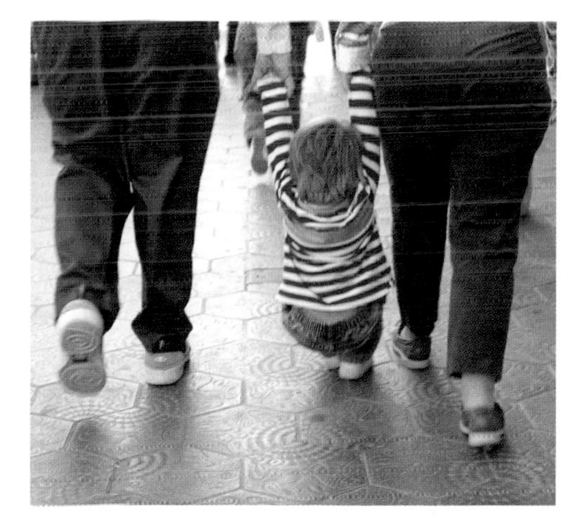

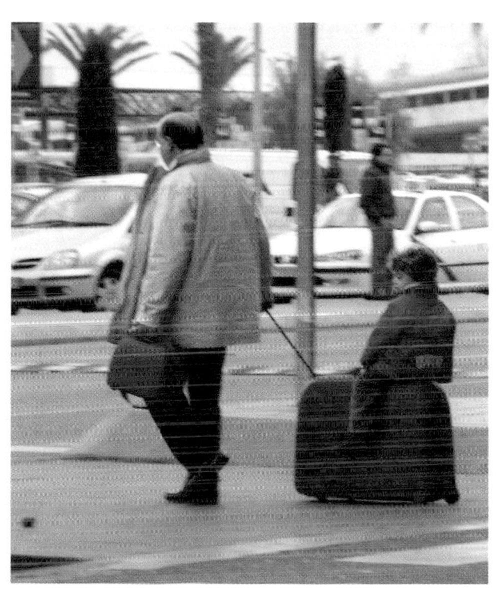

Luggage should be packed sufficiently in advance to avoid forgetting any essential items. It is advisable to first pack items that are not needed for daily use at home. Making a list in advance can be a good way of remembering everything.

When traveling with children, it is particularly important to remember a first-aid kit with anti-pyretic drugs, analgesics, plasters, alcohol, hydrogen peroxide, iodine, a thermometer, scissors, gauze, cotton wool, bandages, and, where relevant, prescribed medication.

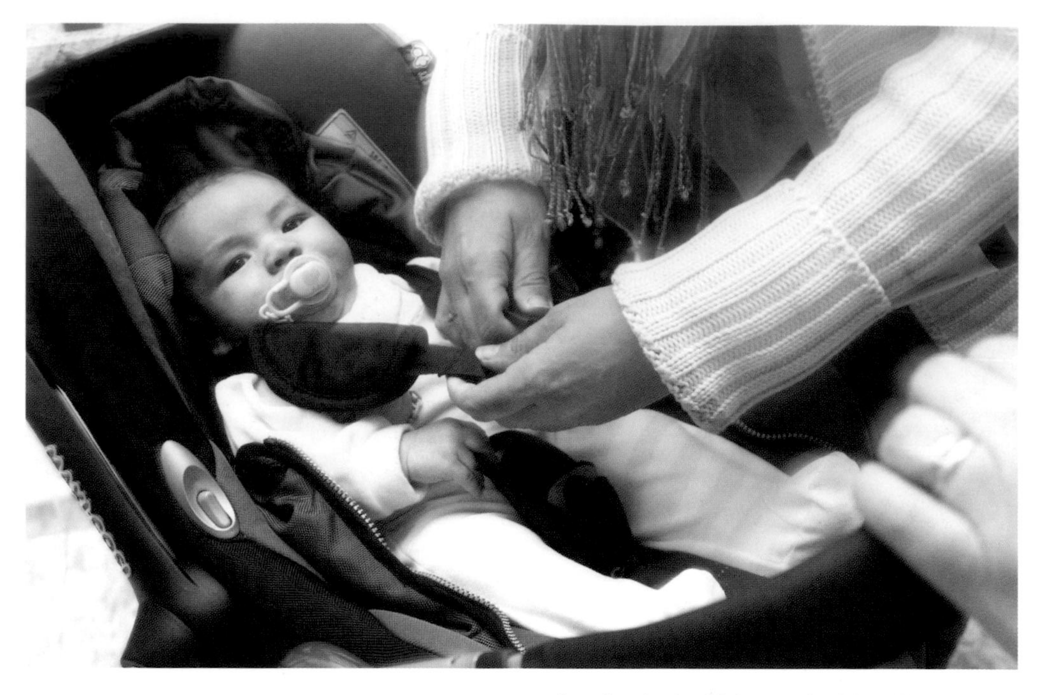

Safety seats

Every child aged under 4 years should travel in an officially approved safety seat. If the child weighs less than 21 lb (9.5 kg) and measures less than 26 in (65 cm), he should travel in a seat looking backward. The seat is attached to the car by means of a safety belt. If you hold a child in your arms, the impact of a crash could make him fly out of your arms into the windshield, or even out of the car altogether.

– Social security or private medical insurance card and vaccination certificates.

– Clothes: pack one outfit for every day of the trip. Babies' and children's clothes do not take up much room, and in this way you will avoid the need to wash too many clothes while on vacation.

Means of transport

• If you choose to travel by car, it is advisable to make frequent stops. The journey will be more relaxed as both children and adults will be able to stretch their legs.

• Always put a child in a safety seat in the back of the car. If he is ill at ease, it is better to stop rather than seat him anywhere else.

• All children under 12 should travel in the back seats and wear a safety belt, in the same way as an adult.

• Do not use a safety seat designed to look toward the rear of the car.

• Avoid leaving any loose objects in the car that could fall on a baby in unexpected circumstances. Leave them in the trunk or on the floor of the car.

• If you travel alone with a baby, put the safety seat in the middle of the back seat, so that, in the case of a robbery or accident, any broken glass from the back windows will be less likely to affect him.

• Check that the security locks on the back doors are in position. The windows should be closed, as there is a risk of children leaning out or throwing out objects that could cause an accident. Children should always get out of a car on the side closest to the sidewalk.

• To avoid travel sickness in children, provide them with good ventilation and light meals during the journey. If necessary, and if your doctor so advises, give them appropriate medication beforehand.

summer and insect bites

Summer beckons children to stroll, play outdoor sports, swim, go on excursions, etc. The beach and the mountains are the favorite destinations of families anxious for a well-deserved break, but these places are also the natural habitat of a host of creatures whose bites and stings demand precautionary measures.

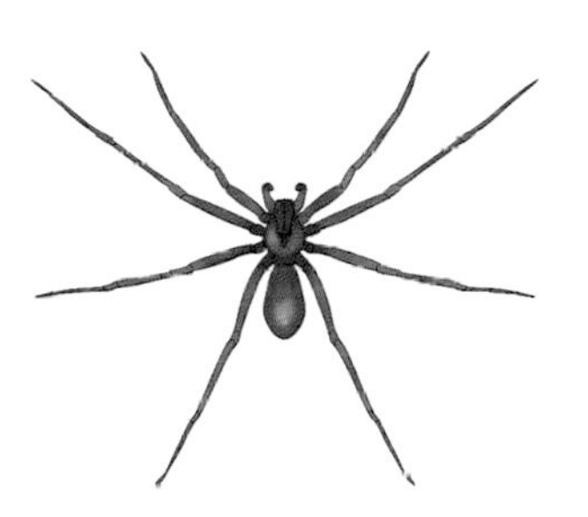

Spider

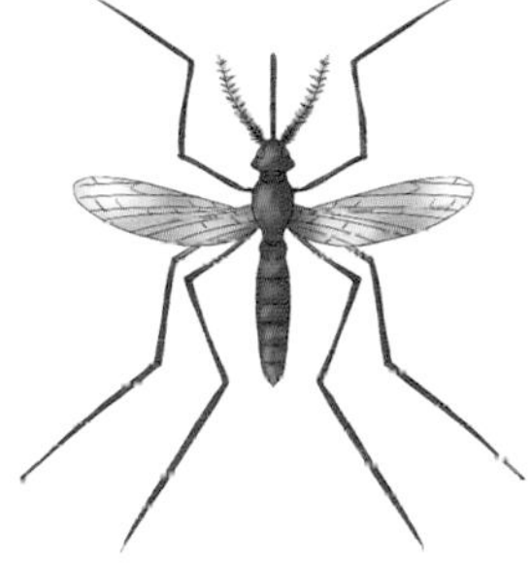

Mosquito

Bee

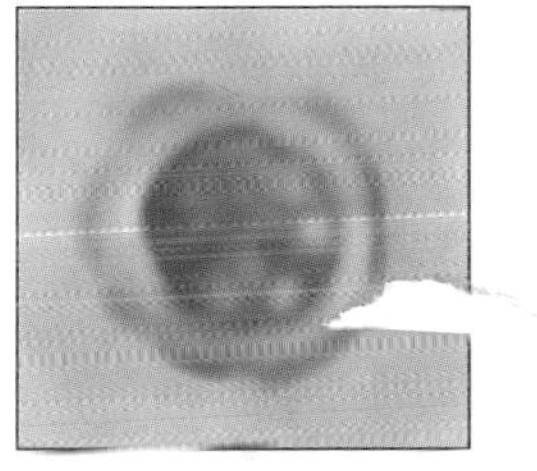

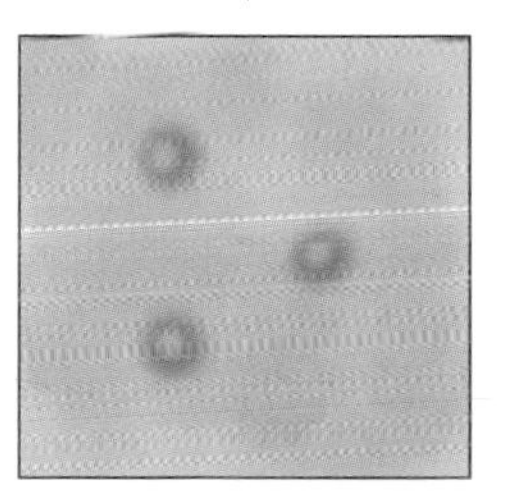

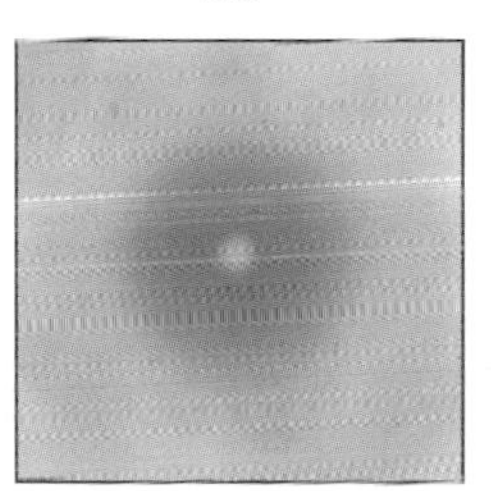

Insects most commonly responsible for bites and stings in summer.

Insect bites and stings

Most people do not realize that they have been bitten until some time later, when they start itching. The skin on the site of the attack may be only slightly irritated or extremely swollen, depending on the degree of allergic reaction.

Insect bites occasionally cause severe allergic reactions that require medical attention. When a child's skin is constantly itchy or in a rash, it is possible that he has insects such as fleas or scabies mites under his skin.

A very small proportion of people who are stung by insects experience an immediate and severe reaction that is potentially fatal. The sting of a yellow wasp is most likely to be the source of this reaction. You need to be alert to urticaria, swelling in the face, breathing difficulties, and general weakness, as these are indicators of a dangerous allergic reaction affecting the entire body, known as anaphylactic shock.

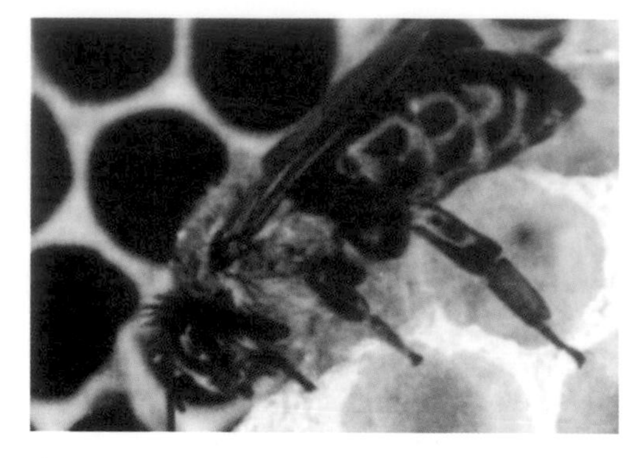

If an insect leaves a sting lodged in the skin, it is likely that it was a bee sting, as wasps don't leave traces of their sting.

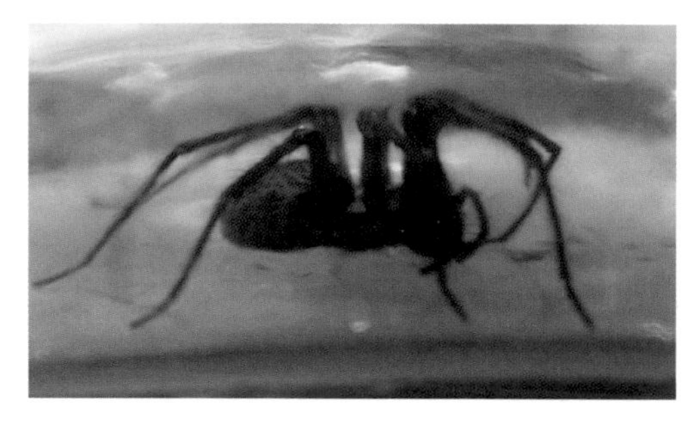

Spider bites can be more burningly painful than those of other insects. Although most spiders are not poisonous, 2 varieties – the black widow and the brown recluse – can trigger generalized reactions that may have fatal consequences.

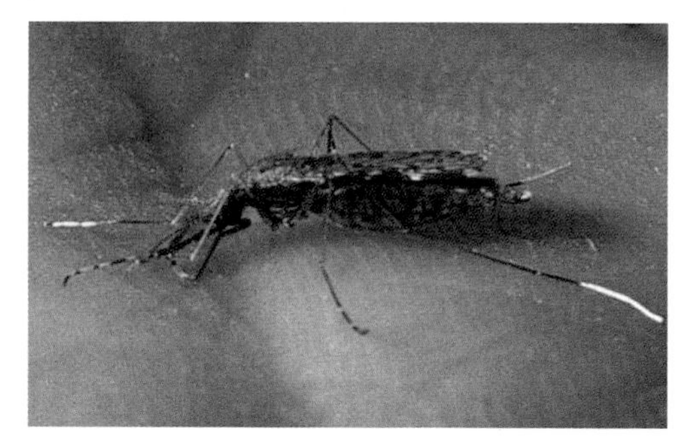

Insects can be carriers of many serious infectious diseases. Mosquitoes, in particular, can transmit malaria, encephalitis, dengue fever, and yellow fever, while ticks can transmit Lyme's disease and fleas can spread plague.

A sting is usually more painful than a bite, especially in children. The discomfort and swelling normally disappear after a few hours, however, and require little treatment.

In some cases, insect stings can trigger more extensive local reactions, with a swelling that spreads over a considerable area for up to a week, sometimes accompanied by nausea and fatigue. This type of reaction requires medical attention.

Spider bites

Young children are at greatest risk. The bite of a black widow is not painful and causes no swelling but, hours later, most victims will experience muscle pains and cramps, inflammation, vomiting, and other symptoms.

The bite of a brown recluse spider causes a red or purplish blister. Both bites require immediate medical attention.

Prognosis for bites and stings

Although any type of skin wound implies at least a slight risk of infection, insect bites are usually a mere irritation.

Although severe reactions only occur in less than 10 percent of cases, it is not possible to know in advance who is allergic before a particular insect bites.

People who have suffered strong reactions to a bite are at great risk of having similar reactions in the future, and they should have skin examinations to assess their sensitivity to venom.

It is very important to have any medicines prescribed for such allergies close at hand.

Preventive measures

Children should not play in places where there could be a lot of hidden insects, such as lumber rooms or stacks of wood.

Bedrooms should be kept clean and free of spider webs.

If you have pets, ask ... p them as free from fleas as ...

Wear clothes ... ection from insects and avoi ... t colors in the countryside. It ... o be well-informed before traveling ... here malaria and other infectious diseases ... ute a health risk.

Treatment

Insect bites

- Calamine lotion containing a local anesthetic, or other ointments containing aloe vera, hydrocortisone, or diphenhydramine, all provide effective relief against insect bites. Avoid scratching the bite, as it can become infected.
- If a child is bitten by a tick that is still clinging to his skin, it should be removed with tweezers or fingernails by grasping its head or mouth area; pull it off with a slow, continuous movement.
- Keep the tick and show it to a doctor, who will assess the risk of contracting any diseases, as ticks can transmit micro-organisms.

Spider bites

- Cold, not heat, should be used to soothe a spider bite.
- The bite should be cleaned and covered with a thin layer of antibiotic cream, in order to avoid infection.
- If a black widow, brown recluse, or any other poisonous spider is responsible for the bite, cold compresses should be applied to the affected area before seeking medical assistance. If possible, kill the spider and take it with you.

Insect stings

- If the sting remains lodged in the skin, it should be removed immediately, without breaking the sac containing the venom because once the sting penetrates the skin, it can continue pumping venom into its victim, especially if the sac is damaged.
- Remove the sting by shifting it sideways, then wash the wound to prevent infection.
- Apply cold compresses or ice to the affected area. Tell the child to rest, and keep an eye out for signs of any severe allergic reaction.
- Oral diphenhydamine can help alleviate any reddening or inflammation around the sting, but this drug requires a doctor's prescription.
- If your child has any breathing difficulties or any rash far removed from the bite itself, it is vital to call the local emergency number or take him to an emergency department immediately.
- If your child is allergic to the insect's venom, an anaphylactic reaction could occur within minutes, although it can sometimes appear up to 2 hours later.

Furthermore, use an insect repellent, preferably one that contains diethyltoluamide (DEET). The use of DEET in products for children is the subject of controversy, however, although many experts consider it safe in a solution of 10 percent or less. Other alternatives are available, but consult your doctor before you use them.

special precautions for vacations

Before setting out on vacation, it is essential to take a number of factors into account, especially when traveling with young children. For example, depending on the area you are going to visit, you must find out if any vaccinations are needed, if it is safe to swim, and if there is any risk of altitude sickness. A few basic preparatory measures can prevent a host of unexpected problems that could ruin a vacation.

Altitude sickness reflects a person's poor adaptation to altitude and is particularly prevalent among people unaccustomed to a reduced oxygen supply, low temperatures, and dehydration. The typical symptoms are nausea, drowsiness, pale skin with cold sweat, tachycardia, and difficulty in breathing.

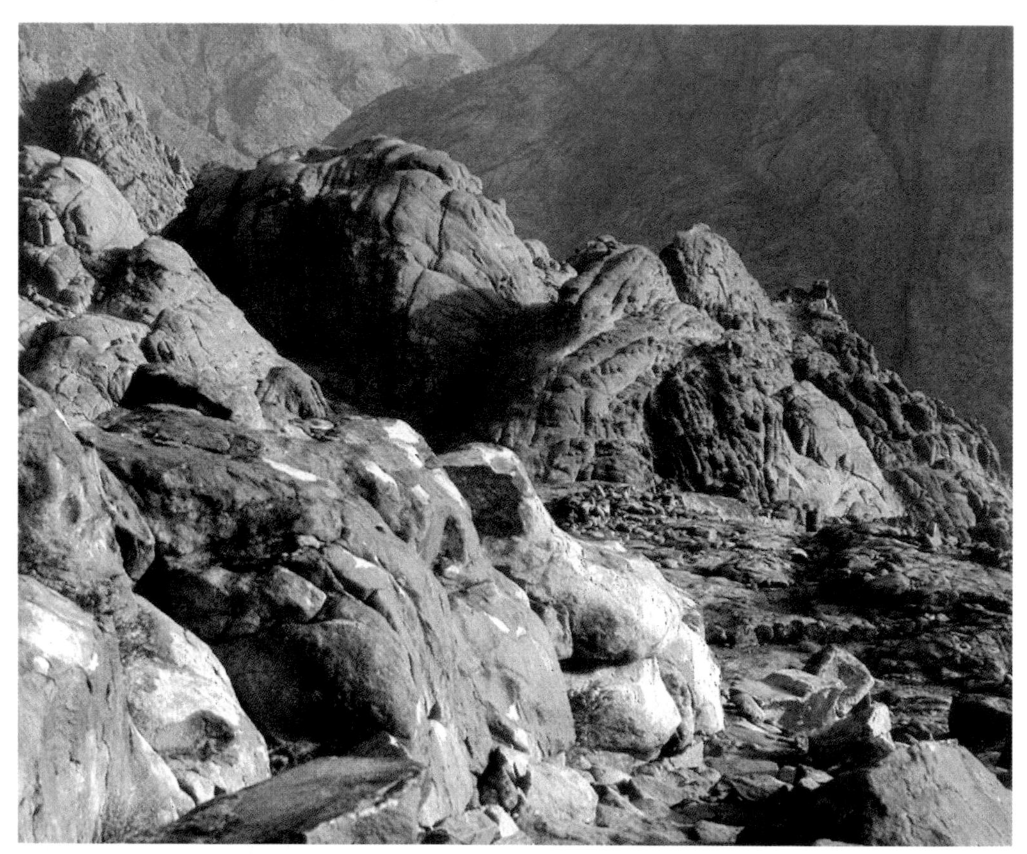

Special precautions for vacations

Altitude sickness

The effects of altitude sickness are usually apparent within a few hours and they can last 2 or 3 days. Some basic preventive measures:

- Consult a doctor before traveling.
- If you arrive in a city at great altitude by airplane, rest for the first 48 hours.
- Drink plenty of liquid.
- Try to progress upward gradually, allowing the body to adapt and avoiding physical exertion.
- If you have a slight headache, take aspirin, paracetamol, or ibuprofen.
- When the first symptoms appear, move down to a lower altitude.
- Coca tea is an Andean remedy commonly offered to tourists at heights of over 10,000 ft (3,000 m). Its analgesic effects and capacity to lower the cardiac rhythm produce euphoria and moderate breathing patterns, thereby alleviating feelings of tiredness.

Swimming

You should avoid swimming in water that could be polluted by human or animal excrement. Polluted water is a transmission route for eye, ear, and skin infections. In contrast, swimming pools with chlorinated water are safer. It is important to be cautious in the sea and obey any signals indicating that is unsafe to swim. In some areas, it is necessary to wear special footwear to protect against bites, stings, cuts, skin complaints caused by corals, or poisonous crustaceans or sea anemones. Also beware of jellyfish, as their bites are extremely painful and irritate the skin.

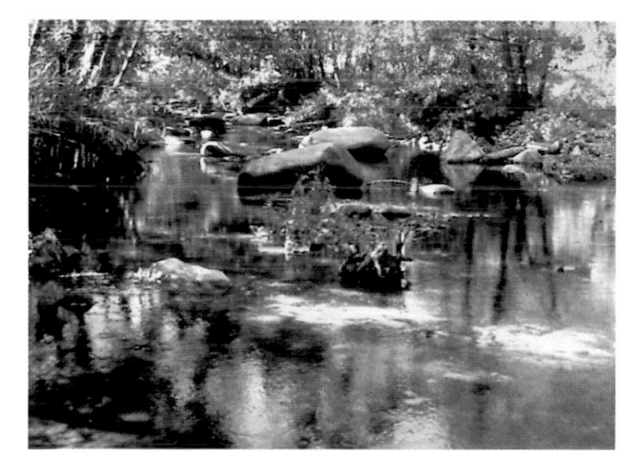

Special care should be taken with water, both for swimming and drinking.

Vaccinations required overseas

A vaccination certificate is an essential requirement for travel to some countries, and can even be compulsory for getting a visa to many African and Asian countries. This type of protection is only available in international vaccination centers authorized by the World Health Organization (WHO), which will provide an international vaccination certificate.

The diseases that most frequently require vaccination are:

- **Yellow fever:** vaccination against yellow fever is compulsory for entrance to many countries in sub-Saharan Africa and Latin America. A single dose provides immunity for 10 years, starting 10 days after receiving the vaccination (which has side effects of muscle pains, headaches, and fever). It is contraindicated in pregnant women, people with an allergy to eggs or those suffering from immune depression, and babies aged under 9 months.
- **Cholera:** Anti-cholera vaccination is no longer obligatory for international travel. It only offers 50% protection, so good hygiene measures provide the best prevention. The risk of cholera is very low for tourists, but an oral vaccine may be recommended in areas where cholera is endemic, such as Asia, Africa, Central and South America, for aid workers, backpackers, and other visitors planning to come into close contact with the local population.
- **Typhoid fever:** the anti-typhoid vaccination provides protection for 3 years, taking effect 3 weeks after receiving it. It is especially recommended for long journeys to countries with suspect hygiene amenities. Typhoid fever is found all over the world; although the incidence is low in developed countries, it is quite common in Africa, Central and South America, the Middle East, and Southeast Asia.
- **Hepatitis A and B:** these preventive vaccinations are very important. The hepatitis B vaccine protects against infection transmitted via the bloodstream; it is recommended for travelers to sub-Saharan Africa and the Far East. Two injections with an interval of 1 month between them are required, along with a booster 6 months and 5 years later. The hepatitis B vaccination requires a booster 6–12 months after the first injection. It is recommended for long journeys and destinations with unhygienic living conditions. A combined vaccine against hepatitis A and B has recently been developed. The recommended administration schedule

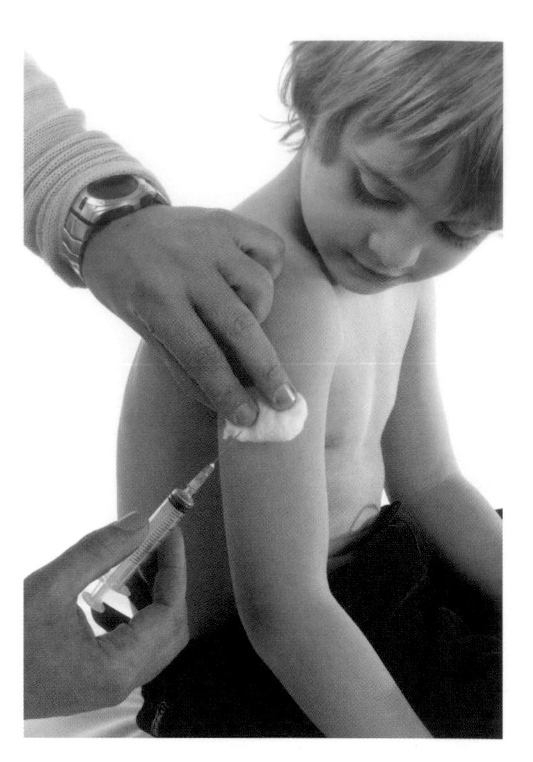

Vaccinations should be given in good time according to individual need.

is 3 doses, the last 2 being given 1 and 6 months after the first, the vaccination is intramuscular and given only at the minimum age of 1 year.

• **Other vaccinations:** other vaccinations are available for travelers; some of these form part of a child's normal vaccination program, such as meningitis, tetanus, poliomyelitis, or diphtheria. Always speak to your doctor before making any decisions regarding any vaccination.

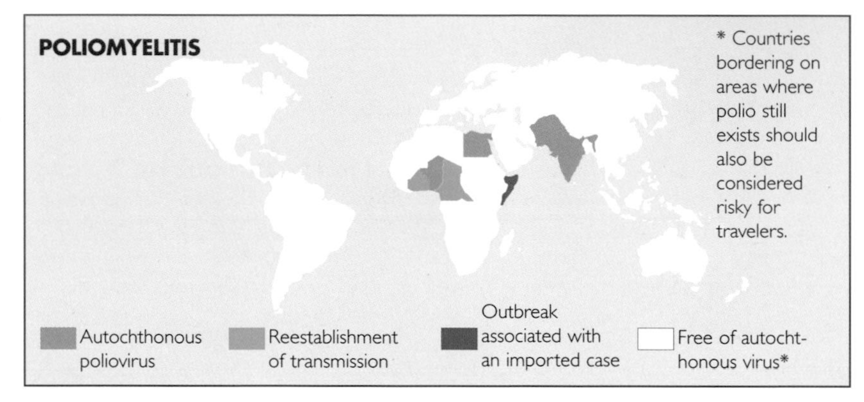

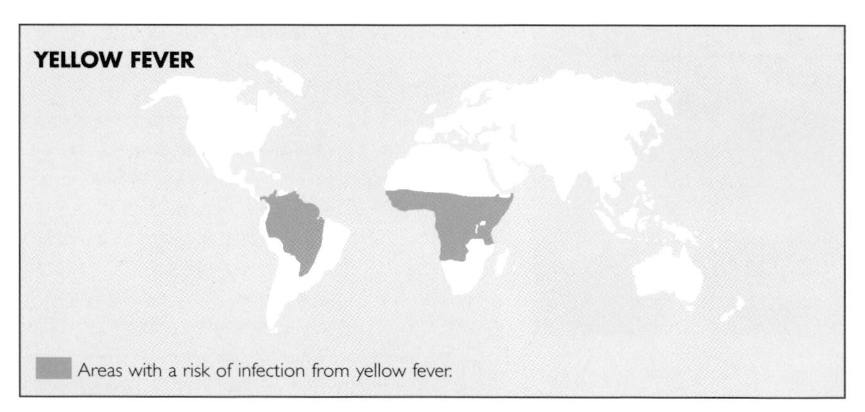

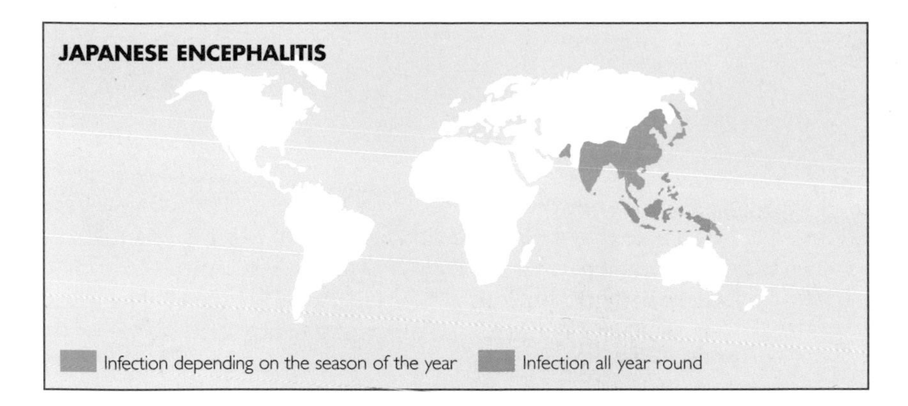
JAPANESE ENCEPHALITIS
Infection depending on the season of the year
Infection all year round

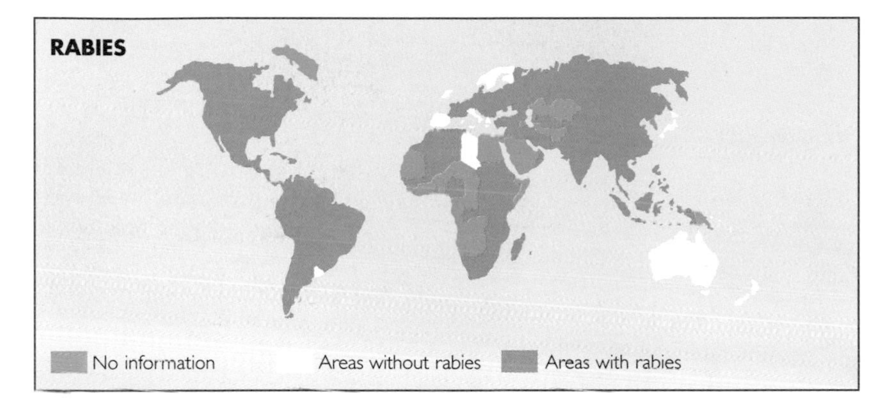
RABIES
No information
Areas without rabies
Areas with rabies

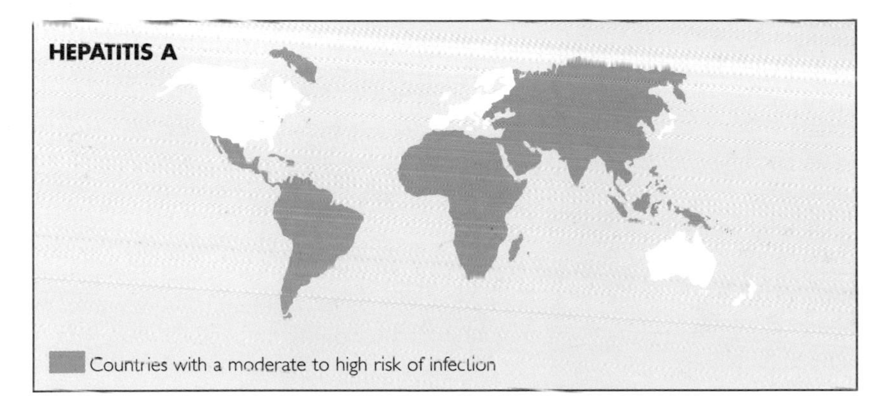
HEPATITIS A
Countries with a moderate to high risk of infection

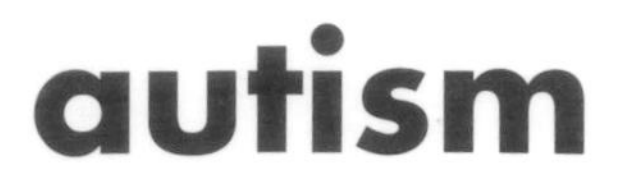

Autism is a syndrome that affects 4 out of every 100,000 children, most usually boys. Even though it has been recognized as a developmental disorder for many years, the causes of autism are still unknown. The growing number of cases diagnosed in recent years could be related to increased recognition of the syndrome, as well as technical advances in its diagnosis.

The causes of autism

The origins of this condition have yet to be clarified, although the latest research suggests that several factors could play a part. The main causes that have been identified are as follows:

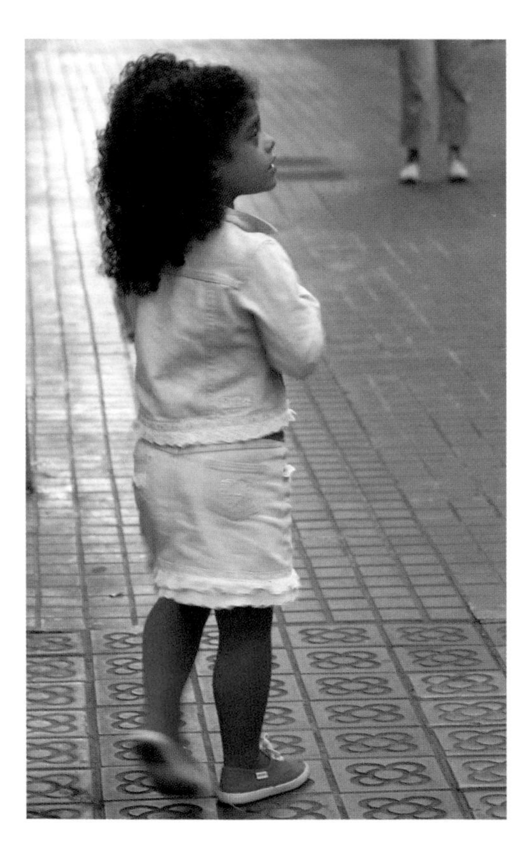

- **Genetic.** It is currently thought that less than 10 genes could be involved in the transmission of autism, and that these could act by multiplying. Weakness in chromosome X has also been postulated as a cause.
- **Neurobiological.** Abnormalities in certain neurotransmitters, particularly serotonin (which is found in high levels in autistic children), could be responsible for changes in the functioning of the brain.
- **Psychological.** There are several theories of causes of a socio-affective, cognitive, or cognitive-affective origin.

Can childhood vaccinations contribute to autism?

Vaccinations such as the MMR (against mumps, measles, and German measles (Rubella)) do not cause autism, although some parents of autistic children suspect that this vaccination, administered at the age of about 15 months, could be related, as it as at that age that children first start to display symptoms of autism. It is probable, however, that the symptoms would appear anyway, even if the child has not been vaccinated.

Another cause for suspicion is that, until recently, some vaccines contained a preservative called thimerosal, which in its turn contained mer-

Autism occurs in all ethnic, social, and ethnic groups, although boys are 4 times more vulnerable than girls. The siblings of an autistic child run a risk – albeit minimal (5%) – of also suffering from autism.

Autism is characterized by changes in cerebral development. The causes of these changes are still not completely clear.

Characteristics of an autistic child

- He avoids physical and visual contact with other people.
- He does not respond to voices and other sounds.
- He does not speak, or he uses language incorrectly.
- He repeats movements, rocks to and fro, and bangs his head or turns it repeatedly.
- He stares at parts of an object, such as the wheels of a toy.
- He does not understand hand gestures or body language.
- He refuses to take part in games which involve pretend play.
- He is very concerned about order, routine, and ritual.
- His face is unexpressive or his voice is monotonous.
- He causes damage to himself and has no sense of danger.

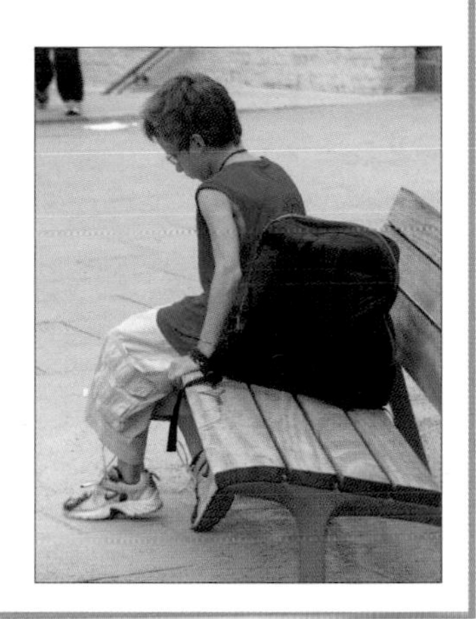

cury. Although high doses of certain forms of mercury can affect cerebral development, research indicates that the mercury content in thimerosal does not reach these levels. In 2001, a group of experts concluded that there was no conclusive evidence that the MMR vaccine, or any other vaccine, increased the risk of developing autism.

Parents of autistic children

Having a physically or mentally handicapped child is very hard to accept and deal with. Parents can feel guilty, confused, and despairing about their child's future. All these emotional reactions are valid and legitimate. This is where the family doctor plays an important role by providing, on the one hand, emotional support and, on the other, professional assistance.

Living with autism

- There is no cure for autism as yet, although progress has been made in its prevention, thanks to the discovery of possible causal factors.
- Pharmacological therapy can be used to treat problems associated with autism, such as insomnia, hyperactivity, convulsions, aggressive behavior, etc.
- Behavioral modification techniques are also used nowadays, in conjunction with specific programs designed to further an autistic child's development by stimulating him, training him to speak

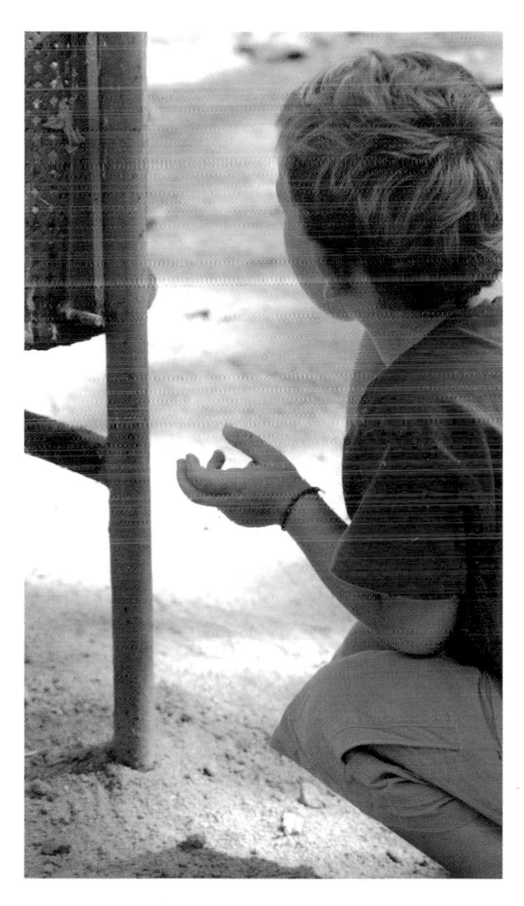

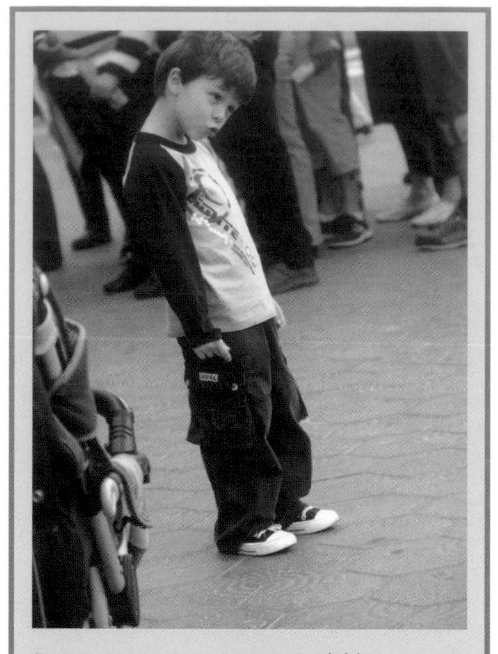

Diagnosing autism. An autistic child is not different from other children as a baby. In the first year of life he may not display any unusual signs, but in the second he may show delayed development in skills such as speech or comprehension, or can even lose abilities that he had previously acquired. Autism is generally diagnosed when a child is about 2 years old, although there is no specific medical test to confirm the diagnosis. Doctors generally observe the child's behavior, sometimes using various techniques that investigate specific traits associated with autism.

Most people know very little about autistic children, and this causes their parents to feel very isolated and misunderstood. This is one of the factors that has prompted the formation of support groups designed to help parents confront the problem and find the most appropriate therapy.

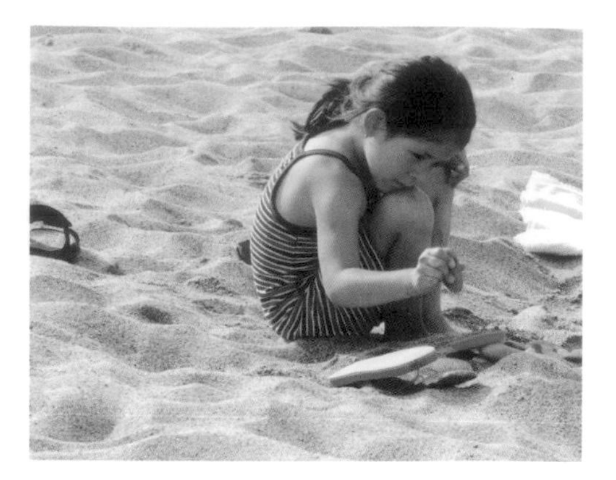

better, improving his capacity for concentration and response, etc; in short, a series of therapeutic strategies aimed at minimizing his deficiencies and enhancing his quality of life and social integration.

- Remember that the parents of autistic children also need help and training, as well as resources to make suitable adjustments to the family home, as autism can lead to disabilities that will persist throughout the child's life.

Special education is fundamental in dealing with autism; this can be imparted in a special school or on an individual basis. Psychotherapy has been used, although with little success, as an autistic child's cognitive and linguistic deficiencies are an obstacle. Family support is extremely useful. Parents should understand that autism is not a result of emotional problems derived from a child's upbringing. It is advisable for them to join a support group specifically formed for parents of autistic children.

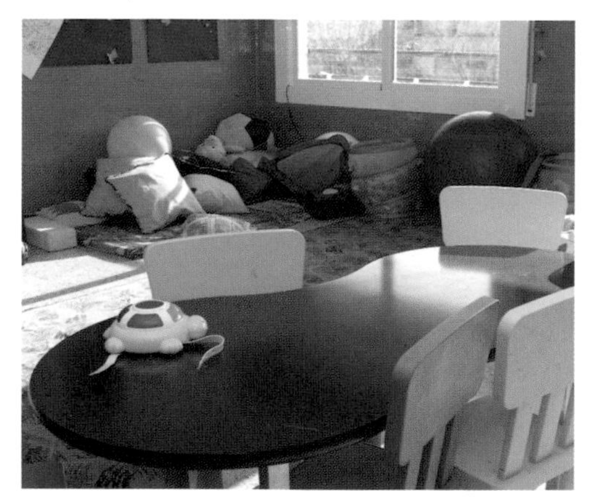

congenital and hereditary neurological disorders

There are a large number of neurological disorders, i.e. anomalies of the central and peripheral nervous system, that are derived from a problem occurring during the development of the embryo, from congenital disease, or from some type of genetic change or hereditary anomaly. The characteristics of this group of diseases, as well as the incidence and degree of disability – which is sometimes life-threatening – are extremely variable.

Congenital and hereditary neurological disorders

Spina bifida

• Spina bifida (myelodysplasia) involves abnormal development of bones in the spine, as well as the surrounding nervous tissue and the sac around the spinal cord containing liquid; it can result in part of the spinal cord and the surrounding structures growing outside the body. This anomaly can occur in any part of the spine.

• Spina bifida is divided into the following categories:

– Spina bifida occulta. This is a mild form, in which the spinal cord and its surrounding structures remain within a baby's body but the bones of

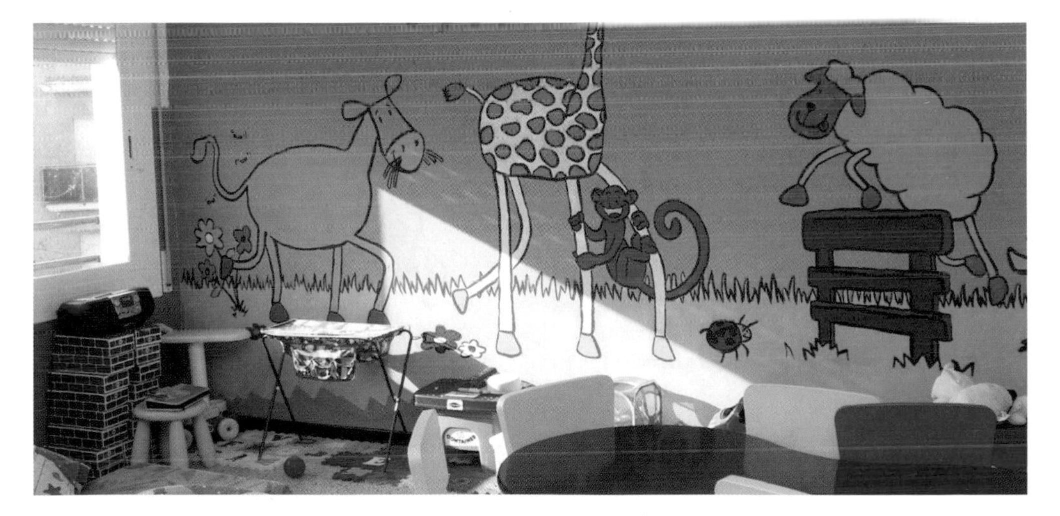

the lumbar region do not grow normally. Sometimes small cavities, birthmarks, or an area covered with hair are visible, but on occasions no sign of any anomaly is noticeable to the eye.

– Meningocele. This is a moderate form of spina bifida in which a sac with liquid can be observed in the spine. This sac does not contain any of the spinal cord or nervous tissues.

– Myelomeningocele. This is a serious form of spina bifida in which the spinal cord and the nervous tissues grow outside the body in a sac of liquid that is clearly visible. Babies who suffer from this type of disorder are usually weak and numb below the site of the anomaly, as well as often suffering from intestinal and bladder problems. Most babies born with myelomeningocele also suffer from hydrocephalia.

Hydrocephalia, microcephalia, and anencephalia

• Hydrocephalia is a disorder involving a lack of absorption, obstructed flow, or excessive production of cephalo-rachidian liquid in the cerebral ventricles. This leads to an accumulation of liquid, which increases the pressure inside the skull, causing the bones to expand beyond their normal size. It can be a congenital disorder or appear later in life. When no genetic cause is apparent, it is believed that a variety of factors, both genetic and environmental, play a role in the development of hydrocephalia.

• Microcephalia is a congenital disorder in which a baby's head is much smaller than that of a normal baby of the same age and gender. Most children with this disorder have a small brain and suffer from developmental disability. Microcephalia can be triggered by exposure to harmful substances during pregnancy, but it may also be associated with hereditary genetic syndromes.

• Anencephalia is a congenital pathology that affects the configuration of the brain and the bones inside the skull. This impairs the development of the encephalon, the area of the brain responsible for thought, sight, hearing, touch, and movement. The rear of the skull is not fully sealed and it is also possible that some bones are missing in the front and sides of the head. The symptoms will depend on the regions that are affected. In serious cases, anencephalia has fatal consequences.

Cerebral palsy

• Cerebral palsy is a wide-ranging term that embraces a group of neurological disorders that affect the communication between the brain and the muscles from birth, leading to a permanent lack of motor and postural coordination. Cerebral palsy usually occurs as a result of an episode that interrupts the supply of oxygen to the brain. Some of the factors that account for its onset are premature birth, very low weight at birth (especially under 2.2 lb/1 kg), some viruses, drug addiction or abuse on the part of the mother during pregnancy, infections, cerebral hemorrhages, injuries, complications during labor and delivery, etc.

• Cerebral palsy has a number of symptoms, including muscular weakness, deficient motor control, trembling, and spasticity in the arms or legs. Muscular rigidity can also be seen, characterized by stiff legs and clenched fists.

Atrophy or muscular dystrophy

• This term groups together a series of syndromes of very diverse origin; some are congenital, while others are caused by hereditary lesions that can appear at various ages. They are characterized by weakness and atrophy of the muscular tissue, with or without degeneration of the nervous tissue. Children suffering from these syndromes are known generically as hypotonic infants.

• Hypotonia is defined as a reduction in the muscle tone, either generally or at a particular point; this has a negative effect on a child's psychomotor capacities. These syndromes are characterized by strange postures and a lack of resistance to passive movements in the joints, along with increased tightness in the joints.

Approximately 80% of cases of spina bifida are located in the lumbar region; the remaining 20% are found in the back of the neck or the upper cervical area. It affects girls more than boys, and in over 95% of cases there is no family history of the disorder.

TYPE	AGE AT ONSET	SYMPTOMS, PROGRESSION, AND LIFE EXPECTANCY
Becker	2–16 years	Symptoms almost identical with those of Duchenne dystrophy, although less serious, and it progresses more slowly; survival up to middle age.
Congenital	At birth	The symptoms include general muscle weakness and deformities of the joints; it progresses slowly, but its victims have a low life expectancy.
Duchenne	2–6 years	The symptoms include general weakness and atrophy of the muscles, affecting the pelvis, upper arms, legs, and all the voluntary muscles; survival beyond the age of 20 is rare.
Distal	40–60 years	The symptoms include weakness and atrophy of the hand muscles, forearms, and lower legs; slow progression; it rarely leads to total disability.
Emery-Dreifuss	Childhood or puberty	The symptoms include weakness and atrophy of the shoulder muscles, upper arms, and scapula, often accompanied by deformities in the joints; slow progression; the health problems associated with it can cause sudden death.
Facioscapulo-humeral	Late adolescence	The symptoms include weakness of the facial muscles, deformity, and a degree of atrophy in the shoulders and upper arms; slow progression, with periods of rapid deterioration; survival is possible for several decades after its onset.
Limb-girdle	After childhood, until middle age	The symptoms include weakness and atrophy, which first affect the scapular area (in men) and the pelvis; slow progression; death usually results from heart and lung complications.
Myotonic	20–40 years	The symptoms usually include weakness in all the muscular groups, accompanied by delayed relaxation of the muscles after contraction; it first affects the face, then the feet, hands, and neck; slow progression; survival until the age of 50 or 60.
Oculopharyngeal	40–70 years	The symptoms affect the muscles of the eyelids and throat, causing weakness that, over time, leads to an inability to swallow, with resulting emaciation through malnutrition; slow progression.

There are 9 types of muscular dystrophy, which all lead, over time, to loss of strength, progressive disability, and sometimes even deformities.

epilepsy

Epilepsy is a brain disorder that causes cyclic muscular contractions, in the form of isolated or generalized seizures. The term usually embraces all types of convulsions of cerebral origin that have no other known cause (fever, injury, etc.); about 0.5 percent of the population suffer from chronic epilepsy, but it may affect up to 10 times that number on a temporary basis. As children quite often go into convulsions with a fever, a diagnosis of epilepsy needs to be confirmed by a series of neurological tests.

Epilepsy

Causes of epilepsy

The most common causes are:

• As a side effect to genetic disorders or problems during birth, in which case the seizures usually begin in infancy.

Internal structure of the brain

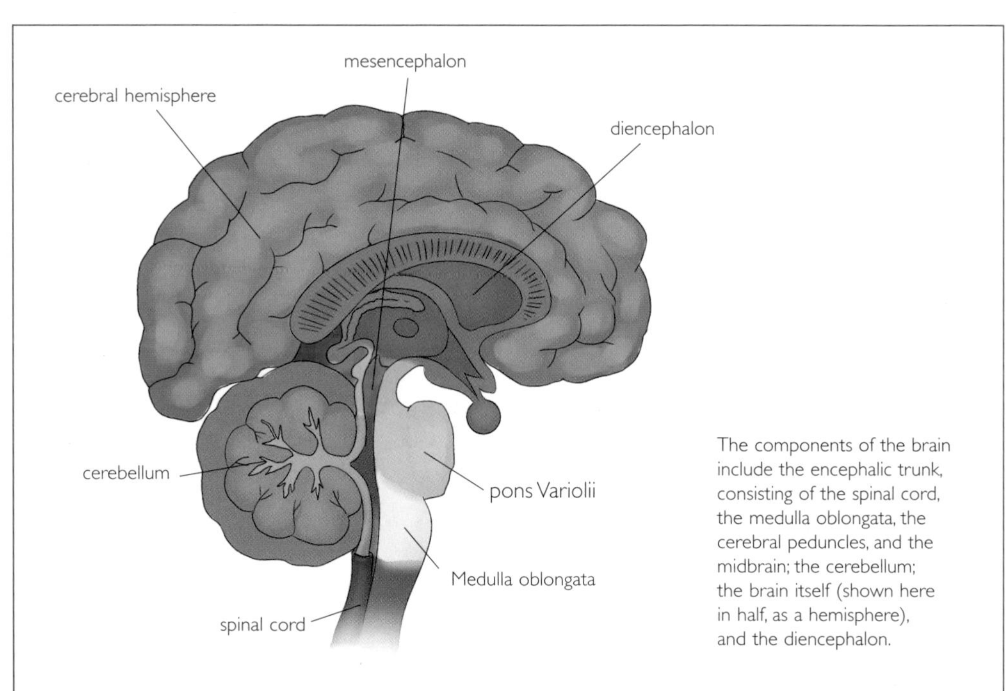

The components of the brain include the encephalic trunk, consisting of the spinal cord, the medulla oblongata, the cerebral peduncles, and the midbrain; the cerebellum; the brain itself (shown here in half, as a hemisphere), and the diencephalon.

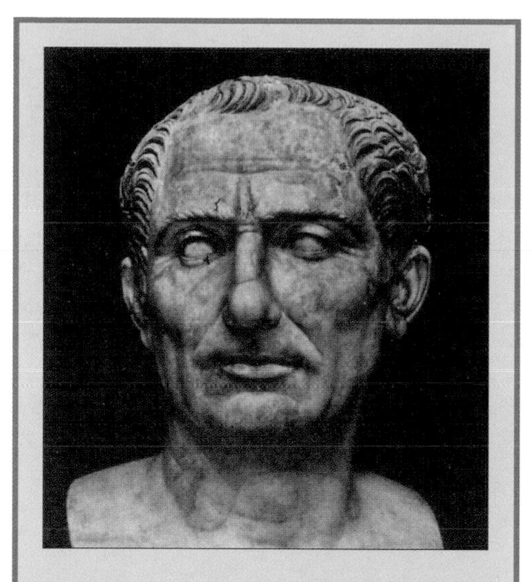

"He fell down in the market-place and foam'd at mouth, and was speechless". This is Shakespeare's description of a fit suffered by the Roman emperor Julius Caesar (Act 1, Scene 2 of his tragedy Julius Caesar). History and literature abound in such descriptions of epilepsy. The great Russian novelist Fyodor Dostoevsky was affected by this disorder, and his work is one of the most striking reflections of the repercussions of epilepsy on the personality.

• If there is no identifiable or idiopathic cause, it starts before the age of 20; it is not normally accompanied by any other neurological problems and is often hereditary.

• Metabolic changes that can appear at any age.

– Diabetes.

Shifts in the electrolytic balance (minerals in the blood).

– Renal insufficiency (increase in urea).

– Nutritional deficiencies.

– Phenylcetonuria (this can trigger seizures in babies).

– Other metabolic diseases.

– Intoxication from alcohol or other drugs.

• Brain damage. Anybody who has suffered from brain lesions (most particularly young adults) can have an epileptic seizure after a latency period of 1–3 years.

• Tumors and other cerebral lesions that occupy space in the skull are more frequent in adults aged over 30. They usually give rise to partial or focal seizures that later affect the whole body.

• Diseases of the blood vessels (stroke, cerebral ischemia, etc.) – the most common cause of seizures over the age of 60.

• Degenerative diseases (Alzheimer's diseases and other similar cerebral syndromes) in elderly people.

• Infections (meningitis, encephalitis, cerebral abscess, complications of AIDS, etc.) can occur at any age and create temporary epileptic crises (once the cause is removed, the seizures do not recur).

Clinical picture

• **Absence or petit-mal seizures.** This is characterized by minimal movements or total immobility, apart from in the eyelids, leading to rigidity in the body and a blank gaze. There is a sudden, brief loss of consciousness, lasting just a few seconds. These are often found in children and are sometimes associated with learning disorders.

• **Tonic-clonic or grand-mal seizures.** This is characterized by violent muscle contractions throughout the body. The affected person is stiff, temporarily loses consciousness, and momentarily stops breathing (apnea), before emitting a loud sigh. Such seizures can be accompanied by urinary incontinence, biting of the tongue or inner cheeks, and injuries resulting from the effects of the convulsions and falling to the ground.

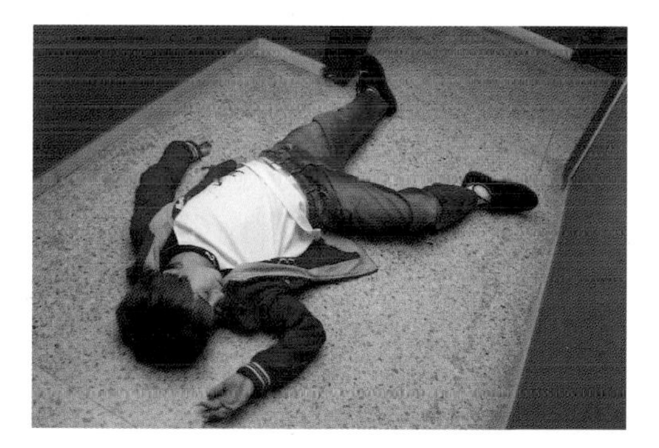

Grand- mal epileptic seizures are very dramatic events that cause great anxiety in both the epileptic child's immediate circles and any passers-by (it is not unknown for seizures to occur in public places).

First-aid measures

Although a child affected by an epileptic seizure must be treated by a doctor, preferably in a hospital, first-aid measures can be useful when the seizure is still in progress, and before the child can see a doctor.

- The first step is to prevent the child from causing himself an injury.
- Put a soft object under the person's head to prevent injury.
- Move aside any furniture or objects that are close by.
- Do not try to impede his movements or help him keep his balance during the seizure.
- If the child vomits or expels large amounts of mucus, prevent him from swallowing or choking on it by turning him on one side, once the seizure has subsided, and keeping him in that position while he sleeps.
- If he turns blue or stops breathing, turn him on one side to keep his airways open and prevent his tongue from blocking them.
- A child usually starts breathing again on his own, once the seizure is over.
- Cardio-pulmonary resuscitation or mouth-to-mouth respiration is rarely needed after a seizure. It should never be attempted during a seizure.

First-aid measures focus on preventing an epileptic hurting himself during the seizure, which normally comes to a halt on its own and rarely requires resuscitation or artificial respiration.

• **Partial seizures.** These form a group of disorders marked by the contraction of a particular part of the body (simple form) or several concurrent symptoms (complex form), such as automatism, nausea, profuse sweating, red skin, and dilated pupils. They are also characterized by fantasies, the reliving of past events, and the perception of phantom smells and tastes; these can all lead to temporary personality changes or reduced mental acuity, maybe accompanied by loss of consciousness.

hip dysplasia

Hip dysplasia or dislocation, which is relatively common in baby girls, is an anomaly in the joint between the top of the femur (thigh bone) and its corresponding cavity in the coxal bone, causing the femur to be dislodged upward and preventing normal movement. This situation prejudices her ability to walk and can lead to arthritis in later life. Early detection and treatment can prevent disabilities that would otherwise blight a child's entire life.

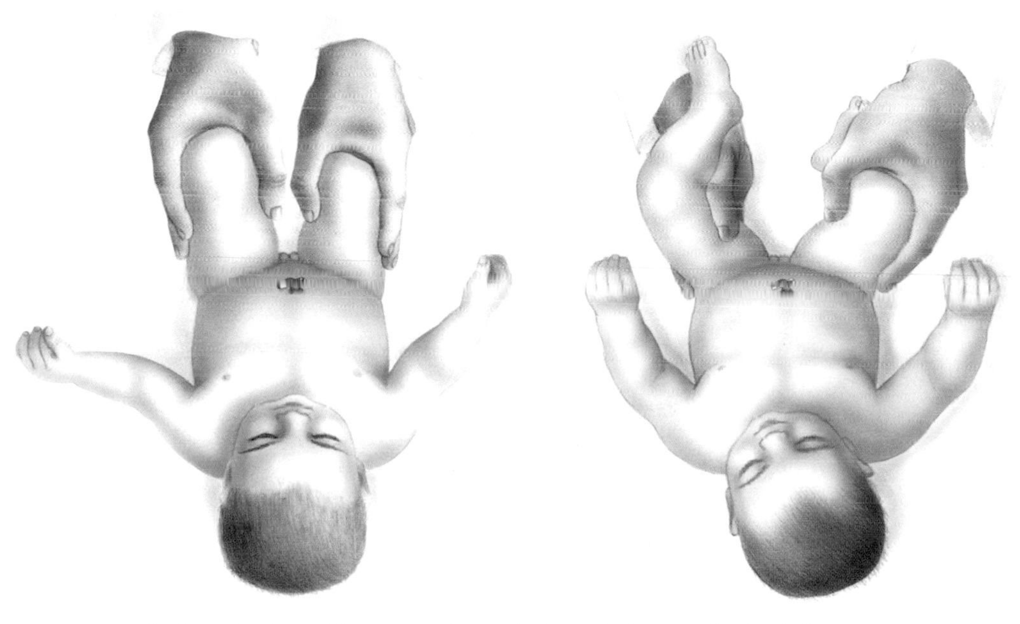

The illustration shows different ways of examining the projection caused by the displacement of the femoral head from its cavity. This protuberance can be found in the front or to the rear, known respectively as the Ortolani sign and the Barlow sign.

Hip dysplasia

Predisposing factors

The most striking of these is gender. Its greater frequency in girls (6:1 with respect to boys) leads us to suppose that the sex of the child must have an influence, even though this still cannot be explained.

Heredity is probably another predisposing factor, as between 20 and 40% of cases – depending on the area studied – have a history of the same disorder in their family.

Hormonal changes have also been suggested as a possible cause. An increase in estrogens would soften the capsule and ligaments of the hip joint, favoring dislocation.

It has also been postulated that bad positioning of the buttocks in the uterus would heighten the propensity to hip dysplasia.

Diagnosis

The Barlow and Ortolani maneuvers are the most reliable diagnosis methods in a newborn child. They now form part of the standard examination undertaken in regular checkups of babies.

The baby is examined lying face up, with one of the doctor's hands holding the pelvis stable. The other hand holds the hip, with the thumb in the groin and the index or middle figure on the greater trochanter (the most prominent protrusion at the back of the femur).

• Barlow maneuver. The hip joint is bent at an angle of 90° and moved toward the midline of the body (adduction), while applying slight pressure outward with the thumb. Any dislocation of the hip can be observed during the adduction (positive Barlow sign).

• Ortolani reduction maneuver. The hip is raised in an effort to put the dislocated femoral head back in its place (hence the alternative name of click maneuver for a positive Ortolani maneuver).

• The hip joint can sometimes be noticeably loose, but without any clearly defined dislocation. At the age of 2–3 months, hip dysplasia can be masked by the baby's muscular tension.

• As the child starts to walk, the clinical signs of hip dysplasia become more subtle, although the folds in her thighs may be asymmetrical and one knee may even be higher than the other (positive Galleazi sign).

• These clinical maneuvers are unfortunately not sufficient to identify all babies with hip dysplasia,

Pavlik harness

The Pavlik harness allows the hip to gradually achieve flexion and abduction, thereby definitively correcting the dysplasia. The illustrations show 2 different types of Pavlik harness.

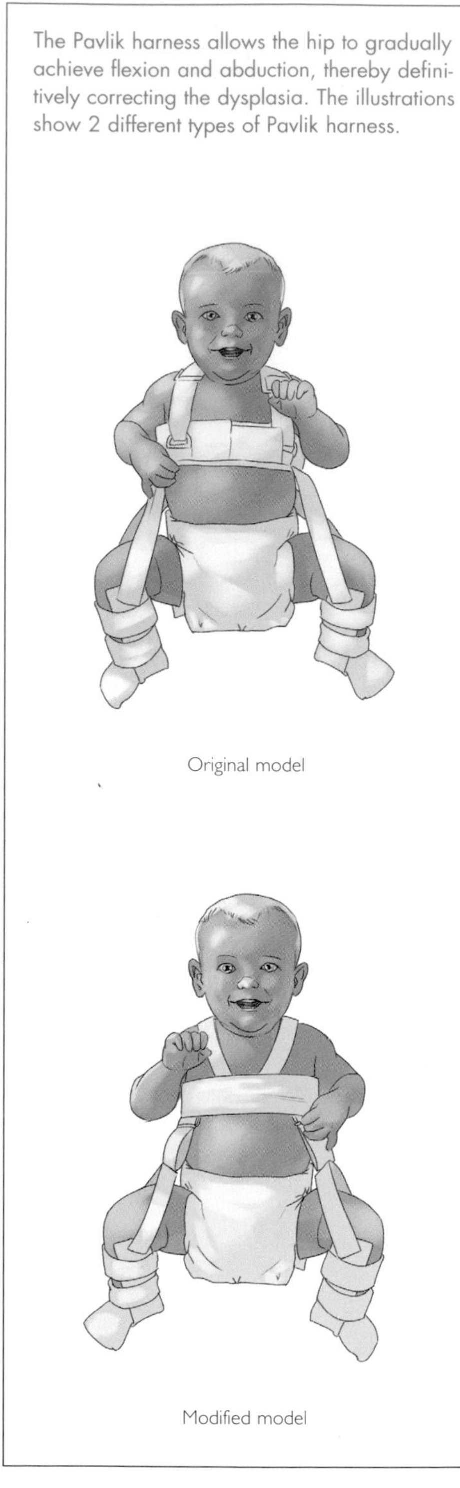

Original model

Modified model

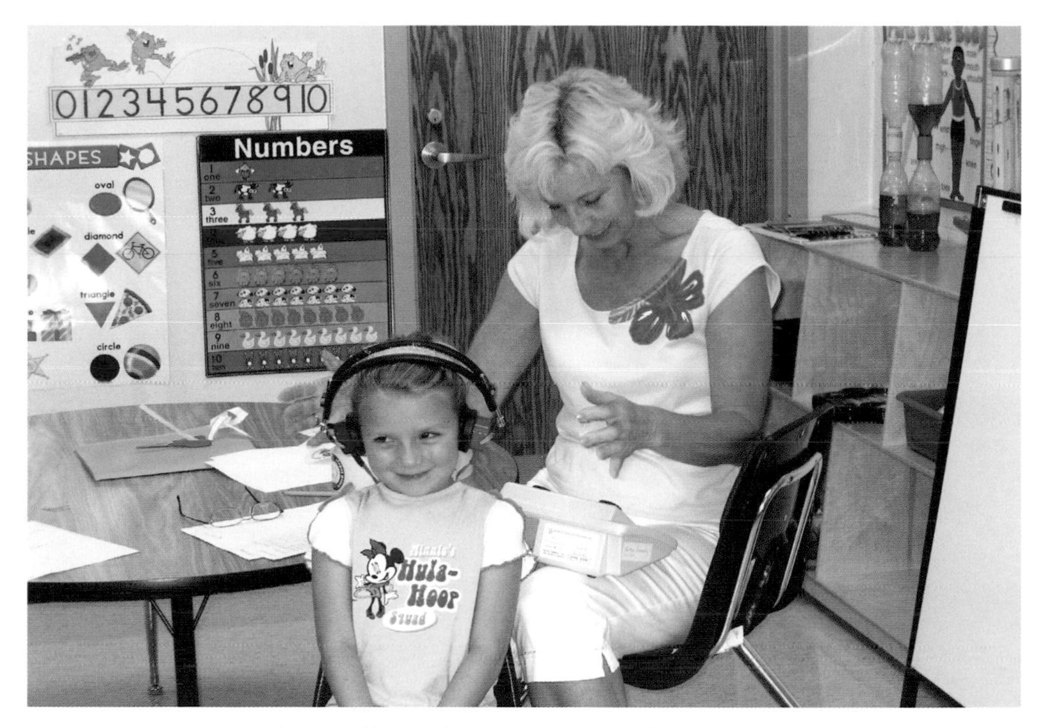

Audiometry is one of the techniques used by specialists to diagnose hearing disorders.

Drugs with toxic effects on the ear (such as aminoglucoside antibiotics).

- Physical damage to the ear.
- Bacterial infections.

Classification of deafness according to hearing deficiency

• It is important to distinguish between deafness and hearing deficiency, which is defined by the hearing threshold in decibels (units for measuring hearing).

– Total deafness: hearing deficiency over 85 decibels.

– Severe deafness: 60–85 decibels.

– Slight deafness: 40–60 decibels.

– Impaired hearing: 25–40 decibels.

– In the last 2 cases, the affected person may be able to speak, albeit with problems in articulation and pronunciation.

Children with hearing deficiency: stimulation and personality

Congenitally deaf children have great difficulties in expressing themselves as they do not have resource to language (deaf mutes). They therefore have great problems interacting with other people. The more severe the deafness, the greater the probability of dumbness. Despite this disability, an appropriately stimulated deaf-mute child will develop a normal level of intelligence.

In contrast, the effects of acquired hearing disorders depend on whether they appear before learning to speak and write, or after. If the child has no language skills, he is in the same situation as a congenitally deaf child; if the problem arises later on, he will have fewer developmental difficulties.

An early diagnosis and implementation of suitable treatment are therefore decisive: early stimulation, hearing aids, acquisition of sign language, lip reading, and/or medical or surgical treatment (implantation of a prosthesis, medication, etc.), according to the assessment of the medical team involved.

The stimulation of a child with a hearing disorder is designed to increase the possibilities of his communicating with other people and fulfilling his overall potential. Initially, the focus is on the motor and sensory capacities: sight, touch, and, where appropriate, sound. For example, stimulatory exercises can call a child's attention to vibrations that can be perceived via touch (a coffee grinder, a washing machine, a deep voice, a vacuum cleaner, etc.).

As regards language, a deaf child should always be spoken to face-to-face, so that he can read the lips of the person addressing him. Parents should avoid being either overprotective and or conveying signs of rejection; most importantly they must talk, sing, and play with the child without thinking, as far as possible , that he cannot hear them.

In cases of severe deafness, there is more chance of finding personality disorders and problems with emotional development. A deaf child is often more undisciplined than other children and is often unable to control his reactions. He can become aggressive, angry, or depressed when he does not get his own way. When a deaf child is confronted with situations he cannot control, he tends to react defensively and withdraw from an environment in which he does not feel secure or comfortable. His hearing disorder also makes him unable to understand instructions in school and at home. All these factors influence his personality and should be taken into account by adults who have to deal with his difficult behavior.

The intervention of a psychologist is advisable to treat a deaf child's emotional problems and attend to the needs of his family. Parents need a great deal of help and dedication to educate a deaf child, and they also need to take care not to neglect the needs of other members of the family, particularly siblings, in the process.

Patience, constancy, and a positive attitude are indispensable if a family is to live together in normal conditions and provide an emotionally stable atmosphere for a deaf child.

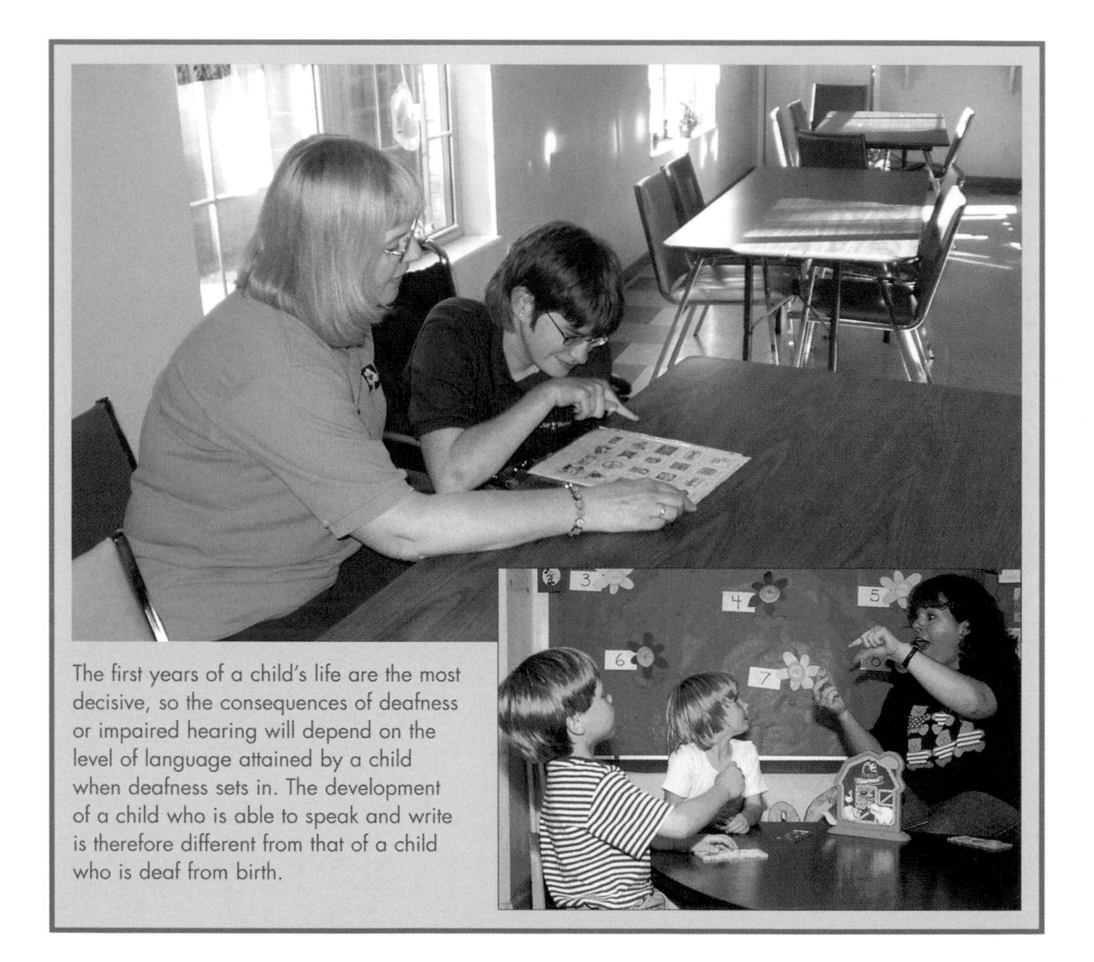

The first years of a child's life are the most decisive, so the consequences of deafness or impaired hearing will depend on the level of language attained by a child when deafness sets in. The development of a child who is able to speak and write is therefore different from that of a child who is deaf from birth.

blindness

Blindness is a disorder characterized by a loss of vision, whether total (zero vision, or merely a minimal perception of light) or partial (enough to be a handicap, despite some capacity to see). It has been estimated that there are currently between 28 and 35 million blind people in the world, the vast majority – almost 90 percent – living in developing countries, particularly Africa and Asia. The risk of being afflicted by blindness is 10–40 times greater in regions with a low socioeconomic level and rural areas than in industrialized countries.

Blindness

Causes of childhood blindness

These can be:

- Hereditary disorders: congenital cataracts, retinitis, degenerative myopia, etc.
- Congenital disorders: atrophy of the optic nerve, loss of visual acuity, German measles during pregnancy.
- Disorders resulting from injury: an excess of oxygen in the incubator, diabetic retinopathy, detached retina, etc.
- Changes caused by tumors, viruses, or toxins; tumor in the retina, inflammation and degeneration of the optic nerve, etc.

Society's attitude to a child with visual impairment is crucial to her integration and sense of self-esteem. A blind child who is well educated and socially accepted can do the same things as other children, only differently. A respectful approach should be adopted as soon as her disability is known. Her potential should not be restricted just because she has a difficulty. On the contrary, she should be given encouragement and shown how she can fulfill her desires.

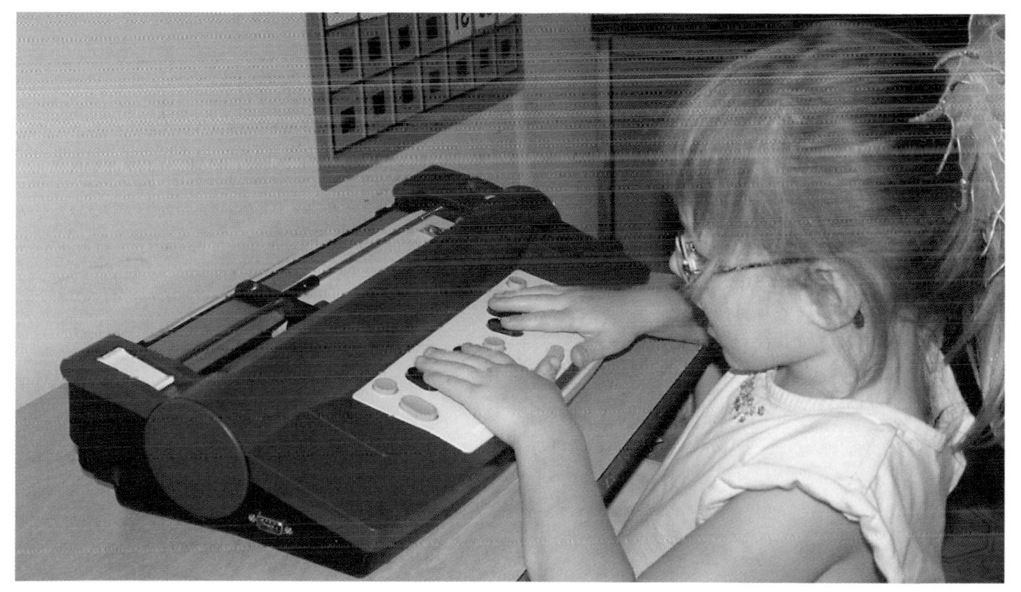

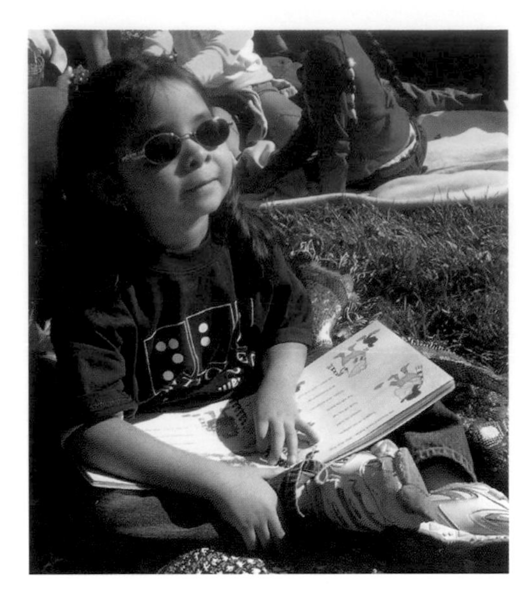

The number of children with blindness through unavoidable causes is constant in both rich and poor countries, but in developing countries, the figures for blindness from preventable causes are much higher. The most frequent causes of blindness in children are cataracts and also a detached cornea. This is an irreversible consequence of vitamin A deficiency, mumps, diarrhea, and malnutrition – all of which are avoidable.

The development of a blind child

• The senses of touch and hearing have to be stimulated and developed in a blind child, as they allow her to get to know her surroundings. For example, the ear can distinguish sounds, detect obstacles, and identify other people's voices.

• The education of a blind baby should be geared to maturing and developing her full potential. Her parents play a crucial role in this respect:

– They should encourage her to explore the various parts of her body.

– They should not stop her moving around out of fear that she may fall or harm herself.

– They should help develop her sense of hearing, as it will allow her to perceive sounds and be able to tell where they come from.

– They should encourage her preverbal expression (smiles, crying, babbling).

– They should stimulate the exploration of her surroundings by giving names to the objects she encounters.

– They should encourage her to undertake everyday activities, such as holding her feeding bottle and pacifier, using cutlery, dressing and undressing alone, urinating in the appropriate place, etc.

• The development of a blind baby is similar to that of a sighted baby in the first weeks of life; differences only start to be apparent in the fourth month. For a blind baby, people exist through the sounds they make. Between the ages of 7 and 9 months, a blind baby starts to look for objects with which she is familiar, and between the ages of 9 and 12 months she knows how to find objects in the place where she left them. A blind baby's postural and motor development usually differs little from that of a sighted baby, although she may start crawling and walking later (12–13 months and up to 19 months, respectively).

A congenital cataract is one of the main causes of blindness in a baby.

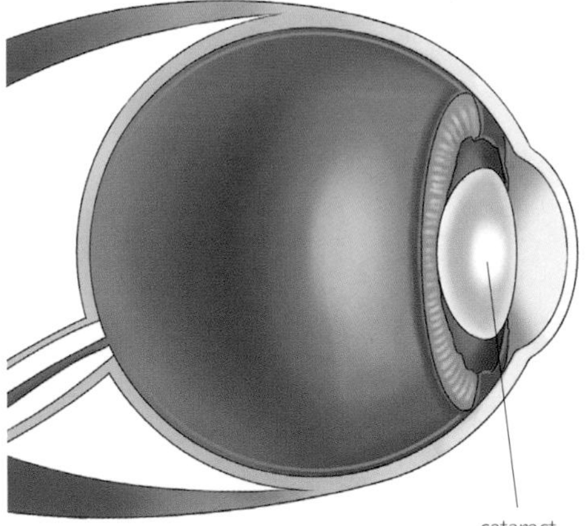

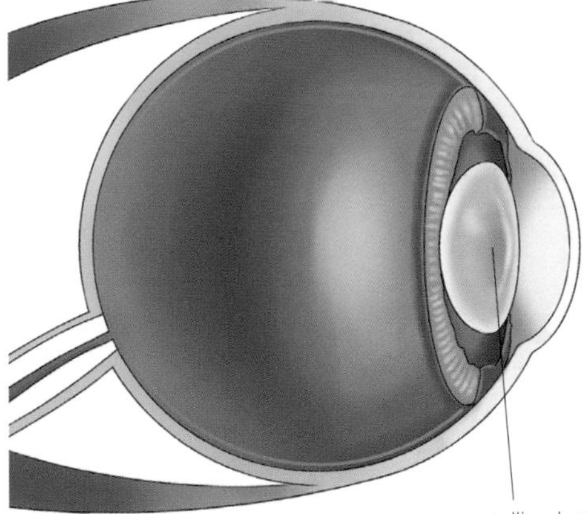

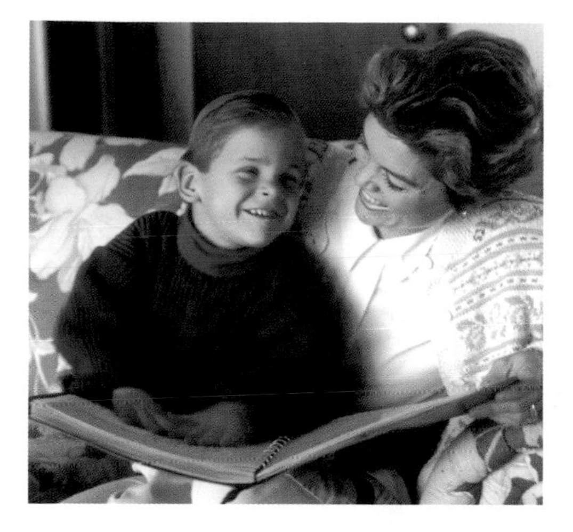

Language plays an essential role in the life of a blind child. If he does not receive sufficient stimulation from his environment, he can become passive and unable to cope with situations that may arise, making him feel inferior and ill at ease with his body.

Recommendations

The children's committee of the World Blind Union has issued the following recommendations for improving the living conditions of blind children:

1. Early identification and referral to specialists, to prevent avoidable forms of blindness in childhood.

2. Prevention by means of education and training, as well as treatment of vitamin A deficiency, river blindness, and cataract surgery.

3. The World Blind Union condemns any eugenic laws or practices that prevent blind women from having children or impede the birth of any child that may be blind.

4. Early-attention services and technical support for families of blind children.

5. Awareness of the profound impact of blind ness on a child's development.

6. Availability and continuity of various types of education, including total and partial integration and special schools for blind children.

7. Equal access to all educational material.

8. Teaching of Braille to all blind children.

9. Provision of books in Braille and assistance for children with visual impairment.

10. Attention for children with additional disabilities.

12. Raised awareness in society as a whole.

The Braille system is a logical system of dots in relief, distributed in 2 columns, with various configurations of dots representing each letter or symbol; using her fingertips, a blind person can read this script, written with an apparatus known as a slate and stylus. In other words, he both reads and writes with his hands.

Braille

• A blind child needs good spatial orientation and a well-trained sense of touch before she can start to use Braille. She needs to have assimilated the concepts of up and down, left and right, etc., as well as being familiar with basic geometric figures and simple silhouettes – and, of course, knowledge of the Braille signs.

• Braille can be written by hand or with a special typewriter. Reading involves placing a book horizontally, then putting the fingers on the lines, pressing down slightly. Both hands are used independently.

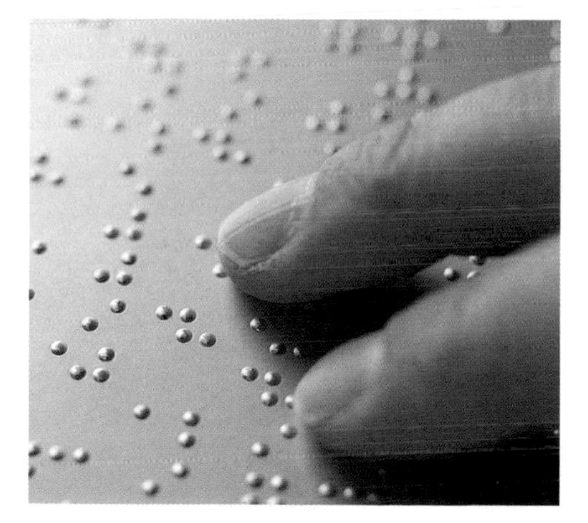

chromosomal syndromes

Under normal conditions, a person has 23 pairs of chromosomes, each with specific characteristics. A chromosomal irregularity can affect the number, size, and form of the chromosomes or the ordering of their component parts, so that, for example, the genetic material of one chromosome can bond with that of another. These irregularities give rise to various signs and symptoms that, together, make up the chromosomal syndromes, some of which have been extensively researched, on account of their relatively high incidence. This is the case, for example, with the Down's, Turner's, and Klinefelter syndromes, and the Cri du chat.

Chromosomal syndromes

Down's syndrome

In 95 percent of cases, this is characterized by a trisomy 21, i.e. an additional chromosome attached to chromosome 21. In other cases, the extra chromosome does not stick to chromosome 21 but to another, resulting in Down's syndrome through translocation.

This irregularity leads to a combination of congenital defects, including a degree of developmental disability – extremely variable, but is usually slight to moderate – distinctive facial characteristics, and, with some frequency, heart defects (35 percent), visual and hearing impairment, and other health problems. The seriousness of these anomalies can vary enormously from person to person.

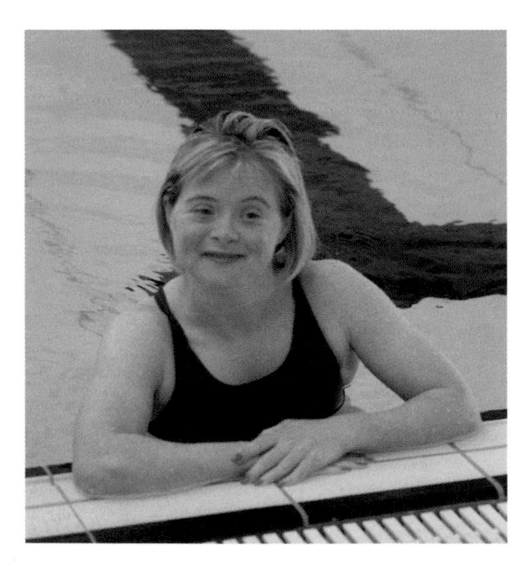

Children with Down's syndrome have a small head, a wide, flat face, a short nose, a large, usually prominent tongue, and slanting eyes. Their ears are small and low-set. Their hands are short and broad, with stunted fingers and a single crease in the palm. In 5% of cases, the fingers have 2 joints instead of 3 and they curve inward. Sometimes there is also a large gap between the big toe and second toe.

The genetic material in the human body cells is distributed by means of 46 chromosomes (23 pairs), except in the cells of the ovules and spermatozoids, which contain half the amount of chromosomes.

Other anomalies

Apart from the physical characteristics described above, children with Down's syndrome can be affected by other anomalies, such as:

- About 40–50% of such children have heart defects. These can be minor and responsive to treatment with medication, while others require surgery. All children with Down's syndrome must be examined by a heart specialist.
- Around 10% are born with intestinal malformations that require surgery.
- Over 50% suffer from some kind of visual or hearing impairment. The most common eye problems include crossed eyes, myopia, hypermetropy, and cataracts. Most of these disorders can be corrected with glasses, surgery, or other treatment. The child must be taken to a pediatric ophthalmologist in the first year of life, for an examination and diagnosis of these anomalies. Impaired hearing may be caused by liquid in the middle ear, a nervous defect, or both. All children with Down's syndrome must have regular eye and ear examinations, to enable any problem to be treated before it affects the development of language and other skills.
- Children with Down's syndrome are at greater risk of being affected by thyroid problems and leukemia. They also tend to catch colds, bronchitis, and pneumonia frequently.
- These children must receive regular medical attention, including vaccinations, as they are more susceptible to infections. Before the age of antibiotics, these infections were one of the most common causes of early death. The life expectancy of children with Down's syndrome has now risen considerably (55 years or more)

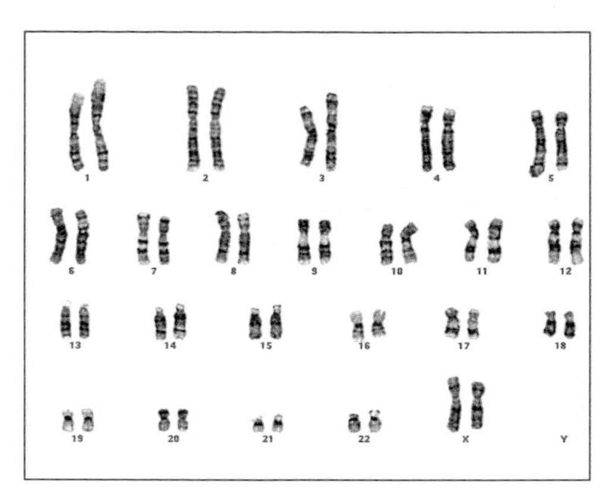

Normal female karyotype

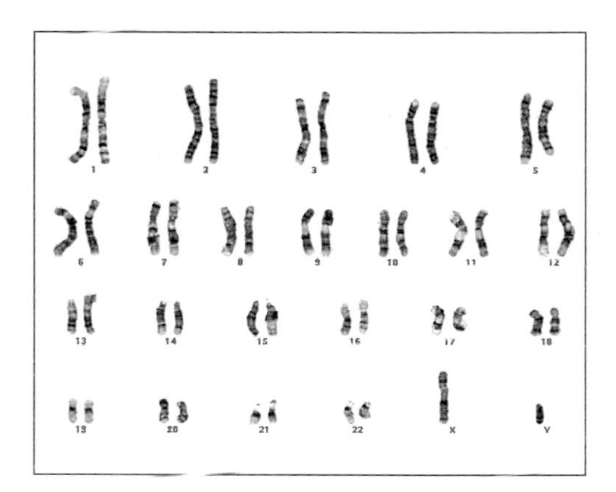

Normal male karyotype

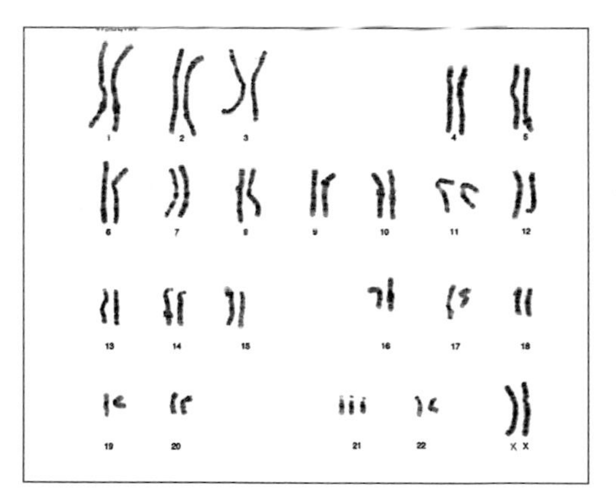

Trisomy 21 karyotype

This syndrome is one of the most common genetic disorders, affecting about 1 in every 800–1,000 children. Over 20 percent are born to women aged over 35, but in about a quarter of cases the extra chromosome 21 comes from the father.

Diagnosing Down's syndrome

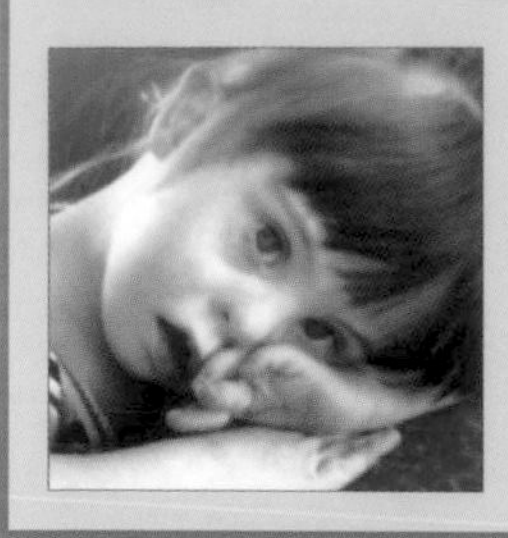

This diagnosis can be made before birth, so it is advisable for pregnant women over 35 years of age to have tests to ascertain whether this anomaly is present. A low concentration of fetoprotein in the mother's blood indicates a greater risk of Down's syndrome in the fetus.

A sample of the amniotic fluid can be taken, via amniocentesis, to confirm the diagnosis. A baby with Down's syndrome has visible signs at birth; the diagnosis will be confirmed by analyzing the child's blood in search of the trisomy 21.

Down's syndrome: educational programs and activities

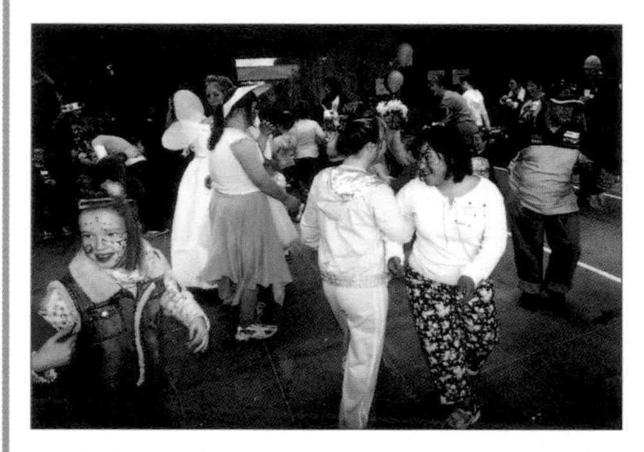

- Children with Down's syndrome can generally carry out the same basic activities as any other child – walking, talking, dressing, and learning to use the toilet – but they normally take longer to learn them. Although it is not possible to predict the exact age at which they will achieve these goals, early intervention programs starting in infancy will help them fulfill their maximum potential.
- Special programs that start in the preschool years have been developed to encourage children with Down's syndrome to further their skills. Apart from allowing many children to benefit from early intervention and a special education, it also enables them to take part in classes with other children, at least to some extent. The outlook for children with Down's syndrome is much brighter than it used to be. Many now learn to read and write, as well as undertake various activities in their school and community; some children with Down's syndrome have even gone on to higher education.
- Special work programs designed for adults with Down's syndrome have allowed many of them to enter the labor market.
- Nowadays, more and more adults with Down's syndrome live semi-independently in communities where they can share domestic chores, form friendships, enjoy leisure activities, and work in and for the community.
- Some people with Down's syndrome form stable relationships and get married. Apart for rare exceptions, the men are unable to have children, while a woman with Down's syndrome has a 50% chance of conceiving a child with the same anomaly. Many such pregnancies end in miscarriages, however.

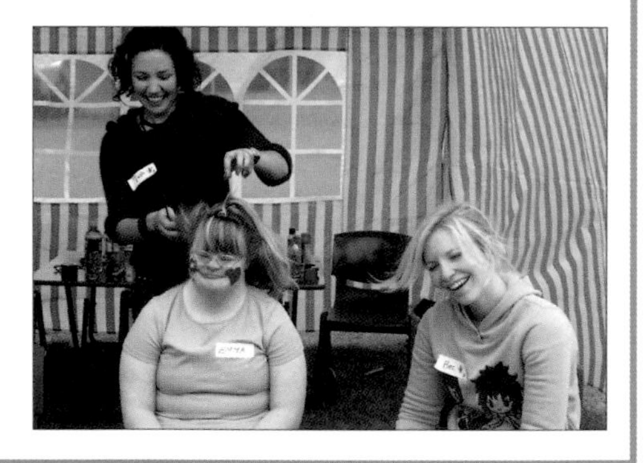

A girl with Turner syndrome is short, has a webbed neck (joined to the shoulders by a large piece of skin) and a very low hairline at the back of the neck. She has drooping eyelids, a broad chest with the nipples wide apart, and a lot of pigmented moles on her skin. Her fingers and toes are short, and her nails are soft.

Turner syndrome

• Turner syndrome, or gonadal dysgenesia, a disorder that affects girls, is characterized by the partial or total absence of one of the X chromosomes (sex chromosomes).

• This syndrome affects 1 in every 3,000 newborn girls. Many have a swelling (lymphedema) on the back of the hands and top of the feet, while folds of limp skin can be found at the back of the neck.

• These girls do not menstruate (amenorrhea) or develop breasts, while their vaginas and vulval lips are underdeveloped. Their ovaries are usually infertile.

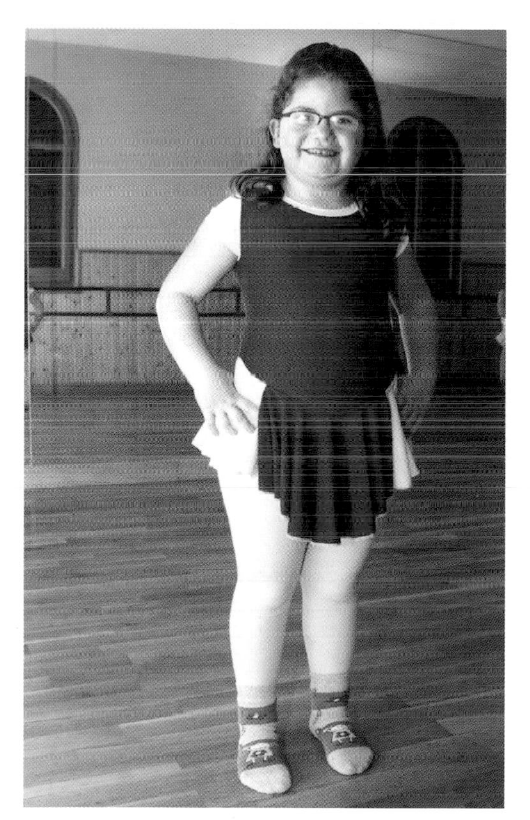

• They have a tendency to high blood pressure, kidney disorders, and small inflammations in the blood vessels. Abnormal blood vessels in the intestine sometimes break and cause hemorrhages.

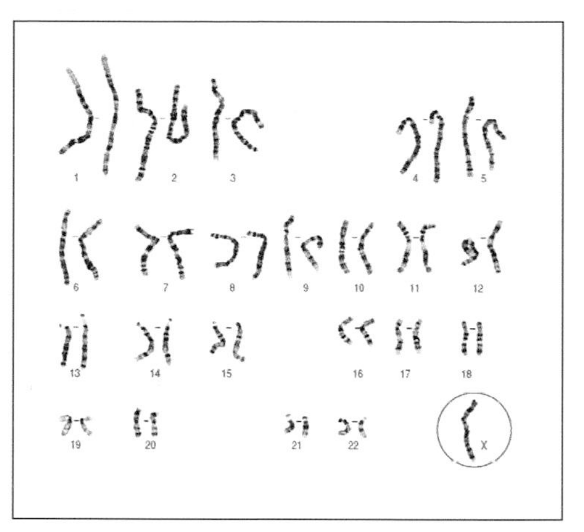

Turner syndrome karyotype

Treating Turner syndrome

Treatment consists of the administration of estrogen, the main female hormone, which encourages the growth of secondary sexual features like the breasts and pubic hair. This treatment cannot be started until adolescence, otherwise it would arrest growth even further. Taking progesterone in conjunction with estrogen will enable girls with this syndrome to menstruate, but their ovaries will remain infertile.

• Many girls with Turner syndrome have difficulty in orientating themselves spatially. They generally achieve poor results in activities that require dexterity and calculation, although their marks in verbal intelligence tests are normal, or above normal. They rarely suffer from developmental delay.

A girl who has not menstruated at the age of 15 should consult a doctor, even if she has no other symptom. Although several factors can

Boys affected by the Klinefelter syndrome usually start puberty normally, albeit with a small penis and testicles, little hair on the face, pubis, and armpits, and larger breasts than normal. They tend to be sterile. Some boys improve with hormonal treatment, which makes their bones denser and gives them a more virile appearance.

cause an absence of menstruation, the possibility of Turner syndrome must be ruled out. After conducting a physical examination and evaluating the girls clinical and family history to determine whether there is a tendency to small stature or problems with menstruation and sexual development in the family, the doctor will ask for a series of blood and urine tests to confirm or rule out the diagnosis.

Klinefelter syndrome

• In this syndrome, boys are born with an extra X chromosome . This relatively frequent chromosomal anomaly (XXY) affects one in every 700 newborn boys.

• Although its physical characteristics can be extremely variable, boys with Klinefelter syndrome are tall and physically unremarkable. Their intelligence is normal, although many have problems with speech and reading.

• They generally improve enormously with speech therapy, allowing them to achieve good academic results.

Complications

This syndrome is associated with an increased risk of tumors in the breast and, less commonly, the germ cells; lung disease; varicose veins, and osteoporosis. There is also a high risk of autoimmune diseases like lupus erythematosus, rheumatoid arthritis, and Sjögren syndrome (reduction in saliva and lachrymal secretion). Despite having an average or high IQ, boys with Klinefelter syndrome often have learning difficulties, resulting from dyslexia, depression, and attention deficit hyperactivity disorder. Taurodontism – teeth with an abnormally large pulp chamber and little enamel – is also very common; it can be diagnosed via a dental X-ray.

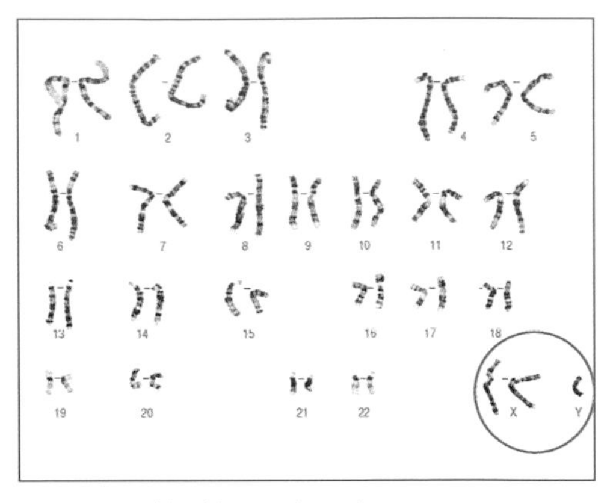

Klinefelter syndrome karyotype.

Most men with Klinefelter syndrome are sterile, although there are cases of patients with an extra X chromosome who have fathered healthy children, sometimes with the help of a fertility clinic.

Deletion syndromes: Cri du chat

• Children suffering from the rare Cri du chat syndrome (or 5p- syndrome) emit a high sound like a mewing cat when they cry, hence its name. This syndrome can be detected at birth.

• Despite the anomalies involved in this syndrome, many children survive into adulthood.

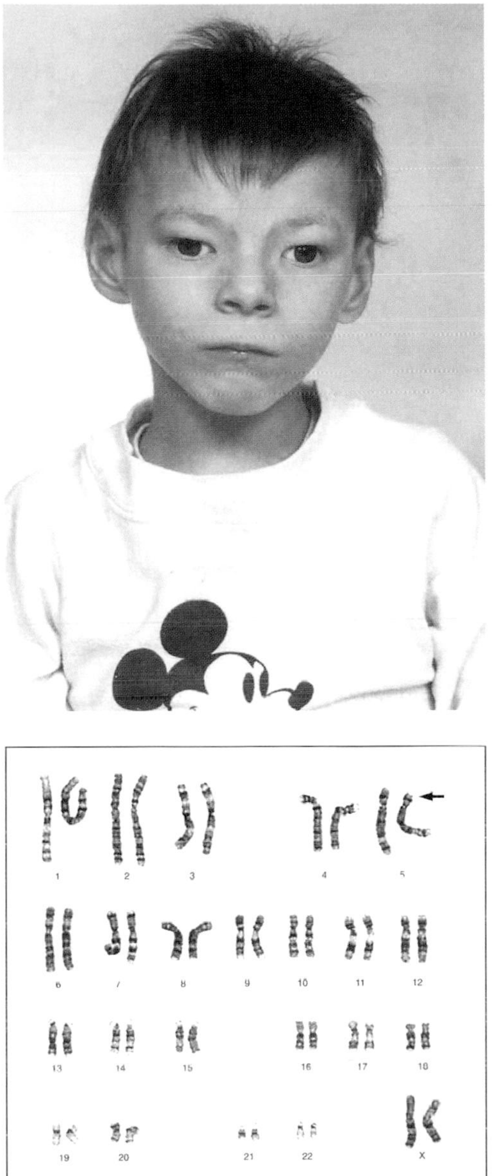

Cri du chat

Structural chromosomal anomalies occur when part of the chromosome is lost (deletion), when there is additional chromosomal material, or when 2 pieces have swapped places. This results in a surplus or lack of generic material in the affected chromosome, which gives rise to genetic defects.

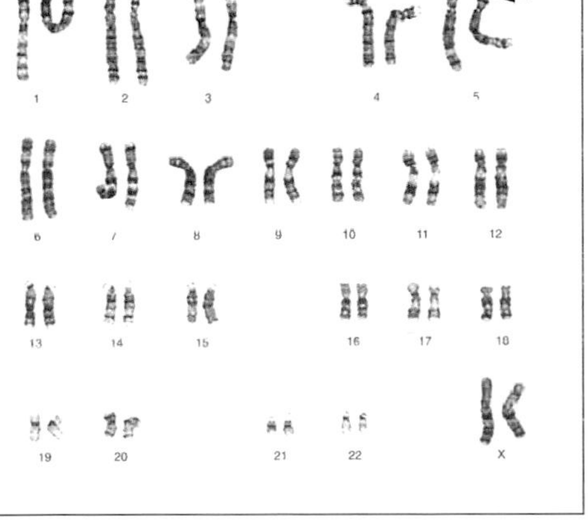

Karyotype of the Cri du chat syndrome

Syndrome 4p-

This even rarer deletion syndrome is similar to the Cri du chat. The developmental disability is substantial, and it may be accompanied by several physical disabilities. Many of the children affected by this genetic disorder die in infancy, and the few that do survive to the age of 20 are severely disabled and very susceptible to infections and epilepsy.

A baby affected by the Cri du chat syndrome is usually underweight at birth and his head is small. He also has an asymmetric face and a mouth that does not close properly. Some babies have a round, moon-shape face with the eyes wide apart. The nose can be broad, while the ears are abnormally shaped and lower-set than usual. The neck can be short and the hands webbed, with extra skin between the fingers. They may also have heart defects. The baby generally has a flaccid appearance and develops little, either physically or mentally.

the celiac child

Celiac disease is a relatively common chronic intestinal disorder caused by a reaction to gliadin, a component of gluten. Gliadin is a protein found in cereals such as wheat, barley, rye, oats, and triticale (a hybrid of wheat and rye). The disorder usually sets in at around the age of 2, after the introduction of cereals in the diet, or later in life, between the ages of 30 and 40. People who suffer from this disorder cannot eat any food that contains these cereals or their flour, as gluten flattens and destroys the tiny protrusions (villi) in the intestinal lining responsible for absorbing nutrients, thereby triggering the symptoms of celiac disease.

The celiac child

Symptoms of celiac disease

In many cases these can pass practically unnoticed, until complications appear.

- The most frequent symptom is chronic diarrhea with malabsorption of nutrients.
- Weight loss.
- Nutritional deficiencies.
- Anemia through iron deficiency.
- Stomach pains, which can recur and be complemented by flatulence, with abdominal distension and abnormal intestinal movements.
- Anemia appears as a result of malabsorption of iron, folic acid, and/or vitamin B12.
- Celiac disease is sometimes complemented by arthritis, characterized by pain, stiffness, and fatigue. Bone lesions can also be found.

Diagnosis

Apart from the clinical picture, the determination of the levels of certain antibodies in the blood and an intestinal biopsy help to confirm a diagnosis.

- The main antibodies involved are:
  - IgG anti-gliadin antibodies, which are specific to celiac disease.
  - IgA anti-gliadin antibodies, which are sometimes not found, as there is an IgA deficit.
- An intestinal biopsy may be necessary; it is usually taken from the duodenum, although the jejunum is much more sensitive. Patients showing improvement or intermittent symptoms can present a normal biopsy and blood test, although they will still be highly sensitive to some types of protein.

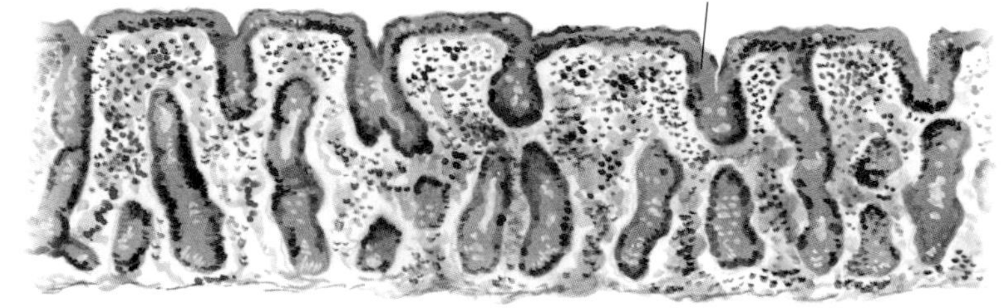

The striking reduction in the height of the intestinal villi is responsible for the malabsorption and chronic diarrhea that characterize celiac disease if gluten is not eliminated from the diet.

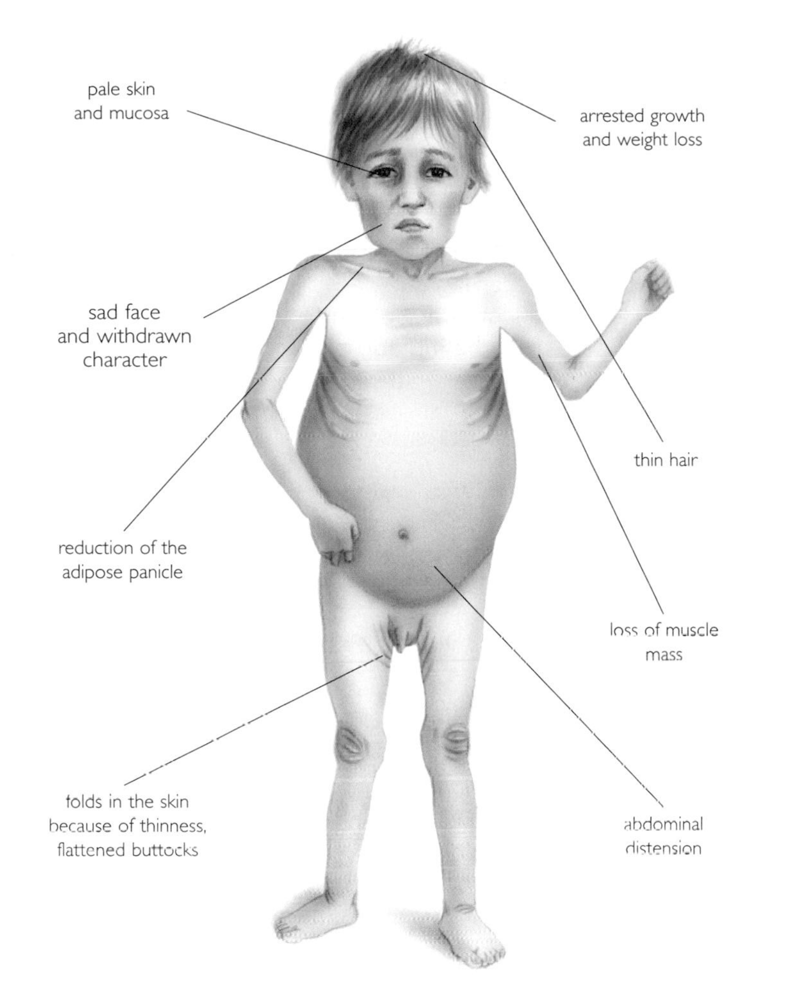

• The nervous system may be affected too, this manifests itself in burning and itching in the limbs, muscle contractions and difficulty in standing upright, irritability, and impaired memory.

Diet – the only treatment

The treatment for celiac disease consists of eliminating food containing gluten from the diet, such as products incorporating wheat flour, barley, rye, oats, and triticale.

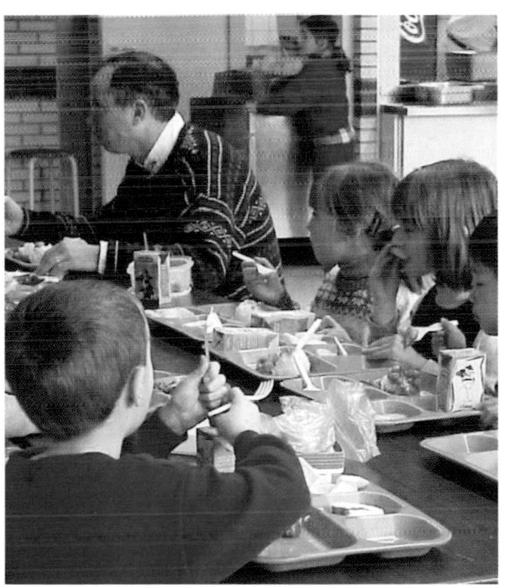

A celiac child should be aware that he can eat food free of gluten, such as meat, fish, milk, eggs, pulses, fruit, tubers, vegetables, fats, and oils, sugar, and cereals that do not contain gluten, such as rice, corn, millet, and sorghum.

When a celiac child eats in a restaurant or school canteen, it is advisable to not only check that all the ingredients of his dishes are gluten-free but also find out how the food is cooked. Gluten-free food can be fried in oil previously used to fry an item containing gluten; potatoes, for example, can be fried in oil left over from preparing croquettes, which normally contain wheat flour and, therefore, gluten.

This means that a child's parents and everybody else involved in feeding him have to grow accustomed to carefully studying the ingredients of packaged foodstuffs to make sure they are gluten-free, as cereals are sometimes used as additives in chocolates, sausages, salad dressing, candies, etc. For the same reason, parents should instil the habit of reading food labels in their child. In some cases, however, it is impossible to know whether a product is gluten-free, but specialist publications are available with lists of products guaranteed to be suitable for people with celiac disease.

Practical advice

Some celiac children cannot understand why they cannot eat the same food as their friends, so it is important for their parents and teachers to explain the disease as fully as possible.

It is best to avoid buying food items that are homemade or sold in bulk, as these are generally not labeled and their ingredients cannot be verified.

Instead of wheat flour, you can use flaked mashed potato, corn flour, or gluten-free breadcrumbs to thicken sauces or coat fried food. A range of other gluten-free substitutes made with rice, soya, quinoa, millet, or amaranth are also available, allowing a celiac child to enjoy a varied diet.

Example of a gluten-free diet for children

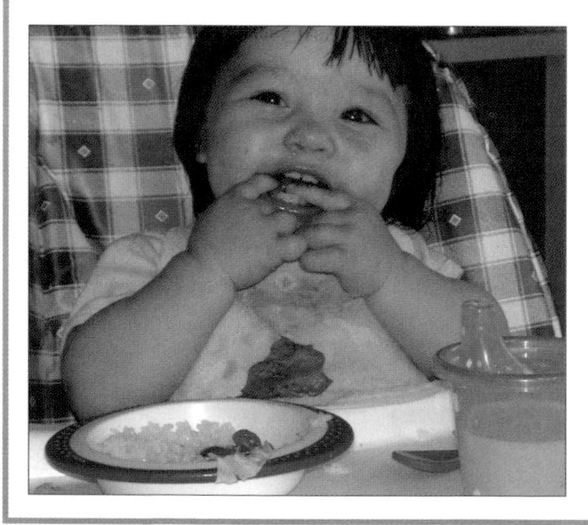

- Breakfast: cornflakes with milk and orange juice.
- Mid-morning break: cheese sandwich (gluten-free bread).
- Lunch: rice with vegetables, grilled pork loin with peppers, and a piece of fruit.
- Tea: a glass of milk and 2 fairy cakes made with corn flour.
- Dinner: Salad of lettuce, tomato, onion, sweetcorn, carrot, and beet; potato omelette, and a piece of fruit.

main congenital heart disorders

Congenital heart disorders can involve anomalies in the organ's walls or valves, or problems with the blood vessels connected to them. Approximately 1 in every 120 newborn babies presents a disorder of this type, but their characteristics, severity, and development can be extremely variable. Generally speaking, they give rise to changes in the normal flow of the blood, which make their presence felt through clinical signs such as a heart murmur (an irregular sound audible through a stethoscope). A series of tests, including an electrocardiogram, chest X-ray, and echocardiogram, are used by pediatric cardiologists to formulate an exact diagnosis and, on this basis, decide on a suitable treatment.

Defects in the atrial and ventricular septa

• Defects in the atrial septa arise between the upper chambers of the heart (atria), which receive blood. In contrast, those in the ventricular septa occur between the lower chambers (ventricles), which pump out blood.

• In both cases, the blood that returns to the heart from the lungs does not complete a full circuit, but is sent back to the lungs instead of being pumped out to the rest of the body. This increases the levels of blood in the lungs and, in some children, causes a feeling of suffocation, difficulty in eating, and excessive sweating, as well as restricting growth.

• These defects can be corrected with surgery.

Persistent arterial duct

Under normal conditions, this duct closes spontaneously 1 or 2 days after birth. If it remains open, some of the blood destined for the body returns to the lungs and overloads its blood vessels. Some babies develop cardiac insufficiency as a result, making it difficult for them to breathe, as well as the heart murmur typical of all these disorders. These babies' cardiac frequency is accelerated and they cannot put on weight. A persistent arterial duct is found more often in premature babies than in full-term ones.

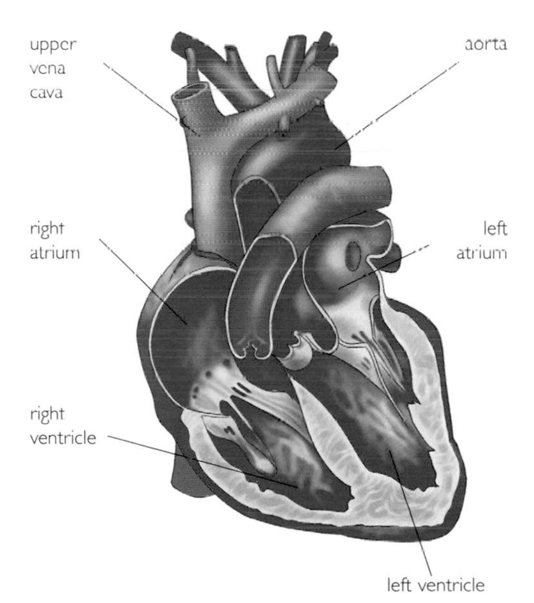

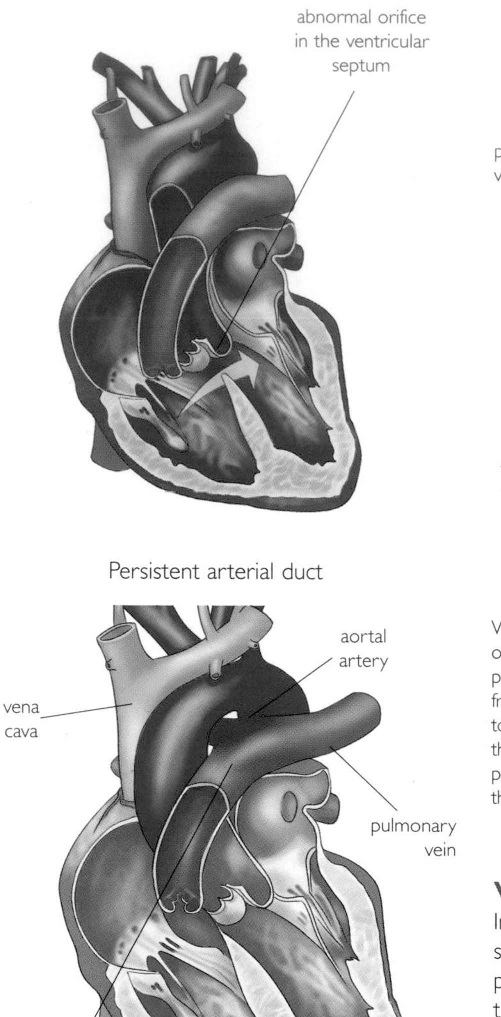

The heart is responsible for pumping blood throughout the body. Once the various organs and tissues have obtained oxygen from the blood and offloaded their waste materials, the blood continues to the upper and lower venas cavas, which pass it on to the right side of the heart (right atrium and ventricle). From there, the blood travels via the pulmonary artery to the lung, where it will be re-oxygenated before beginning the cycle once again; this oxygenated blood flows through the pulmonary veins to the left side of the heart (left atrium and ventricle), from where the aortic artery and its various branches distribute it, thereby supplying oxygen and nutrients to the rest of the body.

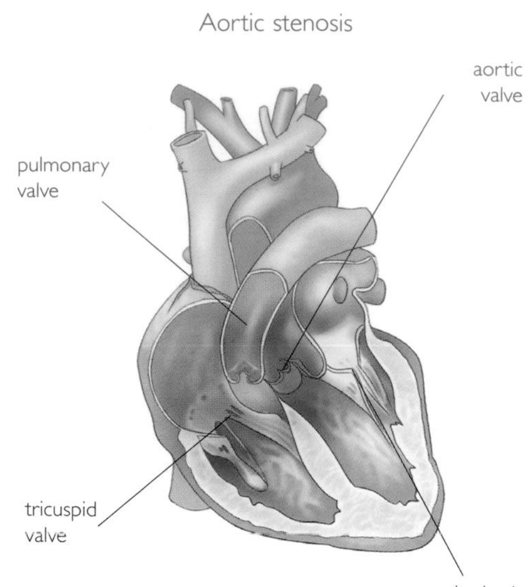

When the great arteries are transposed, there is an inversion of the normal connections linking the aortic artery and pulmonary artery with the lung, leading the blood returning from the body without oxygen to flow from the right ventricle to the aorta, which passes this unoxygenated blood back into the body, without passing through the lungs. The baby has plenty of oxygenated blood, but it stays in the lungs, rather than traveling to the rest of the body.

Valvular stenosis

In aortic stenosis, the aortic valve is partially closed, making the left ventricle exert more energy in pumping blood to the aortic artery and, from there, the rest of the body. In some children, the obstruction is sufficiently serious to need surgical correction. In rare cases, cardiac insufficiency is also found, requiring emergency treatment, usually involving medication and urgent surgery, or a procedure called balloon valvuloplasty.

In stenosis of the pulmonary valve, it is the right ventricle that has to make greater effort to pump blood to the lungs. This stenosis can be so insubstantial that it needs no treatment or, in contrast, so serious that it can require surgery, which sometimes has to be repeated in adulthood.

Aortic coarctation

This is a narrowing of the aortic artery which usually occurs at the point where the arterial duct (ductus arteriosus) joins up with the aorta, which then twists down to the lower chest and abdomen. This results in a reduction in the blood flowing in the lower half of the body; consequently, the pulse and blood pressure are lower than normal in the legs, but higher than usual in the arms.

Coarctation generally causes few problems. The high blood pressure in the arms can cause headaches or nosebleeds in some children, and there can be pain in the legs during exercise on account of the low blood pressure, but in most cases there are no symptoms.

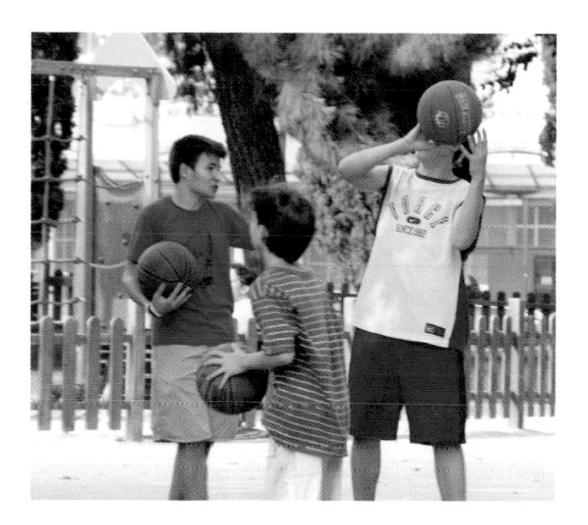

Transposition of the great arteries

Babies born with this anomaly have a very low life expectancy. If they do manage to survive, it is thanks to a small opening between the right and left ventricles that is normally present at birth. This orifice allows a small amount of the oxygenated blood dispatched by the lungs to pass from the right atrium to the left atrium, and then from the right ventricle to the aorta, endowing the body with sufficient oxygen to stay alive. It is now possible to correct this anomaly with surgery.

Fallot tetralogy

This is a combination of several anomalies:

- A major defect in the ventricular septum.
- Abnormal aortic artery that allows unoxygenated blood to flow directly into it from the right ventricle.
- Narrowing of the outlet on the right sight of the heart.
- Abnormally thick wall in the right ventricle.

Babies with Fallot tetralogy usually have a heart murmur that can be heard at birth or shortly afterward. These babies are bluish in color (a condition known as cyanosis), because the blood flowing through their body is insufficiently oxygenated. The symptoms and subsequent complications can be treated with medication, but surgery is the only cure.

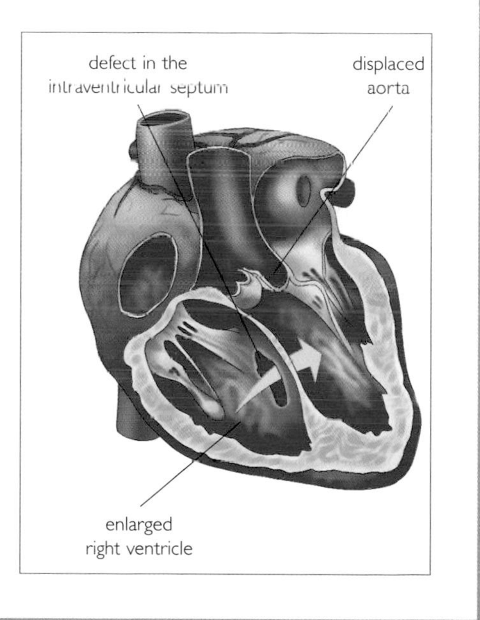